PAEDIATRIC HANDBOOK

PAEDIATRIC HANDBOOK

FOURTH EDITION

By the Staff of the Royal Children's Hospital Melbourne, Australia

MELBOURNE
Blackwell Scientific Publications
OXFORD LONDON EDINBURGH
BOSTON PARIS BERLIN VIENNA

Editorial Offices:
54 University Street, Carlton
Victoria 3053, Australia
Osney Mead, Oxford OX2 0EL
25 John Street, London WC1N 2BL
23 Ainslie Place, Edinburgh EH3 6AJ
238 Main Street, Cambridge
Massachusetts 02142, USA

Other Editorial Offices:

Librairie Arnette SA
2 rue Casimir-Delavigne
75006 Paris
France

Blackwell Wissenschafts-Verlag GmbH
Meinekestrasse 4
D-1000 Berlin 15
Germany

Blackwell MZV
Feldgasse 13
A-1238 Wien
Austria

First published 1992
Reprinted 1993

Designer, Tom Kurema
Set by Semantic Graphics, Singapore
Printed in Australia by Brown Prior Anderson

DISTRIBUTORS

Australia
Blackwell Scientific Publications Pty Ltd
54 University Street
Carlton, Victoria 3053
(*Orders*: Tel: 03 347-5552
Fax: 03 347-5001)

UK and Europe
Marston Book Services Ltd
PO Box 87
Oxford OX2 0DT
(*Orders*: Tel: 0865 791155
Fax: 0865 791927
Telex: 837515)

USA
Blackwell Scientific Publications, Inc.
238 Main Street
Cambridge, MA 02142
(*Orders*: Tel: 800 759-6102
617 876-7000)

Canada
Times Mirror Professional Publishing, Ltd
130 Flaska Drive
Markham, Ontario LBG 1B8
(*Orders*: Tel: 800 268-4178
416 470-6739)

Cataloguing in Publication Data

Royal Children's Hospital (Melbourne, Vic.).
Paediatric Handbook.

4th ed.
Includes index.
ISBN 0 86793 217 1.

1. Pediatrics — Handbooks, manuals, etc.
2. Children — Hospital care — Handbooks, manuals, etc. I. Title.

618.92

CONTENTS

EDITORIAL COMMITTEE

ACKNOWLEDGEMENTS

The information contained is intended to act as a management guide for doctors dealing with paediatric patients. It is not intended that the handbook replace standard texts. This edition of the Royal Children's Hospital *Paediatric Handbook* is the result of the contribution of a large number of consultant and administrative staff. The editorial committee would like to express thanks to all those who supported this project. In particular, thanks are extended to Dr Frank Shann for kindly allowing reproduction of much of *Drug Doses in Paediatrics*, 6th edition. Thanks also to Ms Denise Moore for her part in helping to prepare the manuscript.

Dr M. K. MARKS
Clinical Co-ordinating Editor
Chief Resident Medical Officer, 1991 (currently NHMRC Research Fellow).

CONTRIBUTORS

The editorial committee wish to thank the following people for their direct contribution to the fourth edition of the *Paediatric Handbook*.

R. G. Adler
Professor of Psychiatry, University of Melbourne. Director of Child and Family Psychiatry, Royal Children's Hospital

D. W. Boldt
Director of Radiology, Royal Children's Hospital

A. D. Bryan
Deputy Director, Child Development and Rehabilitation Royal Children's Hospital

N. T. Campbell
Director of Neonatology, Royal Children's Hospital

A. Carmichael
Formerly Director of Regional Paediatrics, Royal Children's Hospital (currently Professor of Paediatrics, University of Tasmania)

A. G. Catto-Smith
Gastroenterologist, Royal Children's Hospital

J. Coakley
Formerly Deputy Director of Biochemistry, Royal Children's Hospital (currently Director of Biochemistry, Camperdown Children's Hospital, Sydney)

W. Cole
Professor of Orthopaedics, University of Melbourne; Chief Orthopaedic Surgeon, Royal Children's Hospital

J. M. Court
Paediatrician, Centre for Adolescent Health, Royal Children's Hospital

H. Ekert
Director of Clinical Haematology and Oncology, Royal Children's Hospital

J. Elder
Ophthalmologist, Royal Children's Hospital

D. E. M. Francis
Senior Dietitian, Royal Children's Hospital

K. Grimwood
Senior Lecturer, Department of Paediatrics, University of Melbourne; Paediatrician, Royal Children's Hospital

G. Hogg
Microbiologist, Royal Children's Hospital

J. Hutson
Senior Lecturer, University of Melbourne; Deputy Director of General Surgery, Royal Children's Hospital

D. James
Paediatrician, Child Protection Unit, Royal Children's Hospital

F. C. Jarman
Deputy Director of Ambulatory Paediatrics, Royal Children's Hospital

A. S. Kemp
Director of Immunology, Royal Children's Hospital

E. J. Keogh
Director of Burns Unit, Royal Children's Hospital

G. Klug
Director of Neurosurgery, Royal Children's Hospital

J. Lucas
Deputy Director of Dentistry, Royal Children's Hospital

M. K. Marks
Chief Hospital Medical Officer, 1991 (currently NHMRC Research Fellow)

P. N. McDougall
Deputy Director of Neonatology, Royal Children's Hospital

Dr T. Nolan
Senior Lecturer, Department of Paediatrics, University of Melbourne; Director of Clinical Epidemiology and Biostatistics Unit, Royal Children's Hospital

R. J. Pepperell
Professor of Obstetrics and Gynaecology, University of Melbourne

P. D. Phelan
Stevenson Professor and Chairman, Department of Paediatrics, University of Melbourne; Chief Thoracic Physician, Royal Children's Hospital

H. R. Powell
Director of Nephrology, Royal Children's Hospital

D. S. Reddihough
Director of Child Development and Rehabilitation, Royal Children's Hospital

F. Shann
Director of Intensive Care Unit, Royal Children's Hospital

L. K. Shield
Director of Neurology, Royal Children's Hospital

M. South
Senior Lecturer, Department of Paediatrics; Paediatrician, Royal Children's Hospital

G. P. Tauro
Director of Laboratory Haematology, Royal Children's Hospital

G. Thompson
Metabolic Paediatrician, Royal Children's Hospital

J. Tibballs
Deputy Director of Intensive Care Unit, Royal Children's Hospital

G. Varigos
Director of Dermatology, Royal Children's Hospital

J. Vorrath
Deputy Director of Otolaryngology, Royal Children's Hospital

G. L. Warne
Director of Endocrinology, Royal Children's Hospital

K. Waters
Administrative Director of Clinical Haematology and Oncology, Royal Children's Hospital

G. Werther
Deputy Director Diabetes and Endocrinology, Royal Children's Hospital

J. Wilkinson
Director of Cardiology, Royal Children's Hospital.

The editorial committee also wish to acknowledge the many people who have contributed to past editions of the Royal Children's Hospital *Paediatric Handbook*.

PREFACE

It is now more than 25 years since the Royal Children's Hospital first produced a handbook for its resident medical staff. It was originally conceived as a ready-reference to give advice to the residents on common paediatric problems and on standard hospital procedures. Over the years the handbook has become widely accepted in Victoria and beyond as a valuable source of information for all medical practitioners who deal with children. It is hoped that this current edition, which has been contributed to by many members of the hospital staff, will continue to be of assistance to the hospital's residents, to residents in other hospitals and to medical practitioners generally who are responsible for the health care of children.

The Royal Children's Hospital is the principal paediatric centre for the State of Victoria, the paediatric teaching hospital for The University of Melbourne and the centre for paediatric education for nurses and the whole range of health professionals. Consequently, it has a major responsibility for the health care of children and adolescents in Victoria. The provision of up-to-date information on the management of common paediatric problems is one way of meeting this responsibility.

This handbook does not specifically cover the very important topics of health promotion and illness prevention. Every time a medical practitioner sees a child and his or her family, there is an opportunity for the provision of advice and counsel on the prevention of illness. Specific attention should be paid to those measures for which there is strong evidence of benefit and which can be easily implemented. From 1992 a Child Health Record Book will be given to the parents of every child born in Victoria. Maternal and Child Health Care Nurses will complete routine growth and development information in the book, various professionals will be encouraged to record details of their encounters with the child and there will be much health promotion and educational material. Hopefully this parent-held record book will become a valuable source of information for parents and for all health professionals who become involved in the child's management.

Childhood immunization remains the single most cost-effective form of illness prevention. It is of vital importance that every child be vaccinated against the common infectious diseases of whooping cough, tetanus, diphtheria, measles, poliomyelitis, mumps and rubella. The immunization status of every child should be checked when he or she is seen by the medical practitioner and if there is any deficiency, the parent should be urged to have their child vaccinated at the earliest opportunity. Complications from vaccination procedures are extremely rare and many, many times less frequent than death or serious complications from these infectious diseases.

Acute respiratory infections are the most common disease in infancy and childhood and asthma the most frequent cause of long-term health problems in children. There is now incontrovertible evidence that passive inhalation of cigarette smoke from parents is a major factor in more troublesome respiratory infections and in asthma. Any parent who smokes is creating an unnecessary health risk for his or her child and medical practitioners should actively encourage all parents to cease this habit in the interests of their child's health as well as of their own.

Accidents are the single most important cause of death in children over 1 year of age and adolescents and a major cause of morbidity. Many can be prevented or the severity of injury reduced. While child restraints are compulsory in motor vehicles, regrettably many parents continue not to insist that their children wear them. The wearing of crash helmets by bicyclists is of proven benefit in preventing serious head injuries. The proper fencing of domestic swimming pools would stop 10–15 deaths from drowning a year in Victoria.

Good nutrition and a healthy life-style with regular exercise are likely to be of considerable value in maintaining optimal health in adult life. Adult eating habits and exercise patterns are to a very large extent the result of childhood experience. Children and adolescents should be encouraged to develop good nutritional and exercise habits and this is best achieved by parent example. Basic information on healthy good nutrition for babies (breast feeding) and for toddlers and younger children is given in the section on nutrition in this handbook.

Victoria has one of the lowest infant and childhood death rates in the world and hopefully our children and their families will continue to have ready access to appropriate health care at a primary and specialist level. Our objective is to reduce current mortality rates, and to control morbidity both by applying principles of illness prevention and by using the advice given in this handbook on the treatment of minor illnesses and paediatric emergencies. The Royal Children's Hospital aims to deliver the highest standard of health care to the children and adolescents of Victoria and adjacent parts of our neighbouring states. It is a major centre for teaching and for research into illnesses of children and without such research further improvement of child health would not occur and the hospital's standards of clinical care and teaching would decline.

PETER D. PHELAN
Stevenson Professor and Chairman
Department of Paediatrics
The University of Melbourne

CHAPTER 1

CONSULTATION

The knowledge and practice of paediatrics is expanding at an enormous rate. The Royal Children's Hospital aims to provide a service beyond the care of children within the institution. The hospital provides a wide range of facilities to medical practitioners and other health care workers who deal with children. In specific areas of the handbook guidelines are set out as to how to seek advice or consultation. Other methods are set out below.

ADMITTING OFFICER (345 5522)

On duty 24 h-a-day for referral of problems to emergency, for advice regarding management or as the first point of referral.

GENERAL CLINIC CONSULTANT (345 6161)

A paediatrician is available for advice and referral. Most sessions are covered Monday–Friday.

SPECIALTY REGISTRAR (345 5522)

On duty 24 h-a-day for advice on the management of diabetes, respiratory, neurological and haematological conditions.

SURGICAL REGISTRAR (345 5522)

On duty 24 h-a-day for consultation about acute surgical or potentially surgical problems.

PAEDIATRIC EMERGENCY TRANSPORT SERVICE (345 5211 OR 345 5212)

Provides a 24 h service for consultation about paediatric intensive care. A patient retrieval service is provided for acutely ill children as well as advice regarding management problems.

NEWBORN EMERGENCY TRANSPORT SERVICE (347 7441)

Based at the Royal Women's Hospital this service provides 24 h-a-day consultation and retrieval service for newborn infants.

COMMUNITY HEALTH NURSES (PAGE THROUGH SWITCHBOARD)

- Maternal and Child Health (345 6163 or page through switchboard)
- Outpatient service (345 5689 or page through switchboard)
- Adolescents (345 5899 or page through switchboard)
- Disabilities (345 5692 or page through switchboard)

Four nurses are available for consultation and referral on matters relevant to their area: infant feeding and infant welfare centre liaison, school problems, sexuality counselling and support and co-ordination of family services, together with information about the full range of outpatient services at the Royal Children's Hospital.

POISONS INFORMATION

- (03) 345 5678 (0900–2200 h)
- (008) 133 890 (0900–2200 h)
- (008) 25 1525 (2200–0900 h)

Provides information on poisons and suspected poisoning including chemicals, medications, poisonous plants, envenomation. Up to date advice on toxic hazard situations, treatment and prevention of poisoning.

CHAPTER 2

EMERGENCIES

CARDIORESPIRATORY ARREST

Cardiorespiratory emergencies in children differ from those in adults. The majority are due to hypoxia or hypotension rather than being primarily myocardial in origin. If cardiac arrest is present the heart is often in asystole or severe bradycardia, but ventricular arrhythmia may, however, be the cause of potentially lethal syncopal states in childhood, even in the absence of other heart disease. The third common arrhythmia is electromechanical dissociation.

DISCOVERY OF EMERGENCY

The first person on the scene should:

CALL FOR HELP

Within the Royal Children's Hospital dial 777. A registrar and nurse will attend from the Intensive Care Unit bringing an ECG/defibrillator.

CARRY PATIENT TO THE TREATMENT ROOM

If this is not possible, place child on firm surface such as a board, or the floor, and bring the resuscitation trolley from the treatment room.

INITIAL MANAGEMENT

Suspect cardiorespiratory arrest when consciousness is lost or the patient appears pale, cyanosed, pulseless or apnoeic. Assess by carotid palpation, or auscultation, or palpation of apex beat. The absence of a pulse, despite heart sounds, indicates inadequate cardiac output. Check respiration by feeling for expired breath at the mouth with the hand, while positioning the head to maintain the airways. Movement of chest, but absent expiration, indicates a blocked airway.

Airways Maintenance and Ventilation

Clear a blocked airway, due to secretions/vomitus, by brief suction of the mouth and pharynx, using a Yankeur sucker. Maintain the airways with backward head tilt, chin lift or forward jaw thrust. If respiration is absent, ventilate the lungs with the Laerdal resuscitator. A high concentration of oxygen is delivered when 8–10 L/min is introduced into the self-inflating bag. Intubation should only be performed by experienced personnel. If unable to ventilate the lungs with Laerdal resuscitator, give mouth to mouth expired air ventilation.

EXTERNAL CARDIAC COMPRESSION (ECC)

If the pulse is still not palpable after establishing a patent airway and giving positive pressure ventilation with oxygen, start ECC. Place the patient on a firm surface. Depress the sternum 2–3 cm using two fingers for a newborn infant, 2.5–4 cm using the heel of one hand for toddlers or small children and 3–5 cm for larger children, teenagers and adults. The site of application is the lower half of the sternum for all ages including newborns. ECC in newborns may be better given by a two-handed technique in which the hands encircle the chest while the thumbs depress the sternum.

Visceral damage (liver, spleen, heart) is much more likely in children than adults, but chest wall damage (e.g. fractured ribs) is less likely. During cardiorespiratory resuscitation employing expired air ventilation or bag-and-mask ventilation, mechanical ventilation and ECC must be given in a co-ordinated manner. With a *single-person rescue*, the ratio of breaths to compressions is 2 : 15. With *two-person rescue*, the ratio of breaths to compressions is 1 : 5 with no interruption of compression. The person compressing the sternum should count aloud so that the person giving ventilation can deliver effective breath between compressions. Proof of adequate ventilation is observation of chest expansion, while proof of adequate cardiac compression is generation of a pulse. During two-person resuscitation, ECC should be given at a rate of 120–150/min for a newborn, 100/min for a small child or infant and a rate of 80–100/min for a large child, teenager or adult. The compression and ventilation rates are given in the following table.

Guide to ventilation–compression rates in basic life support for a large child/teenager, small child/infant and newborn

	Large child/teenager	*Small child/infant*	*Newborn*
Two-person resuscitation			
Ventilation	16	20	24–30
Compression (rate 1 : 5)	80–100	100	120–150
One-person resuscitation			
Ventilation	8–12	12	16
Compression (rate 2 : 15)	60–90	90	120

IF NO RESPONSE TO INITIAL MANAGEMENT, ATTACH ECG TO DETERMINE THE HEART RHYTHM

Within the Royal Children's Hospital ECG monitor and defibrillator are on a trolley available from the Intensive Care Unit. Cardiac rhythm should be defined as soon as these arrive. The rhythm can be determined with the defibrillator paddles or ECG leads.

The success of treatment is dependent on the time delay to treatment and coronary artery perfusion. Insert an intravenous cannula but don't waste time trying to insert an intravenous if the drugs intended for use may be given via the endotracheal tube or intraosseous injection. All drugs may be given by intraosseous injection (upper or lower tibia or anterior superior iliac crest) but only adrenaline, lignocaine, atropine and naloxone can be given via endotracheal tube. Algorithms for sequential management of dysrhythmias are illustrated in the following figure.

ALGORITHMS FOR SEQUENTIAL MANAGEMENT OF DYSRHYTHMIAS

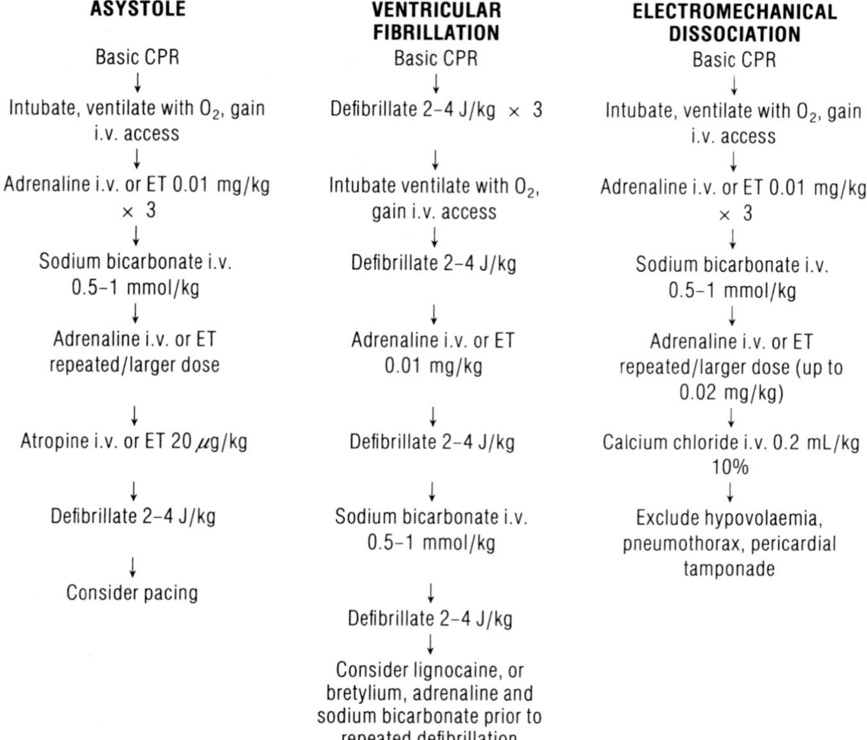

ASYSTOLE-BRADYCARDIA

Adrenaline

As cardiac stimulant and vasopressor.

- Preparation: 1 in 10 000 — 10 mL ampoule; 1 in 1000 — 1 mL ampoule
- Dose: initially 0.01 mg/kg (1 mL/10 kg of 1 in 10 000)

May be given by endotracheal tube. Double the intravenous dose but dilute to a larger volume with normal saline (1 mL neonate, 2–3 mL small child, 5–10 mL large child). Many doses of adrenaline or larger doses (up to 0.2 mg/kg) or an infusion may be necessary.

Sodium Bicarbonate

Give up to 1 mmol/kg (1 mL/kg of 8.4% solution) initially intravenous and then 0.5 mmol/kg every 10 min until recovery. Do *not* give via endotracheal tube. Assess acid–base status with arterial blood gas analysis whenever possible.

VENTRICULAR FIBRILLATION

If ventricular fibrillation is present, apply electrode jelly to the two paddle electrodes. Use the 4.5 cm diameter electrodes for newborns and small children, the 8 cm diameter for all others. When operating the defibrillator, the electrodes are usually held by one person, but may be held one each by two persons. The dose is 2–4 J/kg to defibrillate. Failure to successfully defibrillate may be due to poor electrical contact, inadequate joules, acidosis or the defibrillator not being switched to the defibrillator mode. Refractory fibrillation should be treated with adrenaline (0.01 mg/kg, i.v. or via endotracheal tube), sodium bicarbonate (i.v.), lignocaine (1 mg/kg, i.v. or via endotracheal tube). Bretylium tosylate (5 mg/kg, i.v.) is a useful alternative agent to lignocaine.

ELECTROMECHANICAL DISSOCIATION

Administer adrenaline 0.01 mg/kg, i.v. or via endotracheal tube. If pulse and blood pressure not restored, give further doses of adrenaline and sodium bicarbonate 1 mmol/kg, i.v. Exclude mechanical cause for low cardiac output (hypovolaemia, pneumothorax, pericardial tamponade).

OTHER DRUGS

Atropine

Vagal reflexes are brisk in childhood and may cause asystole and bradycardia. Dose: 10–20 μg/kg, i.v.

Calcium

Used especially for hypocalcaemia, hyperkalaemia and calcium channel blocker toxicity. Dose: 0.2 mL/kg of 10% calcium chloride or 0.7 mL/kg of 10% calcium gluconate. May be useful as inotropic or vasopressor agent. Calcium precipitates with bicarbonate. Calcium has no efficacy in treatment of asystole or ventricular fibrillation and has doubtful benefit in electromechanical dissociation.

FURTHER MANAGEMENT

Continue cardiorespiratory resuscitation until adequate spontaneous function returns. Mechanical ventilation with oxygen, and inotropic and chronotropic cardiac support may be needed for several days.

ENDOTRACHEAL INTUBATION

The internal diameter (size) of the tube selected should be according to the age of the patient. For the newborn, a tube size 3.0 mm is used, a size 3.5 at 6 months and a size 4 at 1 year. For patients over the age of 1 year, the size is determined approximately by the following formula:

$$\text{SIZE} = \text{AGE}/4 + 4$$

Tubes are available with an internal diameter of 2.5–9 mm, with length increasing with size. They have been pre-cut to avoid endobronchial intubation and are only intended for oral use. Insert the tube 12 + age(years)/2 cm and secure it to prevent accidental extubation. Only uncuffed tubes are used in paediatrics. Under the age of 6 months, use a straight-blade laryngoscope, a curved blade for all others.

ANAPHYLAXIS

CLINICAL MANIFESTATIONS

- *Hypotension* results from vasodilatation, capillary leak and loss of plasma volume into the tissues.
- *Bronchospasm* may be severe. Wheezing may not be obvious if the tidal volume is small.
- *Upper airways obstruction* is due to laryngeal or pharyngeal oedema.

The onset of severe clinical manifestations of anaphylaxis is usually rapid; one manifestation may predominate.

IMMEDIATE THERAPY

- *Adrenaline* (1 : 10 000) should be given slowly intravenously as the first line of treatment in all cases in a dose of 0.1 mL/kg of 1 : 10 000, or less if the desired effect is achieved before the full dose is given.
- *Oxygen* should be administered by mask.
- *Hypotension* should be treated initially with colloid solutions [Haemaccel, stable plasma protein solution (SPPS), Dextran 70].
  Crystalloid solutions such as Hartmann's can be used but colloid should be used first if available.
- *Bronchospasm* usually responds to adrenaline infusion. Nebulized salbutamol or intravenous aminophylline may be used as supplementary treatment.
- *Upper airways obstruction.* Oxygen by mask using an airway if necessary. Mild to moderate oedema may respond to an inhalation of adrenaline (0.5 mL/kg) 1 : 1000 (maximum 4 mL), dilute to 4 mL with saline or water if necessary. Intubation of the trachea by an experienced person occasionally will be necessary if obstruction is severe.

SUPPLEMENTAL TREATMENT

- Hydrocortisone. Eight to 10 mg/kg given intravenously. This will not have the immediate effect of adrenaline but should also be given. It reduces capillary leak, oedema and may be beneficial for bronchospasm.
- Antihistamines. These are of little value in the acute situation. Pheniramine (Avil) may be used for urticaria without more severe manifestations of anaphylaxis.

HAEMORRHAGIC SHOCK

Pallor, restlessness and weakness may be the earliest signs of blood loss. A child may compensate for loss of up to half of its blood volume loss without developing hypotension. Measurable hypotension may be a late sign in hypovolaemia shock. Compensation is usually by an increase in heart rate but bradycardia may herald decompensation.

INITIAL MANAGEMENT

Clear and maintain the airways if the patient is unconscious, administer oxygen. Nurse in the horizontal or head down position. Control haemorrhage:

- *Elevate* the bleeding area if practical.
- *Direct pressure dressings.*

- *Tourniquets.* Restore the circulation to the limb by releasing the tourniquet every 20 min.
- *Insert* a large bore intravenous catheter preferably in the upper limb. Two catheters are sometimes required.
- *Withdraw* blood for group and cross-matching.
- *Rapid infusion of SPPS* or Haemaccel up to 20 mL/kg. In decompensated shock a further infusion of 20 mL/kg may be indicated.
- *Blood transfusion* is given as soon as available. If warranted, use urgently cross-matched blood, or if exsanguinating, use O negative uncrossmatched blood. Where an *adequate systolic blood pressure* is maintained, Hartmann's solution may be used until blood is available.
- *Central venous pressure* (CVP) catheter should be inserted if there are difficulties encountered in maintaining the circulation.

Analgesics may be given after full assessment, and providing it does not affect observations (e.g. in head injury). Intravenous morphine may be used.

- Limit movement and splint fractures where necessary
- Prevent heat loss
- Pass a Foley's urethral catheter
- Aspirate the stomach through a large nasogastric tube if there is a danger of vomiting

SUBSEQUENT MANAGEMENT

- Monitoring of the patient's general condition, BP, pulse, peripheral perfusion, respiration and CVP should be carried out every 15 min. Urine output should be measured hourly aiming for 1–1.5 mL/kg per h. A large transfusion may require a blood warmer and calcium gluconate infusion.
- For acute renal failure, mannitol 0.25–0.5 g/kg or frusemide 1–2 mg/kg may be given and repeated if necessary (see also pp. 97).
- Correct any acid–base imbalance.
- Refractory shock may be due to septicaemia. Take blood cultures and give intravenous antibiotics such as a third generation cephalosporin.
- Inotropic support (e.g. Dopamine 5–20 μg/kg per min) is commonly required in septicaemic shock.

MENINGOCOCCAL SEPTICAEMIA/SEPTICAEMIC SHOCK

The diagnosis is usually made clinically on the base of the typical purpuric rash. Immediate and intensive therapy is essential. *Haemophilus influenzae* infection can mimic this condition.

INITIAL MANAGEMENT

- Collect blood for culture if feasible. Give a third generation cephalosporin (e.g. cefotaxime or ceftriaxone).
- In the presence of shock, give intravenous fluids using SPPS 10–20 mL/kg initially. The early use of a catecholamine infusion for inotropic effect is recommended.
- Blood coagulation studies and arterial blood gas may be indicated. After the above measures, CSF examination is usually indicated unless intracranial hypertension is suspected.

- If the diagnosis is strongly suspected in a patient outside the hospital, the antibiotics should be given before transport to hospital, even though this may prevent bacteriological confirmation.

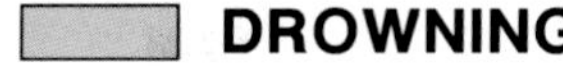

DROWNING

EMERGENCY TREATMENT

- Adequate oxygenation and ventilation is of paramount importance. Ensure an adequate airway. Vomiting and aspiration often occur causing hypoxaemia. Positive pressure ventilation via an endotracheal tube may be necessary. Decompress the stomach with a nasogastric tube.
- Support of the circulation using plasma volume expanders is indicated if shock is present. Infusion of an inotropic agent may be necessary.
- Correct acidosis and fluid or electrolyte disturbances.
- Prophylaxis for and treatment of cerebral oedema (due to hypoxia); use mannitol, 0.25–0.5 g/kg, i.v.
- The differences between salt and fresh water drowning do not affect initial therapy.

ACUTE ADRENAL CRISIS

PRINCIPLES OF MANAGEMENT

- Replace water and electrolytes and administer glucose.
- Administration of adrenocortical hormones.
- Appropriate treatment of precipitating factors such as infection or trauma.
- Gradual reduction of hormone therapy after acute phase has passed.

SPECIFIC THERAPY

- Fluid and electrolytes. Replace fluids in accordance with general principles of intravenous resuscitation. Use isotonic saline for rapid restoration of the circulating blood volume and sodium deficit. Once the circulation has been restored, use 1/2 isotonic saline and 5% dextrose to complete correction of the deficit within 12 h. Maintain with 4% dextrose in N/5 isotonic saline. Correction of hypoglycaemia may be necessary.
- Glucocorticoids. Immediate therapy: hydrocortisone 100–200 mg, i.v. Over next 24 h: hydrocortisone 100–200 mg, i.v. in divided doses. *Note*: In treating patients with adrenal insufficiency, hydrocortisone should be given as a bolus injection either intramuscularly or intravenously, rather than added to the intravenous fluid bottle. This will prevent steroid deficiency occurring in the event of an interruption to the intravenous infusion.

ACUTE LARYNGEAL OBSTRUCTION

COMMON CAUSES

- Epiglottitis
- Laryngotracheobronchitis (croup)
- Foreign body

- Allergy
- Trauma
- For routine management of above list see respiratory section, pp. 78–86.

AIRWAYS MANAGEMENT

Epiglottitis

In general, endotracheal intubation is required. Keep the child in a sitting position and administer oxygen by face mask. If the child becomes unconscious, adequate ventilation may be achieved with well managed bag and mask ventilation. If skilled anaesthetic help is not available and the child cannot be ventilated, attempt orotracheal intubation using a relatively small endotracheal tube with an introducing stylet. If this is not successful, perform tracheostomy or cricothyrotomy; insert a large bore (e.g. 12 gauge) intravenous cannula into the trachea via the cricothyroid membrane, which lies immediately subcutaneously inferior to the thyroid cartilage in the mid-line. Remove needle of intravenous cannula. Connect plastic catheter to resuscitator or bagging circuit via a 2 mL syringe barrel and size 7–8 Portex endotracheal tube connector. Ventilate with oxygen, aid expiration by lateral chest compression.

Laryngotracheobronchitis (croup)

In severe obstruction, give an inhalation of adrenaline (1 : 1000) nebulized with oxygen — in the same way salbutamol is nebulized. This may give transient relief. Obtain anaesthetic help with a view to endotracheal intubation. If help is unavailable, intubate if unconsciousness occurs.

Foreign Body in Airways

If the foreign body cannot be readily removed and respiratory failure is impending, perform tracheostomy. Cricothyrotomy (see Epiglottitis section above) may relieve obstruction at tracheal level. Attempt bag and mask mechanical ventilation if unconsciousness occurs with foreign body in either upper or lower airways.

Allergy

The use of parenteral and inhalational adrenaline is described in the section on anaphylaxis (see p. 7).

STATUS EPILEPTICUS

Any convulsion, with unconsciousness, that does not cease spontaneously in 5–10 min is a medical emergency because of hypoventilation and hypoxaemia. However, most such convulsions will cease with administration of intravenous diazepam or clonazepam. If not, the child should be admitted to an intensive care unit for further anticonvulsant therapy and may need assisted ventilation. Initial care should consist of insertion of an oropharyngeal airway, nursing in semi-prone position and the administering of oxygen by face mask or nasal catheter.

DRUG THERAPY

It should be noted that in meningitis respiratory depression is a common side effect of anti-convulsants.

- *Clonazepam*. Dose: < 1 year, 0.25 mg; 1–5 years, 0.5 mg; > 15 years, 1 mg. Side effects: respiratory depression and hypotension occur rarely.
- *Diazepam*. Dose: 0.1–0.2 mg/kg may be given as an alternative if clonazepam is unavailable. The dose may be administered per rectum if there is no intravenous access (dilute to 5 mL).
- *Phenytoin*. Dose: 15 mg/kg mixed with isotonic saline solution is given intravenously over 1 h. Side effects: Cardiac arrhythmias, and hypotension (negative inotropic agent).
- *Thiopentone*. This should only be used in a situation where facilities for ventilation are available. (In Royal Children's Hospital, it is used by Intensive Care Unit staff only.)

GENERAL SUPPORTIVE MEASURES

Fluid and electrolyte therapy is essential to avoid excess fluid intake and fluids should be given at one-half to two-thirds maintenance rates, except in situations where general circulation and arterial blood pressure are jeopardized. Serum electrolytes should be monitored. Beware of hyponatraemia causing fitting in meningitis (due to inappropriate antidiuretic hormone secretion).

INVESTIGATION

The most common causes of intractable *grand mal* seizures in childhood are metabolic disturbances, poisoning and encephalitis.

ACUTELY RAISED INTRACRANIAL PRESSURE

AETIOLOGY

- Increased CSF volume or obstructed CSF circulation
- Acute brain swelling due to cerebral oedema, e.g. cerebral hypoxaemia, meningo-encephalitis, trauma
- Space-occupying lesion
- Combinations of the above

ASSESSMENT

In addition to usual neurological signs, the following findings suggest an extremely urgent situation.

- Deterioration in conscious state
- Alteration in vital signs such as slowing of pulse, a rise in BP and alteration in pattern of respiration
- Signs of brainstem compression such as pupillary signs, extensor rigidity spasms or extensor plantar responses.

A neurosurgeon should be contacted immediately.

MANAGEMENT

If it is not possible to establish and relieve the cause immediately, the aim is to reduce the volume of the intracranial contents.

Optimize Ventilation

Ensure adequate airways and ventilation. Correct hypoxaemia. Artificial hyperventilation to lower P_{CO_2} to 25–35 mmHg and decrease intracranial blood volume may be necessary. This is the most effective emergency treatment. Nurse the patient 30° head up, with head maintained in the mid-line.

Drug Treatment

- Mannitol. Infuse a dose of 0.25–0.5 g/kg as a 10 or 20% solution. Its effect commences in 20 min and lasts for 3–4 h.
- Steroids. Dexamethasone is given for raised intracranial pressure in association with brain tumours.

Circulatory Support

Correct hypervolaemia with colloid infusion. Use inotropic drugs to raise a low blood pressure to maintain cerebral perfusion. Restrict fluid administration (to reduce cerebral oedema).

CHAPTER 3

POISONS AND ACCIDENTAL INGESTION

PRINCIPLES OF MANAGEMENT

ASSESSMENT

Resuscitate first. Identify the drugs/poison, the quantities ingested and the time of exposure. Relatively non-toxic substances or small quantities of toxic substances may only require reassurance and observation.

In Victoria information can be obtained from the Poisons Information Centre on (03) 345 5678 (0900–2200 h), and Australia-wide (008) 133 890 (0900–2200 h), (008) 25 1525 (2200–0900 h) or from the Royal Children's Hospital Intensive Care Unit on (03) 345 5212 concerning patient management.

Self-administered poisoning in a child over the age of 7 years may be an attempt at suicide.

REMOVAL OF TOXIC SUBSTANCES

Remove from the body as quickly as possible. Ingested substances may be removed from the stomach by induced emesis (preferred method) or by gastric lavage. Emesis can be induced in most children with syrup of ipecac. Both induced emesis and gastric lavage are contraindicated if the patient is not fully conscious, because of the danger of aspiration. Corrosive substances and petroleum products, e.g. kerosene, should not be removed by induced emesis or gastric lavage even in the conscious patient because of the risks of further damage or pneumonitis, respectively. Other methods such as diuresis, dialysis, exchange transfusion, charcoal haemoperfusion, haemofiltration or plasmaphaeresis may be necessary.

Activated Charcoal

Initial dose (suspension) 1–2 g/kg then 0.5–1 g/kg 4 hourly for 12–24 h orally or via gastric tube. This absorbs many toxic substances (except corrosives, metals, petroleum derivatives and turpentine). Charcoal leaches some substances, e.g. theophylline, barbiturates, from the intestinal mucosal circulation when administered on a regular basis. Give a laxative such as magnesium sulfate 0.25–0.5 g/kg per dose orally 4–8 hourly. Most seriously poisoned patients recover with skilled support of vital functions. The most frequent complications of poisoning are aspiration pneumonitis, hypoventilation and hypotension.

MANAGEMENT OF SOME COMMON SPECIFIC POISONS

A few are summarized below. Additional detailed information is available 24 h per day from the Poisons Information Centre (see Consultation p. 2) or from the intensive care unit. Useful references are the Poisindex system, the texts *Handbook of Poisoning* (by R. H. Dreisbach. 11th edn; Large Medical Publications, Los Angeles CA, 1983) and *Medical Toxicology* (by M. J. Ellerhorn and D. G. Barceloux. Elsevier, New York, 1988).

CORROSIVES

Acids, alkalis (including dish-washing powder), ammonia, anti-rust, drain cleaners, floor strippers, oven cleaners, phenol, zinc chloride (soldering flux) and others. Severe oropharyngeal, and oesophageal burns and upper airways obstruction may occur. Ensure adequate airways and ventilation. Admit the patient for observation and oesophagogastroscopy if there is historical or clinical evidence of ingestion. The presence of orophyaryngeal oedema suggests distal damage, but its absence does not exclude damage.

Do not induce emesis or perform gastric lavage.

PETROLEUM DISTILLATES AND TURPENTINE

Kerosene, petrol, mineral oil and other petroleum distillates and turpentine cause vomiting, severe pneumonitis, convulsions, coma and cardiac dysrhythmia. Pneumonitis occurs from fumes or fluid aspirated during ingestion or vomiting. Mortality is associated with pneumonitis.

Do not induce vomiting or perform lavage.

If spontaneous vomiting has occurred and the patient has a cough, aspiration penumonitis is probably present. Oxygen therapy and a chest X-ray are indicated. If the distillate contains toxic additives gastric lavage should only be performed after endotracheal intubation. With CNS depression, ensure adequate airways, ventilation and circulation.

IRON-CONTAINING PREPARATIONS

Admit the patient if there is suspicion of significant iron ingestion (> 60 mg/kg of elemental iron). There are five recognizable stages in iron poisoning.

- *First stage.* Thirty min–2 h after ingestion; lethargy, coma, fitting, vomiting, diarrhoea, haematemesis and malaena. Severe haemorrhagic gastroenteritis with large losses of fluid and blood may cause peripheral circulatory failure. Serum iron levels may be high in this stage prior to hepatic deposition, after which low levels do not exclude significant intoxication.
- *Second stage.* A deceptive quiescent stage may last up to 48 h.
- *Third stage.* Peripheral circulatory failure due to decreased blood volume and myocardial failure. Hypovolaemia is caused by continued fluid and blood loss and increased capillary permeability. Severe acidosis, due to the release of hydrogen ions when ferric ions are converted to ferrous ions and when acids are generated with anaerobic metabolism, may impede myocardial contractility. Hypoglycaemia and other effects of liver dysfunction may occur.
- *Fourth stage.* Hepatic necrosis may occur several days after ingestion.
- *Fifth stage.* Gastric or pyloric scarring may cause gastrointestinal obstruction several weeks after ingestion.

Treatment

General management

Ensure adequate airways, ventilation and perfusion. Peripheral circulatory failure may be an early or late manifestation of significant toxicity. Maintenance of adequate blood volume is essential. Inotropic support and correction of acidosis may be necessary. Renal failure due to hypoperfusion should be treated with dialysis (ferrioxamine is dialysable).

Induced emesis and gastric lavage

Perform according to Principles of Management (see p. 13). Residual ferrous iron may be converted to unabsorbable ferrous carbonate by instillation into the stomach of a diluted solution (1–2%) of sodium bicarbonate to maintain the pH > 5.0. The use of desferrioxamine for lavage or instillation remains controversial. X-rays may help assess the adequacy of removal of tablets. Activated charcoal is not helpful.

Chelation of absorbed iron

If major clinical effects of poisoning are evident, desferrioxamine should be given intravenously at a rate of 10–15 mg/kg per h until the urine ceases to be pink.

SALICYLATES

Neurological effects include coma and fitting. Early manifestations of toxicity are transient tachypnoea (not prominent in children), tinnitus, tremor and hyperpyrexia. Vomiting with severe dehydration and electrolyte disturbance may occur. In addition, bicarbonate is excreted in the urine with compensatory loss of sodium and potassium in the early phase. Later, hydrogen ions are lost to conserve potassium. Carbohydrate metabolism is disturbed resulting in metabolic acidosis, ketosis and hypoglycaemia. Hypoprothrombinaemia, platelet dysfunction and gastritis may cause haematemesis. Non-cardiogenic pulmonary oedema may occur. Plasma salicylate greater than 2.2–2.9 mmol/L is associated with toxicity. A level greater than 7.3 mmol/L is potentially lethal. Ingestion of: less than 150 mg/kg causes nausea and vomiting; 150–300 mg/kg causes hyperventilation, lethargy or excitability; greater than 300 mg/kg causes coma and convulsions.

Treatment

General management

Ensure adequate airways, ventilation and perfusion.

Induced emesis and gastric lavage

Perform according to Principles of Management (see p. 13). Give repeated doses of activated charcoal.

Supportive therapy

Dehydration, electrolyte disturbance and acidosis, should be treated with dextrose electrolyte solution, e.g. 4% dextrose with 1/5 normal saline and sodium bicarbonate according to arterial acid–base status and to plasma and urine electrolytes.

Severe bleeding may require the use of fresh frozen plasma, clotting factors and whole blood. Vitamin K_1 is used in less severe cases to minimize hypoprothrombinaemia.

Facilitation of salicylate excretion

Sodium bicarbonate should be administered to maintain urine pH > 7.5.

TRICYCLIC ANTIDEPRESSANTS

Toxic effects include coma, convulsions, dysrhythmias and hypotension. There may be delayed gastric emptying (anticholinergic effect) and delayed drug absorption.

Treatment

General management

Ensure adequate airways, ventilation and perfusion.

Induced emesis and gastric lavage

Perform according to Principles of Management (see p. 13). Tricyclics may be recovered from the stomach many hours after ingestion.

Activated charcoal

Orally or via gastric tube accompanied by a laxative.

Specific Treatment

- Seizures. Treat with diazepam, clonazepam or phenytoin (see pp. 104 and 110). Beware of respiratory depression.
- Dysrhythmias. All patients with potentially toxic overdoses require admission to intensive care for ECG monitoring. Dysrhythmias are due to anticholinergic, adrenergic and quinidine-like properties of the drugs. ECG changes include tachycardia, prolonged PR interval, widening of QRS complex (> 0.12 s is significant), QT prolongation, ST segment depression and T wave flattening or inversion. Dysrhythmias include heart block, asystole, multifocal ectopics, ventricular tachycardia, flutter and fibrillation.

A patient with no anticholinergic effects with a normal pulse rate and normal QRS duration, is unlikely to be seriously poisoned.

PARACETAMOL

Fatal hepatic necrosis may occur several days after ingestion. Nausea and vomiting usually occur soon after ingestion followed by a quiescent phase before the onset of hepatic dysfunction. Renal damage is rare. Toxic dose is greater than 140 mg/kg.

Treatment

Induce emesis, perform gastric lavage and administer activated charcoal according to Principles of Management (see p. 13). Withdraw blood for paracetamol levels 4–12 h after ingestion (peak level is at approximately 4 h after ingestion). Within the Royal Children's Hospital obtain urgent analysis from the Biochemistry Department. Plot the plasma paracetamol level on the nomogram contained in the literature accompanying *N*-acetylcysteine (Parvolex). If hepatic toxicity is probable, administer *N*-acetylcysteine within 15 h of ingestion; 150 mg/kg over 15 min (beware anaphylaxis) followed by 50 mg/kg over 4 h followed by 100 mg/kg over 16 h (total 300 mg/kg over 20 h) intravenously. Controversy surrounds more delayed administration and greater doses of *N*-acetylcysteine. Monitor liver function: within the Royal Children's Hospital a gastroenterology consultation is recommended.

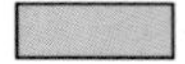

ENVENOMATION

SNAKE BITE

Information should be sought from local authorities regarding snake species in areas outside Victoria. However, the general principles set out here will be of use to those clinicians treating patients with snake bite.

Of the many species of snakes in Victoria, dangerous species are the brown snake, tiger snake, copperhead and red bellied black snake. Venom of these species contains neurotoxins, haemolysins, procoagulants and rhabdomyolysins. Every snake bite should be regarded as venomous and potentially lethal. Fatality may occur due to respiratory failure or haemorrhage following disseminated intravascular coagulation.

Symptoms and Signs

Within an hour of envenomation, important signs are headache, nausea, vomiting, painful regional lymph nodes and transient hypotension causing loss of consciousness. The bite site may be obvious, with fang or scratch marks or with bruising or swelling. It is important to note that the bite may be undetectable and unnoticed by the victim. A state of advanced envenomation is present if at 1–3 h, there are neurotoxic signs such as ptosis, diplopia, blurred vision, facial muscle weakness, dysphonia and dysphagia. Limb, trunk and respiratory muscles become progressively affected. Haemoglobinuria and haemorrhage may occur. The syndrome culminates several hours after envenomation with respiratory and cardiovascular failure. Myoglobinuria may be a late finding. The syndrome may be accelerated in a small child or after multiple bites.

Management

- *Suspected envenomation.* If there is a history of bite but no symptoms or signs, the patient should be admitted for observation, preferably to the intensive care unit. If in place, the first aid bandage and splint may then be removed. In the absence of symptoms and signs, a coagulation profile may indicate envenomation. The presence of venom and species of snake can be determined by the venom detection kit (within Royal Children's Hospital maintained in intensive care unit). Venom in blood or urine (preferred) proves envenomation, while venom on skin or clothing proves a strike.
- *Definite envenomation.* Ensure adequate airways, ventilation and perfusion. Administer appropriate antivenom intravenously (instructions with ampoule). There is a risk of anaphylactoid reaction to antivenom and administration should be preceded by an antihistamine (promethazine 0.25 mg/kg, i.v.) and adrenaline (0.005–0.01 mg/kg, subcutaneously). If there is a history of allergy, hydrocortisone may also be given intravenously.

Brown Snake antivenom is effective only against brown snake envenomation, while tiger snake antivenom is effective against tiger, black and copperhead snake envenomation. In Victoria tiger snake antivenom is used to treat red bellied black snake envenomation. A black snake antivenom is available. If the identity of the snake is known either on the basis of the test with venom detection kit or with irrefutable herpetological evidence, administer one ampoule of tiger snake antivenom or one ampoule of brown snake antivenom. There are initial doses of antivenom irrespective of the patient's weight or age. Additional doses should be given on the basis of clinical and sequential coagulation status. Administer additional antivenom before transfusing blood. In Victoria, if the identity of the snake is not known and the patient is seriously envenomated, administer one ampoule of brown snake antivenom and one ampoule of tiger snake antivenom as initial treatment. In other Australian states, other specific monovalent or polyvalent antivemon may be indicated.

SPIDER BITES

Information should be sought from local authorities regarding spider species in areas outside Victoria. However, the general principles set out here will be of use to those clinicians treating patients with spider bite.

Redback Spider

The only known dangerous spider in Victoria is the redback spider.

Symptoms and Signs

The bite is painful and the site may become red, hot and swollen with sweating over the surrounding skin. The pain may progressively involve the whole limb (occasionally another limb) and is exacerbated by movement. Regional lymphadenopathy, headache, nausea and vomiting may develop over a few hours. Sweating may become generalized and accompanied by pyrexia. Tachycardia and hypertension are common. Many other signs and symptoms may occur and include rashes, arthralgia, paraesthesia and muscle weakness.

Management

If only mild local effects are present after several hours, treatment should be symptomatic. If there are generalized effects, antivenom (500 units) should be given intramuscularly, preceded by antihistamine (promethazine 0.5 mg/kg, i.m.). Adrenaline should be readily available. If the patient has an allergic history, hydrocortisone should be given intravenously prior to antivenom. Occasionally, mechanical ventilation is necessary, in which case antivenom should be given intravenously.

Other Spiders

The white tailed spider and unidentified species have caused local tissue necrosis and systemic effects for which there is no specific treatment.

CHAPTER 4

COMMON MEDICAL PROBLEMS

BACTERIAL MENINGITIS

DIAGNOSIS

Bacterial meningitis is a medical emergency. In infants the signs may be minimal with only lethargy and irritability noted. In older children, headache, vomiting, drowsiness, photophobia and neck stiffness are present.

Diagnosis is confirmed by lumbar puncture. However, when a child is either unconscious, demonstrates focal neurological signs or has signs of raised intracranial pressure, lumbar puncture may result in coning. Under these circumstances, and when meningitis is suspected, lumbar puncture should be delayed. Identification of the organism will then rely upon blood culture and urine antigen results. Antibiotic therapy must be given immediately following the collection of appropriate cultures.

Interpretation of CSF Findings

	Bacterial	*Partially treated*	*TB*	*Viral*
Cells	Polys	Polys or lymphocytes	Lymphocytes	Polys, then lymphocytes
Gram stain or antigen	Usually + ve	May be + ve	– ve	– ve
Glucose	Low	Low or normal	Low	Usually normal
Protein	High	High	High	Usually normal
Bacterial culture	+ ve	May be – ve	– ve	– ve

Up to 5×10^6/L white blood cells in CSF is acceptable. If the CSF is contaminated with blood a ratio of 1 white blood cell to 500 red blood cells is allowable.

The normal CSF protein level is up to 0.4 g/L. Allow 0.01 g/L for every 1000 red blood cells in blood-contaminated CSF. Glucose levels in CSF should be more than 2.5 mmol/L, or 50% the blood glucose value.

ANTIBIOTIC TREATMENT

Age 3 Months to 14 Years

Initial therapy

Cefotaxime 50 mg/kg per Q6 h or ceftriaxone 50 mg/kg per Q12 h.

Continued therapy

Adjust antibiotic treatment according to culture and sensitivity results.

***Haemophilus influenzae* type b:** Amoxycillin 50 mg/kg per Q4 h or cefotaxime or ceftriaxone (dosages as above).

Streptococcus pneumoniae: Penicillin G 30 mg/kg per Q4 h.

Neisseria meningitidis: Penicillin G 30 mg/kg per Q4 h.

Age Less Than 3 Months

Initial therapy

Amoxycillin 50 mg/kg per dose + cefotaxime or ceftriaxone (dosages as above).

Continued therapy

Adjust treatments according to culture and sensitivity results.

Frequency of Intravenous Administration

	Wt < 2000 g		*Wt > 2000 g*	
	< 7 days	*7–28 days*	*< 7 days*	*7–28 days*
Amoxycillin 50 mg/kg	Q12 h	Q8 h	Q8 h	Q6 h
Cefotaxime 50 mg/kg	Q12 h	Q8 h	Q12 h	Q8 h
Gentamicin* 2.5 mg/kg	Q12 h	Q8 h	Q12 h	Q8 h

* Infants < 1500 g may require longer dosing intervals. Monitor gentamicin levels. Between 4 weeks and 3 months of age, the dosage and frequency of antibiotic administration is identical to that of older children. In Gram negative bacillary meningitis, therapy is continued for at least 3 weeks after CSF sterilization.

GENERAL MEASURES

Fluid restriction is an essential principle of treatment because of the risk of inappropriate antidiuretic hormone secretion (SIADH). A patient who is not in shock, and whose serum sodium is within the normal range, is given 50% of maintenance fluid requirements as initial management. If SIADH is present, restrict fluids to insensible losses (250 mL/m^2 per day) plus urine output to a maximum of 50% of maintenance requirements. Control of seizures is vital. Careful attention is paid to the respiratory status of the child, both before the selection, and following the use of an anticonvulsant.

Early consultation with the intensive care unit is necessary for any child who is deteriorating in conscious state, cardiovascular status or experiencing seizures.

Fever persisting for more than 7 days or a secondary fever commonly results from: nosocomial infections, subdural effusions, other suppurative lesions, or immune complex disease (e.g. late onset sterile arthritis). Uncommonly, fever may also arise from inadequately treated meningitis, a parameningeal focus or drugs. Management, including a repeat lumbar puncture, must be individualized.

At the time of publication there is insufficient data to recommend the routine administration of dexamethasone to children with bacterial meningitis.

PROPHYLAXIS REGIMENS

Organism	*Antibiotic*	*Comments*
H. influenzae type b	*Rifampicin 20 mg/kg as a single daily dose (600 mg max.) for 4 days	Give to index case and all family contacts if the index case is younger than 2 years or the household includes other children under 4 years of age If more than one case occurs at a single day care centre, rifampicin prophylaxis is recommended
N. meningitidis	*Rifampicin 10 mg/kg, b.d. (up to 600 mg, b.d.) for 2 days	Give to index case and all intimate, household or day care contacts
S. pneumoniae	None	No increased risks to contacts

* Half dosage in neonatal contacts. *Note:* As rifampicin lowers chloramphenicol levels, children treated with this drug are given prophylaxis at the end of therapy. Rifampicin is contraindicated in pregnancy and decreases the efficacy of oral contraceptives. Pregnant meningococcal contacts may be given ceftriaxone 250 mg, i.m. as a single dose of prophylaxis. However, nasopharyngeal carriage of *H. influenzae* type b is not eradicated by a single injection of ceftriaxone. Any febrile household contact should seek medical attention.

URINARY TRACT INFECTIONS (UTI)

SYMPTOMS

UTI should always be considered in a child who presents with fever, vomiting, or abdominal pain without obvious cause. On the other hand, even when specific urinary symptoms are present, up to one-third will not have a UTI.

SPECIMENS

See Specimens Required for Microbiological Diagnosis (pp. 62–8) and Paediatric Procedures (pp. 178–80).

DIAGNOSIS

See Specimens Required for Microbiological Diagnosis (pp. 62–8).

TREATMENT

Acute Infection

Usual duration of therapy is 1 week. Recommended empirical drugs are: amoxycillin or trimethoprim–sulfamethoxazole. Ongoing therapy is guided by bacterial sensitivity. Further culture of urine after 1 week is indicated.

Recurrent Infection

This can be guided according to past bacterial sensitivity.

Maintenance

Low dose nitrofurantoin or trimethoprim–sulfamethoxazole is indicated in those children with three or more symptomatic infections a year or severe reflux.

INVESTIGATIONS

These should be done for all, i.e. the first, bacteriologically proven UTI, at any age. Paediatric consultation is advised.

- *Less than 5 years of age*. Investigate with MCU and ultrasound.
- *Over 5 years of age*. Investigate with ultrasound. If ultrasound is abnormal proceed to MCU.

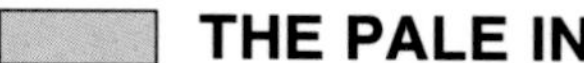

THE PALE INFANT AND CHILD

Pallor is determined by the haemoglobin concentration, haemodynamic status and presence or absence of oedema. Many children appear pale even though they have a normal haemoglobin concentration. Parents may think their lightly complexioned children are anaemic.

Pallor is a well-known manifestation of shock, sepsis, cardiac failure, hypoxia, hypothermia, severe pain and generalized oedema. Other associated features will distinguish these children from those whose pallor is principally due to anaemia.

Anaemia is present when the haemoglobin or haematocrit is less than age appropriate values (see p. 199). The presence of anaemia may be suspected by finding pale mucous membranes or pale palmar creases.

CLINICAL FEATURES

In the history inquire about the onset and duration of pallor, and whether there has been any lethargy, dyspnoea and, in small infants, sweating or feeding difficulties. Ask about the diet (vegetarian, meat and milk intake), bleeding episodes, diarrhoea, weight loss, jaundice, drugs, foreign travel, perinatal history (e.g. prematurity, twins) and family history of anaemia.

As part of the general examination pay particular attention to the presence of pallor, jaundice, petechiae, tachycardia, cardiac murmurs, cardiac failure, lymphadenopathy, hepatosplenomegaly, abdominalmasses, altered conscious state and retinal haemorrhages.

MANAGEMENT

The initial laboratory tests should be a full blood examination (FBE), differential white cell count and reticulocyte count. These tests will provide information on the haemoglobin concentration, haematocrit, red cell indices and morphology, numbers and types of white cells (including the presence of blasts), platelets and reticulocytes.

It will now be possible to investigate and diagnose the type of anaemia present according to the following table.

Red Cell Morphology

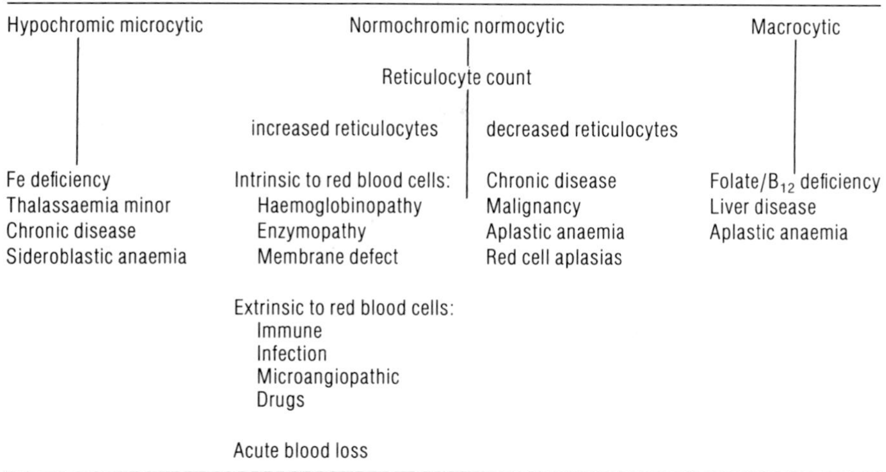

IRON DEFICIENCY ANAEMIA

This is the commonest cause of anaemia in children, and is typically a hypochromic and microcytic anaemia. Causes are age dependent.

1 Less than 6 months: perinatal factors (e.g. prematurity, multiple birth), resulting in low iron stores.
2 Six to 24 months: nutritional (decreased iron intake, excessive milk ingestion).
3 Greater than 24 months: consider blood loss especially from the gastrointestinal tract.

Investigations

Measure serum iron, total iron-binding capacity, ferritin.

Treatment

- Treat underlying cause (e.g. diet, source of blood loss).
- Prescribe 6 mg/kg per day of elemental iron which is equivalent to 1 mL/kg per day of ferrous gluconate. This is best given three times a day, before meals with orange juice, but not with milk or cereals.
- Expect a reticulocyte response in 7–10 days.
- Treat for 3 months to replenish iron stores.

In the otherwise healthy infant aged 6–24 months of age who presents with a mild hypochromic microcytic anaemia and who has compliant parents a therapeutic trial of iron can be administered for 2 weeks without further investigations. If the anaemia responds, the iron is to be continued. Failure of the anaemia to respond to the iron requires further investigation.

Causes of failure to respond to iron therapy include:

- Non-compliance
- Inadequate dosage

- Impaired absorption
- Continued blood loss
- Incorrect diagnosis
- Coexisting disease (e.g. renal failure)

Prevention

Administer prophylactic iron, 2 mg/kg per day of elemental iron, to premature infants, infants of multiple births and those with a history of perinatal blood loss. This is to be started at 3 months of age and continued until the first birthday.

Educate parents to ensure that infants beyond 9 months of age have an adequate iron-containing diet (e.g. meat, green vegetables, eggs), and to avoid excessive ingestion (> 600 mL/day) of milk.

NOCTURNAL ENURESIS

Primary enuresis is rarely due to organic disease. The prevalence in the community at 5 years of age is 10–15%. Secondary enuresis (enuresis occurring after a period of bladder continence at night has been achieved) always requires assessment since an emotional or organic cause may be contributing. Possible organic causes in either primary or secondary enuresis may include:

- Urinary infection
- Systemic illness such as diabetes, renal failure, epilepsy
- Anatomical defects of the urinary tract such as ectopic ureter
- Neurogenic defects

INVESTIGATION

Urine should be examined for protein, reducing substances and evidence of infection.

MANAGEMENT

Referral to medical outpatients should be made if treatment is requested. Conditioning therapy in the form of a buzzer or a pad and bell mattress alarm is the most successful form of therapy. The use of tricyclic antidepressants is of limited value in children, is usually of short term benefit only, and is now considered inappropriate.

TEETHING

Many symptoms including fever, convulsions, cough and diarrhoea have been incorrectly attributed to teething. The diagnosis of many severe illnesses has been delayed because of this. Some increase in day- or night-time restlessness, in finger sucking and gum rubbing, in dribbling and a decrease in feeding may be caused by teething. Examination of the gums reveals no change in the colour of the mucosa in one-third of patients, slight erythema in another third, and marked erythema and small haemorrhages in the remainder. Treatment includes sympathetic reassurance to the parents, softening of the diet if there is reluctance to eat hard foods and a mild sedative such as chloral hydrate in the patient who has trouble sleeping. Consideration should be given to the use of paracetamol to relieve pain. Treatment should not include lancing of the gums or teething powders. Teething rings or baby rusks may offer some relief.

COLIC (INFANT DISTRESS)

Colic or infant distress is the name given to unexplained crying in well infants between 1 and 16 weeks of age. This phenomenon peaks at 4–8 weeks of age and improves spontaneously by 10–16 weeks. If the crying persists, other perpetuating factors should be considered such as maternal anxiety, feeding difficulties or chronic infection. The crying is often worse in the evening and is not relieved by picking the baby up, feeding and the usual comforting measures. If no precipitating or perpetuating factors are present, then this problem resolves spontaneously.

The management consists of:

- Excluding other causes of crying such as feeding problems and pain, e.g. otitis media, anal fissure, cow milk intolerance, oesophagitis and intussusception.
- Identifying and attempting to relieve stresses on the mother, e.g. lack of sleep, social isolation, family tensions or personal emotional difficulties.
- Prophylactic carrying in an infant snuggly (or carrying pouch) has been shown to substantially reduce cry–fuss behaviour in normal babies, but to increase cry–fuss behaviour in babies diagnosed with colic.
- Use comforting measures such as regular rhythmical patting movement or a pacifier. Allow the baby to establish a predictable routine and reduce environmental stimulation by decreasing excessive noise, light and handling. Gently rocking and soft music may help calm a tense baby.

The use of medication is rarely helpful. Mixtures containing anticholinergics are contraindicated.

BREATH HOLDING ATTACKS

These may occur in some young children when they are hurt, annoyed or frightened. In a minor form they are common and consist of a sudden cessation of breathing during the course of a spell of crying. This variety is brief and may be associated with some cyanosis. The severe form may result in unconsciousness and convulsive movements and must be differentiated from true epilepsy by an accurate history. The characteristic sequence of events is provocation, cry, apnoea, cyanosis (sometimes), and *then* loss of consciousness and convulsive movements. Episodes commence between 6 months and 2 years of age and usually disappear spontaneously by 4 years of age. The prognosis is excellent and no drug treatment is needed. These events are often frightening and parents need explanation and reassurance.

APNOEIC EPISODES IN INFANCY

See also Apparent Life Threatening Episodes (p. 59).

Often incorrectly called near-miss sudden infant death syndrome most apnoeic episodes in this age group are associated with choking during milk regurgitation and require no investigation, although management of persistent reflux may be necessary. Other rarer causes include convulsions, cardiac dysrhythmias, respiratory centre abnormalities or systemic disease. Premature infants or infants with other disabilities are more at risk. Admission to hospital is often necessary to observe the nature of these episodes and allay parental anxiety, although detailed investigation is mostly unrewarding. Home apnoea monitoring is of unproven value and should only be considered after consultation with a neonatologist at a tertiary referral centre.

CHRONIC AND RECURRENT HEADACHE

Migraine is the commonest form of chronic or recurrent headache in children and adolescents. In adolescents, muscle contraction (tension) headache also frequently occurs. Common migraine which manifests no focal neurological symptoms, is usually associated with frontotemporal or bifrontal headache, and is frequently accompanied by nausea and vomiting (except in younger children). Migraine is often followed by lethargy or sleep, and is the most frequent form of migraine. Classic migraine is less common.

Migraine has a paroxysmal temporal pattern, whereas tension headache tends to be persistent. If not due to raised intracranial pressure, headaches upon wakening are most likely migrainous, whereas headaches that wake children from sleep are commonly cluster headaches, and are rarely due to migraine or grave CNS disease.

Serious neurological disorders should only be suspected if there are symptoms of focal motor, co-ordination or sensory function which persist in pain-free intervals (although rare migraine syndromes may also present this way), especially if there have been concomitant changes in behaviour, emotional state or school performance.

A careful and detailed history, general physical and neurological examination will permit accurate diagnosis in nearly all cases, and follow-up will confirm this diagnosis. Assessment of growth, head circumference and blood pressure are essential parts of the examination.

Reassurance of the child and parents is a crucial part of management. Children's headaches are real (i.e. not imagined by the child) and common. Laboratory investigations are not usually contributory. If there is a suspicion of, or evidence for, a serious neurological illness; if the pattern of migraine is neither common nor classic (i.e. one of the rarer variants); if there is an unsatisfactory response to simple treatment measures (see below); or if there is extreme parental pressure or anxiety; the most appropriate action is referral to a specialist.

In migraine, trigger avoidance and stress management can be considered as preventative measures. Simple analgesia with paracetamol is very often all the treatment that is required. Abortive treatment includes ergotamine in severe cases. Prophylaxis is indicated only if attacks are severe and frequent enough to cause social, scholastic or occupational dysfunction. Pizotifen, phenobarbitone and propanolol are among the options to be considered, usually in consultation with a specialist. Biofeedback techniques may be of value.

RECURRENT ABDOMINAL PAIN (RAP)

RAP affects about 10% of school age children. It is infrequently caused by organic disorders, and is most often dysfunctional, i.e. physiologically based pain without identifiable pathologic cause. It is also uncommonly psychogenic, i.e. purely the result of emotional or psychological stress. However, in considering the basis for a child's pain it is helpful to remember that emotional factors, life-styles and temperamental characteristics can modulate pain, as well as the child's response to pain, regardless of whether its cause is organic or dysfunctional.

Assessment consists of a careful history including psychosocial details, elicited from parents alone, child alone and the family together. A useful, albeit fallible rule is that the further the pain is away from the umbilicus, the more likely it is to have an organic basis. A thorough physical examination, including blood pressure measurement and rectal examination should be carried out. Full blood count, ESR, urine microscopy and culture and a plain abdominal X-ray are appropriate baseline investigations, to be supplemented by more specific tests only when history or examination finding indicate.

The diagnosis of psychogenic recurrent abdominal pain cannot be made simply in the absence of positive findings for an organic disorder. Positive evidence of emotional maladjustment is separately required, and if present should be managed appropriately.

In the absence of evidence for organic or emotional causes, a provisional working diagnosis of dysfunctional recurrent abdominal pain is made. Parents and child are reassured, and regular follow-up is indicated during which changes in symptoms and signs are monitored. Avoid facile and meaningless diagnoses such as 'allergy', 'prolonged virus' or 'nervous stomach'. Rest and simple analgesia may be useful during episodes. A positive and empathic attitude is required of the physician, and parents need to be encouraged to 'normalize' the child's life as much as possible. Relaxation and visual imagery techniques may be of value in reducing symptoms.

SCHOOL FAILURE

Many factors cause children to have difficulty at school. The aetiology of school problems is rarely straightforward and usually represents the end result of a complex transaction between environmental and child-related factors. The physician needs to rule out physical health problems, medication side effects (e.g. theophylline, anticonvulsants), sensory impairments (hearing and vision deficits), neurological disease, emotional and behavioural disorders, adverse family and social influences, inappropriate classroom environments, and specific cognitive weaknesses, as potential contributors to school failure.

Only a small proportion of children with school failure will have a clearly identifiable medical basis for their difficulties, but a meticulous physical and neurological examination, and formal testing of hearing and vision must be performed as a minimum. Referral can then be made to a paediatrician for more detailed neurodevelopmental testing, which involves assessment of selective attention, spatial organization and visual perception, auditory and visual memory and sequencing, receptive and expressive language, and fine and gross motor function. Referring the child to his or her regional School Support Centre for most detailed cognitive testing and/or psychological counselling is sometimes necessary.

Following assessment, a profile of the child's developmental strengths and weaknesses is obtained, as well as a sense of other constitutional and environmental factors that may be playing a role. An individualized intervention plan is then developed in conjunction with the school. Most importantly, the doctor should act as an advocate for the child in securing needed services.

ENCOPRESIS

Encopresis (see also constipation pp. 95–6) is defined as the involuntary passage of formed or semi-formed stools into the underwear on a regular basis. It is a distressing symptom to the child and family alike, and must be taken seriously. The majority of children with encopresis have inadequate toileting and consequent faecal retention. A plain abdominal X-ray to document the nature and extent of faecal retention, and to serve as a baseline for further treatment is often helpful. The chronic faecal retention is associated with rectal dilatation and insensitivity to the normal urge to stool. This is why a structured toileting programme is the most important aspect of management. It has also been shown that laxative therapy and initial bowel catharsis aids remission from faecal incontinence, and assists the development of a durable toileting routine.

Many regimens are used to clear the bowel of faeces. Often this cathartic regimen is broken down into an initial cleanout which lasts up to 2 weeks (with regular use of home-administered suppositories, enemas, and oral cathartics) followed by maintenance treatment (consisting of oral cathartic only).

Close follow-up is essential with the assistance of a star chart diary to reward regular sitting and successful defecation in the toilet. The treatment regimen should be maintained for several months at a minimum. The aim of treatment is to institute good dietary and toileting habits to ensure that the problem does not recur, and then gradually wean the child from medications. Biofeedback training may be of value in treatment-resistant children. Within Victoria the Royal Children's Hospital Encopresis Clinic provides services for refractory cases.

Sometimes it is clear that a disordered family dynamic exists, or there are emotional factors beyond those which one would expect, given the distressing nature of the symptoms. In these instances there should be careful evaluation of the child and the family, either by the paediatrician or by referral to a psychologist, psychiatrist, or family therapist. However, ongoing psychotherapy has no place in the routine management of children with encopresis.

CHAPTER 5

COMMON SURGICAL PROBLEMS

INGUINOSCROTAL CONDITIONS

The underlying pathological basis of an inguinal hernia, an encysted hydrocele of the cord and a scrotal hydrocele is persistence of the patent processus vaginalis after completion of testicular descent.

INGUINAL HERNIA

The opening of the processus vaginalis is large enough to allow the protrusion of bowel through the inguinal canal and sometimes down to the scrotum. The younger the child the greater is the danger that the bowel will become strangulated. Inguinal hernias always need surgery because of the ever present danger of bowel strangulation and compression of the testicular vessels.

Reducible Inguinal Hernia

- Birth to 6 weeks: Surgical consultation on the day of diagnosis, surgery on the next convenient list, preferably within 2 days.
- Six weeks to 6 months: urgent surgical outpatient appointment with surgery within 2 weeks.
- Over 6 months: surgical outpatient appointment should be within 2 weeks and surgery within 2 months. This is normally done as a day case.

Irreducible Hernia

These should be referred to a surgeon as soon as the diagnosis is made. Normally the surgeon is able to reduce the hernia manually and surgery is performed the following day. The child is admitted overnight and discharged the day after surgery.

SCROTAL HYDROCELE, ENCYSTED HYDROCELE OF THE CORD

In both these conditions the opening of the processus vaginalis is narrow and may close of its own accord in children up to 18 months to 2 years. Important clinical signs are:

- A brilliantly transilluminable swelling
- A narrow cord above the swelling
- The swelling does not empty on squeezing

If any of these features are not present, the swelling may be an irreducible hernia.

If *hydroceles* persist beyond 2 years, surgery is recommended and inguinal herniotomy (i.e. division of the patent processus vaginalis) is performed at a convenient time, usually as a day case.

UNDESCENDED TESTES

When the testis cannot be brought to the bottom of the scrotum it is 'undescended'. Assessment of the undescended testis is easiest between 3 and 6 months of life (avoiding confusion with retractile testis) and early referral to a surgeon is important. The trend in management is for surgery to be performed at an early age. Currently, experienced surgeons perform an orchidopexy at about 1–2 years.

UMBILICAL HERNIA

Umbilical hernia — the protrusion of the umbilicus — is a common finding in newborn children. In most it will resolve spontaneously and not require surgery. If it persists beyond 2–3 years of age then a surgeon should be consulted.

THE ACUTE SCROTUM

A child with a painful tender scrotum should be seen by a surgeon as a matter of urgency. It is usually impossible to differentiate the two common following causes without surgical exploration:

- Torsion of the testicular appendage
- Torsion of the testis

Epididymo-orchitis is a rare disease in prepubertal boys who do not have urinary tract infections. In a boy with acute, but lasting, testicular pain, consider the possibility of intermittent testicular torsion. A testis lying horizontally in the scrotum indicates an anatomical predisposition to torsion.

THE PENIS

THE FORESKIN/PREPUCE

The foreskin is normally adherent to the glans at birth and remains so for a variable amount of time. Usually it is fully retractable by 4 years of age. There is no need to retract foreskins in preschool children.

SMEGMA DEPOSITS

These present as yellow/white firm masses beneath the prepuce in young boys with non-retractable foreskins. It is a normal variant and requires no treatment.

BALANITIS

This is infection under the foreskin with redness, inflammation, swelling and sometimes a white exudate. Immediate treatment with local penile toilet, local antibiotic ointment beneath the foreskin and oral antibiotics is usually sufficient. If the whole penis is red and swollen to the pubis, hospital admission and intravenous antibiotics may be required.

PHIMOSIS

This is scarring of the preputial opening causing:

- Urinary obstruction
- Ballooning of the foreskin on micturition

It is often the end result of recurrent episodes of balanitis. It usually requires circumcision if severe, although mild cases respond to topical 0.05% betnovate cream applied daily for 10 days.

PARAPHIMOSIS

In this acutely painful condition the retracted foreskin is trapped behind the glans and forms an oedematous ring of foreskin proximal to the exposed and swollen glans penis. A surgeon should be consulted immediately if it cannot be reduced manually.

CIRCUMCISION

The indications for circumcision are phimosis and recurrent balanitis. Hypospadias is an absolute contraindication.

It is important to stress to parents that circumcision is not required for cleanliness and that these days less than a quarter of Australian male children are circumcised. It is an unnecessary operation with definite complications of surgery and anaesthesia.

ACUTE ABDOMINAL PAIN

Abdominal pain is a common symptom in children. Appendicitis needs to be distinguished from the other common causes; viral infection, urinary tract infection and constipation.

In the younger child and especially in those less than 4 years of age the diagnosis can be difficult. It is important to refer a child who complains of persistent abdominal pain, even if this is associated with vomiting or diarrhoea. If the child will not allow abdominal examination one should suspect peritonitis.

INTUSSUSCEPTION

In a 3 month to 2 year old infant who presents with intermittent pallor, lethargy, vomiting and abdominal colic, the diagnosis of intussusception should be considered. These are the early symptoms and should be acted upon, rather than awaiting the 'classical' red currant jelly stool, which is a feature of advanced disease. The abdominal mass is central beneath rectus abdominus and is often difficult to feel.

A child with suspected intussusception requires urgent surgical assessment and a contrast enema for diagnosis and/or treatment. If a hydrostatic pressure of 1.2 m fails to reduce the intussusception then emergency surgery is indicated. Contrast enema should not be performed in the presence of peritonitis, significant dehydration or established bowel obstruction. Early diagnosis is the key to easy and successful treatment.

VOMITING IN INFANCY

It is important to determine whether the vomiting is bile stained or not. Green vomiting is an indication for urgent surgical consultation to exclude the anatomical variant of intestinal malrotation and its associated lethal complication of midgut volvulus. Initially there may be no other symptoms or signs of abdominal disease. Abdominal distension is not present and should not be waited for. The twisted intestine may become gangrenous within 6 h after the onset of bile-stained vomiting.

In infants with non-bile-stained vomiting, pyloric stenosis needs to be distinguished from feeding problems, gastro-oesophageal reflux and concealed infections (e.g. urinary tract infection, meningitis). Pyloric stenosis should be suspected if the vomiting is projectile, persistent despite correction of feeding difficulties and/or the use of anti-gastro-oesophageal reflux measures or is associated with failure to thrive.

One should look for gastric peristalsis during test feeding and feel for the pyloric tumour immediately after vomiting. The child should be referred on the basis of symptoms as the demonstration of signs can be difficult.

RECTAL BLEEDING

This is a common symptom and does *not* normally imply a sinister cause. It is usually associated with constipation and is caused by a superficial, acute anal fissure which may not be visible. The constipation should be treated with laxatives with the expectation that the rectal bleeding will resolve.

An intestinal polyp is associated with more persistent rectal bleeding and is not necessarily associated with constipation. The polyp may resolve spontaneously. A large volume of rectal bleeding requires further investigation to exclude the possibility of a Meckel's diverticulum.

CHAPTER 6

INFANT FEEDING AND NUTRITION

BREAST FEEDING

Breast feeding is most desirable and should be encouraged especially for 9–12 months.

Within the Royal Children's Hospital, breast feeding mothers have priority for hospital accommodation, arranged through the Accommodation Officer. Leaflets entitled *Breastfeeding in RCH* and *Collection, Storage and Transport of Expressed Breast Milk* are available. In Victoria mothers wanting advice about lactation can be referred to their Maternal and Child Health Nurse or to the Nursing Mothers' Association (03) 877 5011 (BH), (03) 877 3304 (AH).

ABNORMAL SITUATIONS

- *Inability to suckle.* For example prematurity, comatose patients, heart failure, severe respiratory illness. Mothers can express their milk for feeding via a gavage tube, see Expressing Human Milk (below).
- *Gastro-oesophageal reflux.* Expressed breast milk may be thickened with Carobel, or with cornflour cooked in water to a thick paste. The paste can be given by spoon (2 teaspoons to 50 mL water) during breast feeding.
- *Gastroenteritis* (see p. 91).
- *Hot weather and febrile illness.* Frequency of feeds should be increased. Supplementary water, fruit juice, etc are unnecessary if mother's supply is adequate.
- *Maternal drugs.* Most drugs come through into breast milk to some extent. Drugs that are totally contraindicated for breast feeding mothers include: antineoplastics, bromocriptine, carbimazole, chloramphenicol, diethylstilboestrol, ergots, gold salts, immunosuppressants, iodides, phenindione, radioisotopes, cimetidine, thiouracil, lithium and tetracycline. A number of other drugs are relatively contraindicated. If at all possible breast feeding should be continued.
- *Fluid restriction.* Test weigh the infant or use expressed breast milk.
- *High nutrient requirements*:
  1. Modification of breast feeding technique can increase hind milk intake.
  2. Supplements of an energy dense feed can be alternated with breast feeds.
  3. Expressed breast milk can be fortified with a predigested formula, e.g. Pregestimil 3.5–7 g/100 mL expressed breast milk will increase all nutrients and energy to 25–30 kcal/30 mL (350–380 kJ). When additional energy alone, without extra protein, vitamins and minerals, is needed expressed breast milk can be fortified with either 2–4 g glucose polymer (Polyjoule) and/or 2–5 mL Calogen (fat emulsion)/100 ml expressed breast milk. Fortified feeds should be used with caution in young infants as their concentrated nutrients, high osmolality and solute may exceed the infant's absorption and excreting capacity leading to malabsorption, hypernatraemia, etc.

EXPRESSING BREAST MILK

Milk can be expressed for days or weeks, and this can maintain lactation. Hand expression is cleanest. The KANESON hand pump (appropriately sterilized) is also suitable. These are available from many chemists.

Within the Royal Children's Hospital these are available from the Equipment Distribution Centre Royal Children's Hospital. Electric breast pumps (appropriately sterilized) are available for hospital use in the Departments of Neonatology and Cardiology. For home use electric pumps can be hired from maternity hospitals and commercial agents. The staff on the Neonatal Ward or the Maternal and Child Health Nurse can also give practical advice. The Nursing Mothers Association of Australia can advise on many aspects of breast feeding, including the hiring of breast pumps (phone 877 3304). If expression is performed cleanly, breast milk does not need to be pasteurized or sterilized. A leaflet: *Collection, Storage and Transport of Expressed Breast Milk* is available from the Department of Neonatology or the Maternal and Child Health Nurse.

In general it is best to use fresh human milk (within 48 h of expressing) but if for social reasons it requires storage, it can be refrigerated for up to 48 h, kept in the freeze box section of refrigerator for 2 weeks or kept in a deep freezer for up to 4 months.

The most recently expressed milk should be used first as its composition more closely meets the nutritional needs of the infant. To thaw frozen milk it can be stored in a refrigerator to thaw slowly or placed in a container of water at less than 60°C. Previously frozen milk should be used within 24 h of thawing.

SUPPLEMENTS

Extra fluid is not required for the well infant who is exclusively breast fed. The normal mature breast-fed infant requires no supplementary vitamins or iron for the first 6–9 months, by which time solids should provide the iron requirement. Premature infants are given extra Vitamins C, D, folate and iron. The iron supplements should not be commenced until at least 3 months of age.

ARTIFICIAL FEEDING

Infants

If breast feeding ceases and expressed breast milk is not available, commercially prepared iron fortified infant formulae are to be used. These are modified milk preparations based on cow's milk with added vitamins and minerals usually including iron.

Term infants less than 6 months: use whey predominant formulae such as Nan 1, S26, Enfalac or Karitane Infant Formula. Low iron formulae are not recommended. Formulae within the same generic group can be interchanged (see table on pp. 40–41).

Premature infants and those with high nutrient requirements or low fluid needs, require high nutrient feeds such as Enfalac-Prem, Low Birth Weight S26 or PreNan.

From 6–12 months iron fortified formulae such as Nan, S26, Enfalac, Enfamil, Similac and Lactogen are recommended.

Children Over 6 Months

'Follow on' formulae are available for children over 6 months and include S26 Progress, Nan 2, Enfapro 6, Karitane follow on milk food. 'Follow on' formulae should never be given to infants under 6 months. The higher levels of protein and electrolytes in these formulae could impose a high renal solute load leading to dehydration and other problems.

Infants should stay on breast milk or iron fortified infant formula until they are 12 months old and on a wide range of solids, at which point full cream cow's milk can be introduced. Cow's, evaporated and dried, are not recommended as the primary milk drink for infant feedings until after 12 months of age, but can gradually be introduced in custards, yoghurt and cheese from about 8–9 months.

Sweetened condensed milk is never appropriate.

Soy

If cow's milk formulae cannot be used a nutritionally adequate formulae should be used, e.g. Prosobee, Infasoy or Isomil are suitable alternatives (see table on pp. 40–1). There are other soy drinks available which are not suitable for infants and young children.

FREQUENCY OF FEEDING

Demand feeding is recommended. The number of feeds will vary in the well baby from four to eight per day, determined by the individual's needs. If the infant appears hungry and growth rates are satisfactory the infant may be thirsty so extra boiled water should be first offered. Extra water is also useful in the infant who tends to be constipated.

FLUID REQUIREMENTS

Fluid requirements vary with gestational and postnatal age and other aspects of management, e.g. patients on mechanical ventilation require less water, patients under phototherapy or gastroenteritis may require more, as do those with pyrexia and during heat waves.

Zero to 6 Months

Recommended intake for normal infants is about 150–200 mL/kg bodyweight per day. This is usually graded up from day 1 as follows:

Day	*mL/kg (divide into 3 or 4 hourly feeds)*
1	30
2	60
3	90
4	120
5 and thereafter demand feed	150–200

Six to 12 Months

Offer 100–150 mL/kg per day and divide into four to five feeds.

One Year and Over

Offer 750–1200 mL fluid/day to meet thirst.

SUPPLEMENTS

Vitamins

No vitamin or mineral supplementation is necessary for normal infants being breast fed or receiving a commercially manufactured formula provided it is fortified and includes iron. Although not recommended should cow's milk be used before 12 months of age it should be boiled and Vitamins A, D, C and iron supplements are recommended. Babies with special requirements for supplements should be given them from a teaspoon or by medicine dropper.

Fluoride

Administration of fluoride is recommended to protect teeth from caries where the mains water supply is not fluoridated. *Note:* Melbourne's mains water supply is fluoridated and supplementation is not required.

ABNORMAL SITUATIONS

Feeding the Infant in Hot Weather

Fluid requirement is increased in hot weather and extra boiled water should be offered. Diluted fruit juices can be introduced from about 3 months. Large quantities of fruit juice can deter milk intake and cause diarrhoea.

Feeding the Sick Infant

It is usually unnecessary to change the generic type of formulae but it may need to be given in smaller quantities more frequently. It may be temporarily necessary to offer the feeding in a more dilute form, e.g. half strength. In order to meet nutrient requirements the infant should proceed to full strength feeding as soon as possible, and appropriate solid foods for age should be given.

Gastro-oesophageal reflux (see p. 95)

Thickened feeds can be helpful:

- Cornflour one teaspoon/100 mL is cooked in the water used for making the formula
- Precooked cornflour (Douglas instant food thickener) two teaspoons/100 mL
- Instant Carobel 0.1–0.3% is added to the prepared formula (one scoop = 0.3 g)
- Infant Gaviscon one-half to one teaspoon/120 mL is added to the prepared formula

Cornflour is recommended. Infant Gaviscon has a high sodium (4 mmol sodium per 2 g dose) and is high in aluminium content, therefore it is not recommended. Carobel is expensive.

Constipation (see pp. 95–6)

- Increase fluid intake with cool boiled water or dilute fruit juice
- Encourage fruit, vegetable and cereals once the child is taking educational diet solids

- If the above fails 1% Maltogen (1/2–1 teaspoon) may be temporarily added to formula or fruit juice once or twice daily
- Bran is not recommended

Fluid Restriction and High Nutrient Needs

Fluid restriction for more than a day or two will compromise the infant's nutrient intake unless a nutrient dense feed is used. Infants with poor weight gain or increased requirements, e.g. oxygen dependency also benefit from nutrient dense feeds. Normal infant formulae contain 270–280 kJ (65–70 kcal)/100 mL, i.e. 20 kcal/30 mL.

Feeds of 25 kcal/30 mL

The following will increase the energy to 365–380 kJ (87–90 kcal)/100 mL

- 4.2 g (2 × 5 mL level teaspoons) glucose polymer, e.g. Polyjoule to each 100 mL formula; or
- 5 mL Calogen (fat emulsion) or Liquigen (MCT emulsion) to each 100 mL formula.

All nutrients can be increased by the cautious addition of extra powder or use of a 'low birth weight'/'prem' formula. The concentrated nutrients, high osmolality and solute may exceed the infant's absorptive and excreting capacity particularly in those under 6 months and those with renal or liver impairment resulting in malabsorption or hypernatraemia, etc.

One hundred and twenty-five per cent powder to the same volume of water or 85% water to the normal quantity of powder, e.g. instead of one scoop of powder to 30 mL of water use one scoop of powder to 25 mL water.

FLUORIDE SUPPLEMENT

Natural fluoride in drinking water (parts/10^6)	*0–2 years*	*2–3 years*	*Over 3 years*
Less than 0.3	0.25 mg fluoride ion	0.5 mg fluoride ion	1.0 mg fluoride ion
0.3–0.7	No supplement	0.25 mg fluoride ion	0.5 mg fluoride ion
Over 0.7	No supplement	No supplement	No supplement

Fully breast-fed babies 0.25 mg fluoride ion. Partially or fully bottle-fed babies – dosage depends upon natural fluoride concentration in water supply and age of child. *Note:* 2.2 mg sodium fluoride is equal to 1 mg fluoride ion.

One tablet (all brands) contains 2.2 mg sodium fluoride. Dosage in drops refers to Fluret Liquid Fluoride drops (Cooper Laboratories Pty Ltd) the only drops available. 1 mL (16 drops) contains 2.2 mg pure sodium fluoride equal to 1 mg fluoride ion.

SOLID FOODS – EDUCATIONAL DIET

Introduce from 4 to 6 months; initially a teaspoon of one of the pre-cooked rice cereals mixed with human milk, formula or water is given before a feed, and the amount and frequency is gradually increased.

Other foods are then introduced one at a time, e.g. fruits and vegetables then from 7–8 months meats, egg, different cereals, rusks, bread, custard, etc. The consistency of foods changes from smooth purees to mashed, minced then diced foods to encourage chewing. By 12 months the well child should generally be taking a diet similar to that of the family. Milk intake should be reduced to 600 mL (900 mL maximum)/day. Fluid should be taken from a cup and bottle feeding largely discontinued by this age. A change to full cream milk is recommended and other fluids including water should be offered.

NUTRITION FOR CHILDREN

The diet should be selected from the basic food groups. Once solids have been introduced and the child is on a mixed diet, bread and cereals, fruit, vegetables, milk, cheese, lean meat, poultry, fish and eggs should form the major dietary sources of nutrients and energy. Butter, mono- or polyunsaturated type margarines and oils should be included but used sparingly. A wide variety of foods should be included. Whole nuts should be discouraged in children under 5 years due to the risks of inhalation, and other hard foods should be given under supervision.

ABNORMAL SITUATIONS

- *Food refusal* is common in toddlers and unwell children. Provided it is of short duration and growth failure does not occur it is of little consequence.
- Children with *chronic illness and/or long-term food refusal* require investigation and a dietary assessment, particularly if growth failure occurs.
- *Diets* excluding major sources of nutrients, e.g. milk and/or wheat require dietary assessment. An appropriate milk substitute should be recommended for children (especially those < 2 years). A calcium supplement may suffice for older children.
- *Constipation.* Increase the intake of fluids, food, fibre and recommend a reduction of milk (if excessive) to 600 mL/day.
- *Overweight.* Discourage energy dense foods containing added sugars and fats and encourage a diet selected from the basic food groups.
- *Sick children* who eat insufficiently for their growth needs require concentrated sources of nutrients or supplements such as fortified milkshakes, Sustagen supplements or enteral feeds such as Pediasure, Osmolite, Ensure Plus. Those with special needs require therapeutic formulae and diets to be prescribed, and advice from the dietitian.
- *Gastroenteritis* (see section p. 91).

Within the Royal Children's Hospital nutrition education leaflets are available from the Department of Nutrition and Dietetics.

NUTRITIONAL RICKETS

The great majority of children with nutritional rickets are recent immigrants. It is also occasionally seen in premature and Aboriginal infants. The diagnosis is usually made when the child presents with a respiratory infection and suspicious clinical and radiological signs are found. Occasionally a baby presents with hypocalcaemic tetany. Frequently these children are having inappropriate nutrition. Infants of breast feeding Muslim mothers (fully covered by clothes) may be at higher risk.

The differential diagnosis includes familial hypophosphataemic rickets, malabsorption syndromes, renal tubular acidosis and uraemic renal disease.

All patients with rickets should be admitted or referred to medical outpatients. When a diagnosis of nutritional rickets is confirmed initial therapy is usually 3000 units of calciferol daily for 1 month by which time there is radiological evidence of healing. This is followed by 1000 units daily for 6 months. Advice should be given to correct inappropriate nutrition.

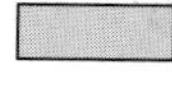

RECOMMENDED FORMULAE AND MILKS FOR DIFFERENT AGE GROUPS

INFANTS 0–6 MONTHS

Breast feeding is the preferred form of infant feeding. Where breast feeding is not possible select from the following generic group an iron-fortified formula.

Whey-Dominant Modified Cow's Milk

Enfalac; Karitane Infant; Nan 1; S26

- *Six to 12 months.* All of the above plus: Enfapro-6; Karitane Follow on milk; Nan 2; S26 Progress.
- *Two years and over.* All of the above plus semi-skimmed milk, e.g. Rev.

Casein-Dominant Modified Cow's Milk

Enfamil; Lactogen; Similac; SMA.

- *Twelve months and over.* All of the above plus full cream cow's milk and full cream goat's milk.
- *Five years and over.* All of the above plus skimmed milks, e.g. Skinny and Physical.

WHEN NON-MILK FORMULAE ARE REQUIRED

- *Soy modified*
  - **a** Infants: Infasoy; Isomil; Prosobee.
  - **b** Children: So-Good; Soy Fresh; Other calcium fortified soy.
- *Goat's milk formula* Karitane Goat's milk formula.
- *Hydrolysate formulae* Alfare; Nutramigen; Pregestimil.

SPECIALIZED FORMULAE FOR PAEDIATRIC NUTRITION

- *Pre-term and low birth weight:* Enfalac Prem; Low Birth Weight S26; Similac Special Care; Pre-Nan
- *Enteral:* Pediasure; Osmolite; Ensure (powder); Ensure Plus; Enrich; Jevity; Isocal; Sustagen; Traumacal
- *Low lactose:* Delact Infant; Digestelact; Balance Low Lactose
- *Energy supplements:* Polyjoule (glucose polymer); Polycose (glucose polymer); Calogen (LCT); Liquigen (MCT fat emulsion)
- *Oral rehydration:* Gastrolyte
- *Other special products:* Portagen (MCT); Ross Carbohydrate Free (selected CHO must be added); 3232A very low carbohydrate (selected CHO must be added) Neocate (infant elemental amino acid formula); Protein Free Powder 80056 (+ appropriate protein source)
- *Low phenylalanine:* Lofenalac; Maxamaid XP; Maxamum XP; Aminogran food supplement and minerals
- *Thickeners:* Cornflour; Instant Carobel; Infant Gaviscon

COMPOSITION PER 100 mL OF GENERIC FORMULAE AVERAGE

Further details from manufacturer or Dietetic Department, Royal Children's Hospital.

		Human milk mature	*Infant formula*			*Follow-on formulae*	*Premature and low birthweight*	*Low lactose, e.g. Delact infant*
			Whey dominant	*Case in dominant*	*Soya*			
Energy:	kcal kJ kcal/30 mL	70 297 20	67 280 20	67 280 20	67 280 20	67 280 20	80 340 24	72 300 20
Protein:	g Casein: whey Type	0.9–1.2 20–4 : 80–60 Human	1.5 30–40 : 70–60 Cow	1.5 80 : 20 Cow	2.0 – Soya isolate + methionine	2.2 80 : 20 Cow	2.2 40 : 60 Cow	1.8 80 : 20 Cow
Carbohydrate:	g Type	7.6 Lactose	7.2 Lactose	7.2 Lactose	6.8 Varies, lactose free ± sucrose	7.4 Lactose	8.6 Lactose + glucose polymer	8.1 Glucose galactose + glucose polymers
Fat:	g Type	4.0 Human	3.8 Vegetable oils	3.6 Vegetable oils	3.6 Vegetable oils	3.2 Vegetable oils ± 'butter'	4.1 Vegetable oils + MCT	3.6 'Butter' + peanut oil
Sodium:	mmol	0.6	0.75	0.7–1	0.9–1.4	0.8–1.6	1.4	1.7
Potassium:	mmol	1.4	1.6	1.8	1.8	2.0	2.2	1.8
Solute (by calc):	mmol	8.7	9.8	9.8	12.9	15	16	12.9
Calcium:	mg	32	48	50	65	68	70–144	69
Phosphorus:	mg	15	28	36	46	47	46–72	59
Age suitability:		From birth	From birth	From birth but preferably 6 months	From birth	From 6 months	Prems & LBW	From birth
Comments and supplements:		Recommended	Iron fortified formula recommended	Iron-fortified formula recommended	Iron-fortified formula recommended	Iron-fortified formula recommended	Supplements of vitamins and iron may be required	Selected low lactose solids for age

Plus gradual introduction of solid foods from 4 to 6 months and at least by 8 months

COMPOSITION PER 100 mL OF GENERIC FORMULAE AVERAGE (Continued)

		Hydrolysate formula	*Cow's milk full cream*	*Goat's milk liquid*	*Soya beverage (Calcium fortified) e.g. So Good*	*Enteral formulae*		
						e.g. Pediasure	*e.g. Osmolite*	*e.g. Ensure Plus*
Energy:	kcal	67	67	67	62	100	100	150
	kJ	280	280	280	260	420	420	627
	kcal/30 mL	20	20	20	20	30	30	45
Protein:	g	2.0	3.4	3.2	3.4	3.0	3.7	5.5
	Casein: whey	–	80 : 20	–		82 : 18	–	–
	Type	Casein or whey hydrolysate	Cow	Goat	Soya isolate	Cow	Cow + soya 88 : 12	Cow + soya 88 : 12
Carbohydrate:	g	7.7	4.6	4.6	4.7	11.0	14.5	20
	Type	Glucose polymers	Lactose	Lactose	Lactose-free contains sucrose	Glucose polymer + sucrose	Glucose polymer	Glucose polymer + sucrose
Fat:	g	3.2	3.8	4.0	3.5	5.0	3.8	5.3
	Type	Vegetable oil ± MCT	'Butter'	'Goat'	Vegetable oils	Vegetable oils + MCT	Vegetable oils + MCT	Corn oil
Sodium:	mmol	1.6	2.4	1.5	1.7	1.7	2.4	5.0
Potassium:	mmol	2.0	3.8	4.6	3.5	3.4	2.6	6.0
Solute (by calc):	mmol	15	26	25	24	22	29	48
Calcium:	mg	62	115	126	112	97	53	63
Phosphorus:	mg	41	97	106	115	80	53	64
Age suitability		From birth	From 1 year	From 1 year	From 2 years	From 1 year but preferably 2 years	From 2 years but preferably 5 years	From 5 years
Comments and supplements:		Selected low allergen solids for age	Variety of solids providing Vit. A, D, C, B_{12}, folic acid + iron	Variety of solids providing Vit. A, D, C, B_{12}, folic acid + iron	Variety of solids for age	–	–	–

CHAPTER 7

FLUID AND ELECTROLYTE THERAPY

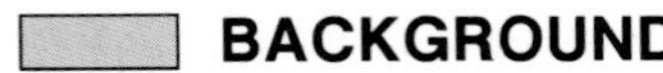

BACKGROUND

FLUID DISTRIBUTION

- Water constitutes approximately 750 mL/kg of bodyweight in the full-term newborn infant and approximately 500–600 mL/kg of bodyweight in the normal adult
- Intracellular water constitutes approximately 350 mL/kg of bodyweight in the infant
- Extracellular water constitutes approximately 400 mL/kg of bodyweight in the newborn infant decreasing to approximately 300 mL/kg by 9 months of age
- Whole blood constitutes approximately 70–80 mL/kg of bodyweight in children and 80–90 mL/kg in infants
- Plasma constitutes approximately 40 mL/kg of bodyweight in children

CONVERSION FACTORS

Sodium Chloride

- 1 g contains 17 mmol Na and 17 mmol Cl.
- 58 mg contains 1 mmol Na and 1 mmol Cl.

Potassium Chloride

- 1 g contains 13 mmol K and 13 mmol Cl.
- 74 mg contains 1 mmol K and 1 mmol Cl.

Sodium Bicarbonate

- 1 g contains 12 mmol Na and 12 mmol HCO_3.
- 84 mg contains 1 mmol Na and 1 mmol HCO_3.

Molarity — Definition

Osmolarity denotes the molar concentration per litre of solution of osmotically active particles in a solution.

Osmolality denotes the molar concentration per kilogram of water of all osmotically active particles in a solution.

NORMAL VALUES

- Plasma osmolality = 2 Na + glucose + urea
- Osmolality of plasma = 270–295 mmol/kg water
- Osmolality of urine = 50–1400 mmol/kg water

MAINTENANCE FLUID REQUIREMENTS

Bodyweight	*Requirements*
3–10 kg	100 mL/kg per day
10–20 kg	1000 mL + (50 mL/kg per day for each kg over 10 kg)
20 kg and over	1500 mL + (20 mL/kg per day for each kg over 20 kg)

Fever increases the requirement by approximately 12% for each degree Celsius rise in body temperature. At all ages, the daily requirement of sodium, potassium and chloride is approximately 2 mmol/kg.

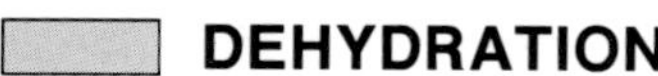

DEHYDRATION

INITIAL ACUTE MANAGEMENT

Circulatory failure due to diminished plasma volume requires re-expansion of circulatory volume as rapidly as possible with a solution containing normal plasma electrolytes.

In general, an isotonic saline solution containing sodium bicarbonate, or Hartmann's solution, 10–20 mL/kg depending on response, is suitable. If other factors, such as septicaemia or blood loss are involved, stable plasma protein solution or blood may be required. Five per cent dextrose with low sodium concentrations (e.g. 5% dextrose in 0.225% NaCl) must not be used for rapid infusion as severe hyponatraemia with fitting may occur.

In states of hyponatraemia or hypernatraemia, correction of serum sodium towards normal should not occur at more than 1–2 mmol/L per h.

REPLACEMENT THERAPY

Three basis aspects are considered:

1 Existing deficit.
2 Continuing losses during therapy.
3 Maintenance requirements.

Existing Fluid Deficit

This is calculated from the bodyweight according to the degree of dehydration estimated by the clinical features:

- Decreased peripheral perfusion
- Deep (acidotic) breathing
- Decreased skin turgor
- Increased thirst

A history of oliguria, restlessness, lethargy, sunken eyes, dry mouth, sunken fontanelle, and the absence of tears are poor signs of mild to moderate dehydration in children. In general:

- 0–4% bodyweight loss: no clinical signs

- 4–10% bodyweight loss: clinical signs present; and the severity of the signs is a guide to the degree of dehydration
- 10–15% bodyweight loss: peripheral circulatory failure

Electrolyte Deficit

The type and amount of electrolyte deficit depends on the diagnosis, e.g. in gastroenteritis, loss of base leads to acidosis; in pyloric stenosis, loss of acid and chloride leads to hypochloraemic alkalosis. The rate of infusion of potassium must not exceed 0.5 mmol/kg per h. Concentrations of potassium greater than 40 mmol/L should be used with extreme caution. Electrocardiographic monitoring should be considered in massive replacement. Infusions of concentrated solutions should be controlled with the use of a pump.

Continuing Losses

It is essential to have an accurate recording on a fluid balance chart of volumes of vomitus or gastric aspiration, drainage from fistulae, diarrhoea, urine output and other fluid losses. These will determine both the volume and type of fluid and electrolyte replacement required.

Maintenance Requirements (See Above)

These are given in addition to replacement fluids for existing deficit and continuing losses. In general, fluids to replace existing deficit are given over the first 24 h. In hypernatraemic dehydration, at least 48 h should be taken for replacement.

ACID–BASE PROBLEMS

The maintenance of pH within narrow limits is by two mechanisms.

1. Buffer systems: the bicarbonate system is quantitatively the most important in plasma (70% of the total)
2. Excretory mechanisms: via the kidneys and lungs

Acidosis (low pH) and alkalosis (high pH) may be respiratory or non-respiratory ('metabolic') in origin. Respiratory disorders result from changes in the excretion of volatile carbon dioxide, and consequently in the levels of carbonic acid. Metabolic disorders occur with changes in concentrations of non-volatile acids, and consequently in the concentration of buffer base — mainly bicarbonate.

The four primary disorders are:

1. Metabolic acidosis. This arises from: increased production of non-volatile acid, e.g. ketoacids and lactic acid; failure of the kidney to excrete non-volatile acid or conserve base; excess loss of buffer base, e.g. gastroenteritis or intestinal fistula.
2. Metabolic alkalosis. This arises from: excess loss of non-volatile acid, e.g. pyloric stenosis; excess intake of buffer, e.g. bicarbonate infusion or ingestion; potassium depletion, where an extracellular alkalosis occurs as hydrogen ions are lost in the urine, e.g. renal tubular syndromes, pyloric stenosis or diuretic therapy.
3. Respiratory acidosis. Hypercapnoea is the result of alveolar hypoventilation from any cause e.g. central, neuromuscular, pulmonary or cardiac.
4. Respiratory alkalosis. This arises from hyperventilation.

INDICATORS OF ACID–BASE STATUS

pH

This reflects the actual hydrogen ion concentration and alters in response to both respiratory and metabolic changes.

P_{CO_2} (Partial Pressure of Carbon Dioxide)

In arterial and capillary blood samples, this represents the P_{CO_2} in blood leaving the lungs. Alterations reflect disturbance in the respiratory component of acid–base state.

Base Excess

This is an estimate of the change in total buffer base that would be present if the P_{CO_2} were normal (40 mmHg). Changes in base excess reflect disturbance in the metabolic component of acid–base. In metabolic alkalosis, total buffer base is increased, and thus base excess is positive. Other calculated measures of the metabolic component are the standard bicarbonate and the total buffer base.

Actual Bicarbonate

This is the plasma concentration of bicarbonate. As with base excess, the plasma concentration of actual bicarbonate is influenced by metabolic components. The bicarbonate excess is slightly less that the total base excess.

Theoretical Changes in Variables in Arterial or Capillary Blood (Before Compensation)

Reference range	*pH* 7.36–7.44	*P_{CO_2} (mmol/L)* 36–44	*Base excess (mmol/L)* – 5 to + 3	*Actual bicarbonate (mmol/L)* 18–25
Metabolic acidosis	Decrease	Normal	Decrease	Decrease
Metabolic alkalosis	Increase	Normal	Increase	Increase
Respiratory acidosis	Decrease	Increase	Normal	Increase
Respiratory alkalosis	Increase	Decrease	Normal	Decrease

In practice, isolated metabolic and respiratory disorders are uncommon. Most disorders have a metabolic and a respiratory component. Usually one is the primary disorder, the other occurs secondarily, and tends to correct the change in pH. However, sometimes primary metabolic and respiratory disturbances occur together, e.g. in respiratory distress syndrome, when hypoxia leading to lactic acid accumulation produces metabolic acidosis, and carbon dioxide retention produces a respiratory acidosis.

The interpretation of changes in base excess and P_{CO_2} as primary or secondary changes must be made clinically.

Changes in Indicators of Acid–Base Status Seen in Combined Disorders

	pH	*P_{CO_2}*	*Base excess*	*Actual bicarbonate*
Primary metabolic acidosis + 'compensatory' respiratory alkalosis, e.g. gastroenteritis, diabetic ketosis	Decrease or normal	Decrease	Decrease	Decrease
Primary metabolic alkalosis + 'compensatory' respiratory acidosis, e.g. pyloric stenosis	Increase or normal	Increase	Increase	Increase
Combined primary respiratory and metabolic acidosis, e.g. respiratory distress syndrome	Decrease	Increase	Decrease	Normal

CORRECTION OF METABOLIC ACIDOSIS

A guide to the amount of bicarbonate required is given by: mmol of HCO_3 required = base deficit (mmol/L) × weight (kg) × 0.3. The factor (weight × 0.3) represents the volume of extracellular fluid through which the base deficit (negative base excess) is distributed. In babies less than 5 kg, the factor is weight × 0.5 due to the greater percentage of extracellular fluid. Biochemical reassessment is required to confirm the clinical response to therapy after half this calculated dose has been given.

The rate of administration of bicarbonate will be determined by the cause of the metabolic acidosis and the clinical state of the patient, e.g. in cardiac arrest, infuse rapidly; in gastroenteritis, correction should be undertaken over at least 6 h. Rapid correction of metabolic acidosis will cause a fall in extracellular potassium.

The principles of correction of metabolic alkalosis are discussed in the section on pyloric stenosis (p. 47).

COMMONLY USED INTRAVENOUS SOLUTIONS

	Na^+ (mmol/L)	*Cl^- (mmol/L)*	*K^+ (mmol/L)*	*Lactate (mmol/L)*	*Ca^{2+} (mmol/L)*	*Glucose (g)*
Isotonic saline (0.9% NaCl) 'Normal saline'	150	150	–	–	–	–
1/2 isotonic saline with 5% glucose	75	75	–	–	–	5
1/5 isotonic saline with 4% glucose	30	30	–	–	–	4
1/5 isotonic saline with 4% glucose and KCl 20 mmol/L	30	30	20	–	–	4
Hartmann's solution	130	110	5	30	2	–
Hartmann's solution with 5% glucose	130	110	5	30	2	5

SALINE BICARBONATE

This solution is made up by adding 60 mL of sodium bicarbonate to each litre of 1/2 isotonic saline and 2.5% dextrose. The solution is stable for only 24 h.

STABLE PLASMA PROTEIN SOLUTION

In addition to 5% plasma proteins, this solution contains:

- Na 130–150 mmol/L
- K 4–6 mmol/L
- Ca 1.5–2.5 mmol/L

ALBUMIN (20%)

This solution contains sodium (85–130 mmol/L)

ADDITIVES

- molar potassium chloride 1 mmol/L of K^+ and Cl^-
- molar sodium chloride 1 mmol/mL of Na^+ and Cl^-
- molar sodium chloride 1 mmol/mL of Na^+ and HCO_3^-
- molar sodium lactate 1 mmol/mL of Na^+ and lactate$^-$
- calcium gluconate 10% 0.22 mmol/mL of Ca^{2+}, which is 8.9 mg/mL of Ca^{2+}
- magnesium chloride for intravenous (5 mmol in 5 mL) 1 mmol/mL of Mg^{2+}, which is 120 mg/mL of $MgCl_2$.

MANAGEMENT OF SOME SPECIAL CONDITIONS

PYLORIC STENOSIS

Hydrogen ion and chloride loss predominate, with consequent hypochloraemic alkalosis. There may be substantial potassium loss because of H^+/K^+ exchange in the renal tubules. The duration and severity of vomiting will, to a large extent, determine the degree of fluid and electrolyte imbalance.

Assessment

All patients require biochemical assessment, but not all will require intravenous therapy. Any child who is clinically dehydrated or has significant biochemical derangement requires intravenous therapy.

Intravenous Therapy

In *severe dehydration* (> 10%), commence with isotonic saline until adequate circulation has been established and then continue with 1/2 isotonic saline and 5% dextrose.

In *moderate dehydration* (5–10%), commence with 1/2 isotonic saline with 5% dextrose. Await electrolyte results before commencing therapy if only mildly dehydrated.

Adequate potassium and chloride replacement is necessary for correction of the acid–base status. As soon as urine flow is established, potassium chloride is given up to a maximum of 0.3 mmoL/kg per h. Usually 20–40 mmol/L is adequate.

ACUTE OLIGURIA AND ANURIA

The definition of severe oliguria is a urine output of less than 0.5 mL/kg per h.

Initial Management

Three clinical situations occur:

1. Sudden and complete anuria should arouse suspicion of urinary obstruction, provided the catheter is correctly placed and not blocked.
2. Renal hypoperfusion causing oliguria should be suspected in the presence of clinical dehydration or septicaemia leading to hypotension. Blood volume expansion is necessary.
3. Renal tissue injury, e.g. acute post-streptococcal glomerulonephritis or secondary to hypoperfusion or nephrotoxin. Frusemide (1–2 mg/kg) should be given intravenously and, if there is no response, treatment for continuing anuria should be instituted.

Continuing Anuria

Fluid intake is restricted to the previous 24 h loss from stools, urine and other losses. Fluid of approximately 20 mL/kg per day must also be given to replace insensible water loss less endogenous water production.

Calories as carbohydrate are given to spare tissue protein from catabolism for energy, which accentuates the rise in blood urea. Ten to 20% glucose, i.v., or oral Caloreen or Polyjoule are suitable.

Peritoneal dialysis or haemofiltration will be required for hyperkalaemia, severe uraemia (blood urea > 50 mmol/L), acidosis, or water overload leading to hyponatraemia, oedema, or hypertension, and should always be considered if anuria persists for more than 24 h

HYPERKALAEMIA

The management of hyperkalaemia depends on its cause. In acute oliguric renal failure, if urine is not formed after intravenous frusemide (see above) the presence of hyperkalaemia (> 7.0) is an indication for dialysis. High values not requiring treatment may be found in the neonatal period.

If cardiac arrhythmias are present, rapid but temporary benefit may be achieved by:

- Sodium bicarbonate 2 mmol/kg, i.v.
- Regular insulin 0.1 unit/kg given with 2 mL/kg of 50% dextrose, i.v.
- Calcium gluconate 10% 0.5 mL/kg given intravenously slowly
- Sodium polystyrene sulfinate (Resonium) 1 g/kg, p.r.

Management of Specific Conditions

- Acute infectious diarrhoea (see p. 91).
- Haemorrhagic shock (see p. 7).
- Burns (see pp. 159–64).
- Diabetes mellitus (see pp. 136–41).
- Meningococcal septicaemia (see p. 8).

Useful Formulae

- Anion gap = Na − (Bicarbonate + Cl). Normal < 12
- Number mL/h, i.v. = microdrop/min = 4 × drop/min
- No. mmol = mEq/valence = mass (mg)/mol. wt
- Sodium deficit mL 20% NaCl = wt × 0.2 × (140 − serum Na)
- Water deficit (mL) = 600 × wt (kg) × [1 − (140/Na)]

INTRAVENOUS NUTRITION

Within the Royal Children's Hospital advice on intravenous nutrition can be obtained from Dr Frank Shann (Intensive Care Unit), the intravenous nutritionist on call in pharmacy, Dr Neil Campbell (Neonatology), Dr Arnold Smith (Gastroenterology), Dr Julie Bines (Gastroenterology) or Mr Alex Auldist (General Surgery). The following section is a description of the details of intravenous nutrition within the Royal Children's Hospital.

Details will vary in other institutions; however, the general principles remain the same.

THE REQUIREMENTS IN INTRAVENOUS NUTRITION

In addition to minerals and vitamins, a patient's nutrition depends on the amount per kilogram he/she receives of water, protein (amino acids) carbohydrate (dextrose) and fat (e.g. Intralipid). Amounts usually administered are shown in the table on p. 46.

THE SYSTEM OF ORDERING

Orders to nursing staff for administration of intravenous nutrition fluid should be expressed in mL/h on the green intravenous medical record. A pale yellow form entitled 'Intravenous Nutrition Orders' is available for ordering from pharmacy. All prescriptions must be expressed in terms of amount required per kg per day.

Weight

Must be included to enable calculation by pharmacy of the actual volumes of nutrient solution and fat emulsion required. In a very malnourished child, use the ideal weight for the child's actual height, rather than the actual weight.

Nutrient Volume

Refers to the volume of the combined amino acid, dextrose, electrolyte and vitamin solution, but excludes fat emulsion. Volumes should be rounded to 40, 50, 60, 70, 80, 90, 100, 110, 120, 130, 140, 150, 175 or 200 mL/kg per day.

CONTENTS OF NUTRIENT SOLUTION

- Protein: Vamin – patients under 5 kg; Synthamin – patients over 5 kg
- Dextrose: ordered as g/kg per day
- Potassium: ordered as mmol/kg per day (av. req. = 3 mmol/kg per day)
- Sodium: ordered as mmol/kg per day (av. req. = 3 mmol/kg per day)
- Calcium: under 5 kg as ordered to max. 12 mmol/L; over 5 kg 7.5 mmol/24 h (max. 12 mmol/L) or as ordered
- Phosphate: under 5 kg as ordered to max. 12 mmol/L; over 5 kg 7.5 mmol/24 h (max. 12 mmol/L) or as ordered
- Magnesium: 4 mmol/L or as ordered
- Heparin: 1 unit/mL

Trace Elements

- Chromium: 0.005 μmol/kg
- Copper: 0.5 μmol/kg
- Iodide: 0.04 μmol/kg
- Manganese: 0.2 μmol/kg
- Zinc: 3.0 μmol/kg

} or as ordered

- Selenium added for patients receiving TPN for over 3 months.

Vitamins

- B group and C vitamins: 4 mL/kg of solution containing: thiamine 10 mg/2 mL, riboflavin 5 mg/2 mL, sodium pantholene 5 mg/2 mL, nicotinamide 50 mg/2 mL, pyridoxine 2.5 mg/2 mL and ascorbic acid 50 mg/2 mL
- Vitamin K: 2 mg/L
- Cyanocobalamin: 20 μg/L
- Folic acid: 100 μg/24 h

} or as ordered

Oil Soluble Vitamins

For patients receiving total parenteral nutrition for more than 7 days, the addition of oil soluble vitamins and biotin should be considered. These will be added on 5 days per week (Monday–Friday).

- Patients < 1 kg: MVI Paediatric 1.5 mL/24 h
- Patients 1–3 kg: MVI Paediatric 2.5 mL/24 h
- Patients > 3 kg and < 12 years: MVI Paediatric 5 mL/24 h
- Patients > 12 years: MVI12 10 mL/bag

MVI Paediatric 5 mL contains Vitamin A 2300 U, Vitamin D 400 U, Vitamin E 7 U, thiamine 1.2 mg, riboflavin 1.4 mg, pyridoxine 1 mg, nicotinamide 17 mg, cyanocobalamin 1 μg, ascorbic acid 80 mg, pantothenic acid 5 mg, folic acid 140 μg, biotin 20 μg, Vitamin K 200 μg.

MVI12 10 mL contains Vitamin A 3300 U, Vitamin D 200 U, Vitamin E 10 U, thiamine 3 mg, riboflavin 3.6 mg, pyridoxine 4 mg, nicotinamide 40 mg, cyanocobalamin 5 μg, ascorbic acid 100 mg, pantothenic acid 15 mg, folic acid 400 μg, biotin 60 μg (also add Vitamin K 2 mg/L).

Fat Emulsion

Ordered as 1–3 g/kg per day. Not included in the nutrient volume. Very close monitoring is required with administration of 3 mg/kg per day of fat. Serum samples should be examined for lipaemia.

Fat emulsion 20% (2 cal/mL)	*ml/kg per h*	*Cal/kg per day*
1 g (5 mL)/kg per day	0.21	10
2 g (10 mL)/kg per day	0.42	20
3 g (15 mL)/kg per day	0.63	30

Total calories are calculated by the resident from the amount of protein, carbohydrate and fat. This figure is not required by the pharmacy but the column is included here for convenience, so that the intravenous nutrition orders form contains a complete record of the patient's intravenous nutrition.

Contents of the Nutrient Solution

The pharmacy will list on each bottle of nutrient the concentration (in amount per litre) of amino acids, dextrose, potassium and sodium. The nutrient solution will also provide:

- mmol/L: Ca^{+} 6, PO_4^{+}6, Mg^{2+} 4. For children under 3, larger amounts may be added.
- μmol/kg per day: Mn^{2+} 0.2, Zn^{2+} 3, Cu^{+} 0.5, I 0.04, Cr^{+} 0.005.
- B_{12} 20 μg/L, Intravite 4 ml/L, Vitamin K 2 mg/L, folic acid 0.1 mg/day.

If Vitamins A, D and E cannot be given orally, children on intravenous nutrition for longer than 1 week should be given intravenous fat soluble vitamins (Dayamin or MVI); discuss with pharmacy.

GENERAL PRINCIPLES IN INTRAVENOUS NUTRITION

Give appropriate replacement (in addition to nutrient solution) for fluid losses. Always introduce and withdraw intravenous nutrition gradually (over about 3 days). A dislodged intravenous cannula should be replaced immediately in a patient on intravenous nutrition. If nutrient solution is not available at any time, it should be replaced with an infusion of a similar concentration of dextrose in water (e.g. 10% dextrose in N/4 saline with potassium).

Beware of hyperglycaemia (with glycosuria and dehydration), hypoglycaemia, sepsis, extravasation of nutrient and fat emulsion from veins, thrombocytopenia, hypoproteinaemia, electrolyte imbalance, acidosis, anaemia, lipaemia and uraemia.

Monitor:

- Daily: inspect intravenous site, electrolytes, acid–base, serum lipaemia (reduce fat emulsion rate if lipaemia +, + +, + + +). Very close monitoring is required with administration of 4 g/kg per day of fat.
- Twice weekly: (transfuse blood p.r.n. for anaemia), platelets, proteins.
- Weekly: creatinine, Mg, Ca, phosphate
- Dextrostix (or BM test) of blood 8 hourly
- Clinitest (or BM test) of urine 8 hourly (reduce dextrose intake if more than trace)
- Weigh frequently (daily if possible)

Monitoring can be less frequent once the child is stabilized on intravenous nutrition.

Patients on restricted fluid intake: The maximum dextrose intake in g/kg per 24 h (providing Na^{+} and K^{+} not more than 4 mmol/kg per 24 h) is calculated from the table below.

MAXIMUM DEXTROSE INTAKE

Fluid intake (mL/kg per 24 h)	*Intake of amino acid (g/kg per 24 h)*			
	1.0	*1.5*	*2.0*	*2.5*
Vamin (7% solution)				
20	2	–	–	–
30	9	4	–	–
40	15	10	6	–
50	22.5	17.5	12.5	7.5
60	29	24	19	14
70	36	31	26	21.5
Synthamin (10% solution)				
20	5	15	–	–
30	11	7.5	5	–
40	18	15	11	7.5
50	25	20	17.5	14
60	32	27.5	25	20
70	39	35	30	27.5

For example a child restricted to 40 mL/kg per day of nutrient solution being given 2 g/kg per day of amino acid (as Synthamin 10%) can be given no more than 11 g/kg per day of dextrose.

TPN TYPICAL COMMENCEMENT REGIMEN

	**Neonates*	*< 10 kg*	*10–15 kg*	*15–20 kg*	*20–30 kg*	*> 30 kg*
Total fluid (mL/kg per day)	100	100	90	80	70	50
Amino acids (g/kg per day)						
Day 1	1.5	1.5	1	1	1	1
Day 2	2	2	1.5	1.5	1	1
Day 3 +	2	2	2	1.5–2	1–2	1–2
Dextrose (g/kg per day)						
Day 1	10	10	5	5	5	5
Day 2	10–15	10	10	10	10	5–10
Day 3	15–20	15–20	15	10–15	10–15	10
Fat (intralipid; g/day)						
Day 1	1	1	1	1	1	1
Day 2	2	2	2	2	1.5	1.5
Day 3	3	3	3	2	2	1.5
Day 4 +	3	3	3	3	2.5	2
Total calories needed/day†	100/kg	100/kg	1000 + (50/kg) > 10 kg	1500 + (20/kg) > 20 kg		

* Neonates: day 1 of life 60 mL/kg, day 2 90 mL/kg, day 3 120 mL/kg.

† Total calories/kg per day = g/kg per day of amino acids × 4 + g/kg per day of fat × 10 + g/kg per day dextrose × 4.

Administration

Solutions containing Vamin are *incompatible* with fat. If there is only one line available for infusion, run the nutrient solution for 3 h and then the fat emulsion for 1 h and so on. The line should be flushed with 0.5 mL of isotonic saline between solutions. This gives 18 h of nutrient and 6 h of fat per day. Solutions containing Synthamin are *compatible* with fat emulsion providing the combined concentration of calcium and magnesium does not exceed 10 mmol/L. These solutions may be mixed in the intravenous line if the lines meet close to the patient. Synthamin solutions with more than 10 mmol/L of calcium and magnesium must be cycled in the same manner as Vamin solutions.

To calculate rates of administration determine whether or not the nutrient solution will be run with the fat. Multiply the mL/kg per 24 h nutrient volume by the weight and divide by the number of hours over which the solution will be infused (18 h for cycled nutrient/fat). For the rate of fat emulsion, multiply the g/kg per 24 h of fat by the weight by five and then divide by the number of hours over which the solution will be infused (6 h for cycled nutrient/fat).

Example

For a child weighing 10 kg who requires a total fluid intake of 1100 mL/day, comprising parenteral nutrition and 2 g/kg per day of fat emulsion (this is equivalent to 110 mL/kg per day): 2 g/kg per day of *fat* (20%) = 10 mL/kg per day of fat emulsion. This leaves 100 mL/kg per day. This child will receive 100 mL/kg per day × 10 kg = 1000 mL/day of *parenteral nutrition* solution. In this 1000 mL she/he will receive 7.5 mmol of Ca^{2+} and 4 mmol of Mg^{2+}. This will require cyclic nutrient/fat administration. Therefore, she/he will receive: 1000 mL of nutrient over 18 h = 55.5 mL/h for 3 h in 4; 100 mL of fat over 6 h = 16.7 mL/h for 1 h in 4.

INTRAVENOUS NUTRITION (IMPLIED DEXTROSE CONCENTRATION)

Fluid mL/kg	*Dextrose g/kg per day*											
per day	*2.5*	*5*	*7.5*	*10*	*12.5*	*15*	*17.5*	*20*	*22.5*	*25*	*27.5*	*30*
40	6.3%	12.5%	18.8%	25%	31.3%	37.5%	43.8%	50%				
50	5	10	15	20	25	30	35	40	45%	50%		
60	4.2	8.3	12.5	16.7	20.8	25	29.2	33.3	37.5	41.7	45.8%	50%
70	3.6	7.1	10.7	14.3	17.8	21.4	25	28.6	32.1	35.7	39.4	42.9%
80	3.1	6.3	9.4	12.5	15.6	18.8	21.9	25	28.1	31.3	34.4	37.5%
90	2.8	5.6	8.3	11.1	13.9	16.7	19.4	22.2	25	27.8	30.6	33.3%
100	2.5	5	7.5	10	12.5	15	17.5	20	22.5	25	27.5	30%
110	2.3	4.5	6.8	9.1	11.4	13.6	15.9	18.2	20.5	22.7	25	27.3%
120	2.1	4.2	6.3	8.3	10.4	12.5	14.6	16.7	18.8	20.8	22.9	25%
130	1.9	3.8	5.8	7.7	9.6	11.5	13.5	15.4	17.3	19.2	21.1	23.1%
140	1.8	3.6	5.4	7.1	8.9	10.7	12.5	14.3	16.1	17.9	19.6	21.4%
150	1.7	3.3	5	6.7	8.3	10	11.7	13.3	15	16.7	18.3	20%
175	1.4	2.9	4.3	5.7	7.1	8.6	10	11.4	12.9	14.3	15.7	17.1%
200	1.3	2.5	3.8	5	6.3	7.5	8.8	10	11.3	12.5	13.8	15%

The table shows the concentration of dextrose implicit in a prescription. If a patient received nutrient 150 mL/kg per day, dextrose 15 g/kg per day, and Intralipid 4 g (20 mL)/kg per day. From the above table, there would be 10% dextrose in the nutrient solution. Concentrations of dextrose over 25% should rarely be necessary and concentrations over 15% should only be given through a central line.

CHAPTER 8

NEONATAL PAEDIATRICS

This chapter aims to provide the clinician with information about some of the important conditions found in the newborn infant. Feeding and intravenous nutrition is covered in other chapters of this handbook.

In Victoria, the Royal Children's Hospital Department of Neonatology offers a 24 h consultative service for neonatal problems. Advice is also available through the Neonatal Emergency Transport Service (NETS) by telephoning 347 7441.

JAUNDICE

Jaundice commonly occurs in the newborn period and is most frequently due to unconjugated hyperbilirubinaemia. The significance of the jaundice depends to a large degree on the age of its onset.

THE FIRST 36 h

Any degree of jaundice with its onset in the first 36 h is abnormal and may cause kernicterus.

The most likely cause is haemolytic disease of the newborn due to either Rh or ABO incompatibility between mother and fetus.

Investigations

- Serum bilirubin (SBR)
- Maternal and baby's blood group
- Direct Coombs' test
- Full blood examination

Further investigations are indicated if there is no evidence of haemolysis or if conjugated hyperbilirubinaemia is present.

Management

Any baby with jaundice in the first 36 h should be admitted to hospital immediately. Paediatric advice should be sought.

There are standard indications for treatment available from most major neonatal hospitals. At this age the following are guidelines for therapy for the term baby with no other illnesses.

- SBR < 150 mmol/L = *observe*
- SBR 155–250 mmol/L = *phototherapy*
- SBR > 250 mmol/L = *exchange transfusion*

Frequent monitoring of serum bilirubin levels is essential.

DAYS 3–5

The jaundice is most likely physiological if the following criteria are satisfied.

- The jaundice had its *onset* on day 3 or 4
- The jaundice is clinically minimal being confined to the head, neck and upper trunk
- The baby is not preterm or low birthweight (< 2500 g)
- The baby is well (afebrile, feeding well, alert)
- The baby is passing normal bowel actions and urine
- No other abnormalities

No investigations at all are necessary if the above criteria are fulfilled. Up to 50% of babies become visibly jaundiced by 3–4 days of age. This usually occurs when the SBR rises above 85–120 mmol/L. In 97% of these babies the SBR does not exceed 220 mmol/L. In a well term baby kernicterus does not occur at or below these levels.

If the baby clinically appears more extensively jaundiced, a SBR is indicated. If the SBR is greater than 220 mmol/L further investigations are needed. Sepsis needs to be considered. Treatment (well term baby):

- If SBR > 285 = *phototherapy*
- If SBR > 340 = *consider exchange transfusion*

PROLONGED JAUNDICE (AFTER 14 DAYS)

This needs investigating. A sudden onset at this age is suggestive of either sepsis, or haemolysis due to a red blood cell enzyme abnormality. The baby would need urgent admission to hospital. If the jaundice was a prolongation of the neonatal jaundice the infant could be investigated as an outpatient. The presence of pale stools and dark urine is highly suggestive of *conjugated hyperbilirubinaemia* and needs to be investigated in hospital.

Causes

1 Raised conjugated SBR.
- **a** Biliary atresia.
- **b** Neonatal hepatitis.
- **c** Choledochal cyst.

2 Raised unconjugated SBR.
- **a** Hypothyroidism.
- **b** Sepsis.
- **c** Red cell enzyme abnormalities.

If all the above are excluded, the baby is well and feeding by breast, the likely diagnosis is breast milk jaundice which occurs in 2–4% of breast feeding infants. This is not associated with kernicterus and does not need any treatment. Careful reassurance that breast feeding should continue is very important.

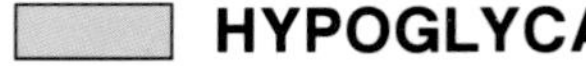 HYPOGLYCAEMIA

See also p. 143.

DEFINITION

A true blood glucose of less than 2.5 mmol/L in any baby. 'Dextrostix' or 'BM stix' are useful for screening purposes. However, if a screening test suggests hypoglycaemia a true blood glucose should be performed before starting any invasive therapy.

Blood glucose measurement should be done on infants with the following conditions:

- Infants of diabetic mothers
- Small for gestational age infants
- Preterm infants
- Large for gestational age infants
- Asphyxiated infants
- Infants with seizures
- Infants receiving intravenous infusions

CLINICAL FEATURES

There are no specific clinical features of hypoglycaemia. The infants may be asymptomatic or exhibit symptoms of apathy, hypotonia, poor feeding, temperature instability, jitteriness or convulsions.

TREATMENT

For well, asymptomatic infants with a true blood sugar in the range of 1.5–2.5 mmol/L it is reasonable to institute early and frequent enteral feeds. However, if there is no response within 2–4 h parenteral dextrose is indicated.

Intravenous dextrose infusion is indicated for symptomatic hypoglycaemia or if the true blood glucose is less than 1.5 mmol/L. An initial intravenous bolus of 25% dextrose 2–4 mL/kg should be followed by an infusion aiming to provide 5–10 mg/kg per min of glucose. The response to therapy should be monitored by frequent blood glucose estimations.

For a 'large-for-dates' infant who has severe hypoglycaemia (< 1 mmol/L) it may be very difficult to insert an intravenous line. In these circumstances give 0.05 units/kg of glucagon intramuscularly.

Further investigation and treatment is necessary for severe intractable hypoglycaemia.

NEONATAL SEPSIS

Bacterial sepsis is one of the most common preventable causes of neonatal mortality and morbidity. Bacterial infections may be acquired before or at birth (*early onset*) from the mother's birth canal, or postnatally from the environment by droplet spread or handling (*late onset*).

The most frequently encountered organisms are:

- Group B β-haemolytic *Streptococcus*
- *Escherichia coli*
- Listeria monocytogenes
- *Staphylococcus aureus* — usually a nosocomial infection

The early symptoms and signs may be minimal, but if ignored rapid progression to overwhelming sepsis may occur. The following are important warning signs:

- A change in an infant's behaviour is usually the first warning sign of serious neonatal infection
- Respiratory distress is frequent in early onset sepsis
- Fever: rectal temperature of > 37.5°C
- A sudden history of poor feeding
- Apnoea
- Seizures

A careful examination is essential. Special attention should be given to:

- Cardiorespiratory system: signs of respiratory distress
- Abdomen: distension, tenderness with or without cellulitis of the abdominal wall may indicate necrotizing enterocolitis
- The fontanelle may be bulging in meningitis
- Skin: poor circulation or rashes
- Skeletal system: septic arthritis or osteomyelitis

MANAGEMENT

Investigations

If one or more of the warning signs are present it is mandatory to perform a complete septic work-up. This includes:

- Blood culture — arterial or venous — at least 2–4 mL.
- Urine — suprapubic aspiration (SPA). If one SPA fails do not keep attempting. A catheter specimen should be obtained by inserting a 5 French gauge catheter under aseptic technique. Discard the first two to three drops. A bag specimen is of little value.
- Lumbar puncture — 2–4 mL is required. Exercise caution in an extremely sick baby with a bulging fontanelle.

Treatment

Any neonate with a rectal temperature of greater than 37.5°C should be investigated and treated in hospital. Broad spectrum antibiotics given parenterally are indicated. Usually this will start with penicillin and gentamicin for septicaemia or amoxycillin and cefotaxime for meningitis. The antibiotics are then manipulated when cultures are available.

Careful attention to temperature stability, ventilation, fluid and electrolytes, blood pressure, blood glucose and haematology is essential.

PROBLEMS OF THE EX-VERY LOW BIRTHWEIGHT INFANT

While it is not the intention of this handbook to discuss all the problems of management of VLBW infants it is important to be aware of some of the potential problems that frequently occur after discharge from the neonatal unit.

BRONCHOPULMONARY DYSPLASIA (BPD)

BPD is a common chronic lung disease occurring in infants who have survived mechanical ventilation. It is characterized by prolonged oxygen dependency. The majority of infants are able to be weaned out of oxygen within 4 weeks of the time that they were due to be born. A small number require oxygen therapy for months and some are managed at home in oxygen.

These babies are particularly susceptible to respiratory infections in the first 18 months of life. Warning signs and symptoms:

- Cyanotic episodes
- Poor feeding
- Apnoeic episodes
- Crackles on auscultation

The presence of one or more of these signs is an urgent indication for admission to hospital. If a baby with BPD has a respiratory infection without the above, management at home is reasonable but the parents need to be informed of the warning signs and the child reviewed frequently.

NECROTIZING ENTEROCOLITIS (NEC)

NEC is an acquired gastrointestinal disease due to infection in the immature small and/or large intestine which has suffered vascular compromise. The result is transmural inflammation of the gut. While many babies recover after conservative management (nil orally, intravenous alimentation, antibiotics) some develop bowel necrosis necessitating bowel resection.

The risks to these babies after discharge from hospital are:

Stricture Formation

This can present up to months after the initial NEC episode. The presenting features include: constipation, failure to thrive and vomiting.

Gastroenteritis

This can produce severe dehydration very rapidly particularly in a baby who has had a bowel resection. It is not appropriate to manage these infants at home with oral rehydration therapy. Admission to hospital is essential.

HERNIAS

Umbilical hernia is common and does not require treatment. *Inguinal hernias* are also common and require surgical repair as there is a significant risk of strangulation.

OTITIS MEDIA

This is common and should be considered in babies presenting with fever.

IMMUNIZATION

An infant should receive the first three doses of Triple Antigen and Sabin at 2, 4 and 6 months from the actual date of birth, irrespective of the degree of prematurity. There are no grounds for delaying immunization based on size or prematurity.

APNOEA

Apnoea is a very common problem in the VLBW infant up to 34 weeks gestation. Any ex-VLBW infant is at risk for significant apnoea up until 3 months of age past the due date; particularly with surgical procedures requiring general anaesthesia and with respiratory infections (especially respiratory syncytial virus (RSV) infection). Careful monitoring is essential in infants with these conditions.

SUDDEN INFANT DEATH SYNDROME (SIDS)

SIDS is the major 'cause' of death between the ages of 1 and 12 months. The incidence of SIDS in Victoria is 1 per 500 live births. The causes of SIDS are unknown. It is likely that SIDS occurs as a result of an adverse trigger in a baby who is susceptible. No investigations, including pneumograms, have been able to identify susceptible infants.

Although the incidence of SIDS is slightly higher in subsequent siblings of a SIDS infant when matched for birth order there is no difference in incidence from controls.

Risk factors have been identified which increase the chances of SIDS:

- *Prone sleeping position.* Extensive studies have concluded that this is not the desirable position for babies in the first months of life. It is advised to lie babies on their side or supine except in the case of significant gastro-oesophageal reflux.
- *Hyperthermia* — from over-wrapping — should be avoided particularly in a baby with an infection. The sign of sweating around the head and neck suggest the baby is too hot.
- *Parental smoking* should be avoided.
- *Artificial feeding.* Breast feeding should be encouraged.
- *Extreme prematurity* (< 32 weeks) — a low threshold for admission to hospital during infections.
- *Parental narcotic or cocaine abuse* increases the risk of SIDS.
- *Viral infections.* Close review of young infants needs to be given.

APPARENT LIFE THREATENING EPISODE (ALTE)

Previously known as 'near-miss SIDS' it is defined as a combination of apnoea, colour change or choking, which is frightening to the observer. At least 10% of these infants will have another episode. Admission to hospital for investigation and monitoring is essential.

The awareness of parents and medical practitioners may be of assistance in reducing the incidence of SIDS. Any baby under the age of 6 months presenting to a doctor or infant welfare nurse needs to be given very careful attention.

HOME APNOEA MONITORING

No study has been able to demonstrate that widespread home apnoea monitoring programmes reduce the incidence of SIDS. The Neonatal Department at the Royal Children's Hospital has monitored over 350 babies in the last 6 years. Analysis of our data have drawn the following conclusions:

- A significant number (13%) of infants have received successful resuscitation by their parents
- An overwhelming relief of parental anxiety particularly in parents of subsequent siblings of SIDS infant, infants who have had an ALTE, and infants who have been extremely premature
- A very low incidence of false alarms
- Six per cent of our families referred have had pre-existing psychiatric disturbance including Munchausen by proxy

We do not recommend widespread home apnoea monitoring. However, the following are our recommendations for consideration of home apnoea monitoring.

- Subsequent siblings of SIDS victims
- ALTE
- Twin of SIDS victim
- Extremely premature infants

Within the Royal Children's Hospital and in Victoria advice regarding home monitoring is available through the Department of Neonatology.

NEONATAL SEIZURES

CLINICAL FEATURES

- Subtle — deviation of eyes, abnormal sucking, apnoea
- Tonic — usually all limbs frequently associated with apnoea and eye deviation
- Multifocal clonic — migratory clonic movement of limbs
- Focal clonic
- Myoclonic

These should be distinguished from 'jitteriness' which is a movement disorder or tremulousness. This has no ocular phenomena, is stimulus sensitive, and is stopped with gentle passive flexion of the limbs.

AETIOLOGY

An aetiology can usually be found for neonatal seizures.

1. Hypoxic ischaemic encephalopathy — the seizures occur within 48 h of the hypoxic event.
2. Intracranial haemorrhage.
3. Metabolic.
   - a Hypoglycaemia.
   - b Hypocalcaemia/hypomagnesiaemia.
   - c Hypo- or hypernatraemia.
   - d Local anaesthetic intoxication.
   - e Amino acid/organic acid/hyperammonaemia.
   - f Pyridoxine dependency.
   - g Kernicterus.
4. Infection.
5. Drug withdrawal.
6. Developmental brain abnormalities.
7. Autosomal dominant neonatal seizures.
8. Unknown.

MANAGEMENT

Admission to hospital is mandatory.

Investigations

Aimed at recognizing and treating the cause.

- Lumbar puncture
- Blood glucose
- Electrolytes, Ca, Mg
- Cranial ultrasound
- Metabolic screen — if indicated
- Cranial CT scan — if focal seizures, birth trauma, uncertain aetiology
- EEG – to detect seizure activity and to aid prognosis

Treatment

Anticonvulsants

- Phenytoin — 20 mg/kg, i.v. stat in not less than 20 min.

- Phenobarbitone — 20 mg/kg, i.v. stat over 10 min. A further 10 mg/kg may be given for refractory seizures.
- Clonazepam — up to 0.25 mg. This may cause apnoea. Careful monitoring and the availability of mechanical ventilation are essential.

Other anticonvulsants, including Thiopentone, may be necessary.

Most infants are able to be weaned off anticonvulsant therapy within 2 weeks of the last seizure. Some infants who have residual seizures or abnormal neurological signs with an abnormal EEG are treated for months.

General treatment

Attention to optimal ventilation, blood pressure control, fluid and electrolyte balance and normoglycaemia are essential.

SURGICAL CONDITIONS OF THE NEONATE

IMPORTANT WARNING SIGNS

- Excessive drooling of frothy secretions from the mouth may suggest *oesophageal atresia*. A 10 French gauge catheter should be pressed through the mouth.
- *Bile (green) stained vomiting is always abnormal.* Malrotation may present with minimal bile stained vomiting at any age. Admission to a paediatric hospital is essential.
- *Delayed passage of meconium* — beyond 24 h is abnormal.
- *Inguinal hernias* need urgent attention.

CHAPTER 9

INFECTIOUS DISEASES

SPECIMENS REQUIRED FOR MICROBIOLOGICAL DIAGNOSIS

The following information covers the safe and efficient collection of appropriate specimens for the identification of infective organisms. Much of this information reflects practice at the Royal Children's Hospital; however, many procedures are applicable to other centres.

URINE

Collection of Specimens

- Midstream specimen urine. *Males:* wash penis with warm water, retract prepuce and collect sample in a sterile container. *Females:* wash the perineum and labia with warm water. The child should be sitting or standing with legs apart. It is recommended that before voiding, the labia should be parted by the nurse, the mother or the child.
- Bag specimen. Wash perineum and genitalia with warm water. Dry, attach bag and inspect at least every 20 min. A urine collected in a bag and left on the patient for a longer period, will probably produce a result that cannot be interpreted.
- Suprapubic aspiration (SPA) — see Paediatric Procedures pp. 178–80.
- Catheter specimen — see Paediatric Procedures pp. 178–80.

Dipslide Culture

The dipslide provides the means to inoculate the culture immediately after collection and prevents the overgrowth of contaminating bacteria that occurs with stored urine specimens. The dipslide is removed from the container and held by the cap. The agar surfaces are fully immersed (once only) in the urine collected in the universal container. The inoculated dipslide is drained free of excess urine and placed back in its container and the universal container is recapped. Outside laboratory hours the inoculated dipslide is incubated and the urine for microscopy refrigerated. It is important that the method of specimen collection be indicated clearly on the request card, and on the dipslide label, e.g. (MSU), (SPA), (BAG).

Mycobacterium tuberculosis Culture

All of the first early morning specimens of urine passed should be collected on 3 consecutive days and sent to the laboratory in special bottles which can be obtained from the laboratory on request. The results of culture should be available in 4–6 weeks.

Urine for Viral Culture

Approximately 5 mL urine should be sent in a virus transport tube.

Urine Microscopy

Within the Royal Children's Hospital urines are screened initially with a reagent strip (Nephur test plus leucocytes) which can detect the presence of pus cells, red cells/haemoglobin, protein and nitrate reducing organisms. If all four parts of the screening test are negative, or if they clearly indicate an infection, microscopic examination will not be done. Microscopy will be performed only on those with a positive screening test (for blood, protein or nitrate reduction) or if it is specifically requested, usually for assessment of red cell morphology and the presence of casts.

The usual normal upper limit of 10 white blood cells/mm^3 (10 × 10^6/L) may be exceeded in otherwise normal children during episodes of fever. More commonly an excess of white blood cells in the urine in the absence of bacteriuria is due to antibiotic treatment of urinary tract infection. Persistent 'sterile' pyuria in absence of antibacterial activity requires further investigation.

Report of Urine Cultures

Within the Royal Children's Hospital a negative culture report is available approximately 24 h from the time of delivery of the specimen to the laboratory (Monday–Friday). A full report on positive cultures requires an additional 24 h. A laboratory opinion of the interpretation of the culture results is indicated on the report form.

FAECES

Requests for examination of faeces should be accompanied by appropriate clinical information — particularly duration of symptoms (usually diarrhoea), associated abdominal pain or vomiting and any clues to the source of infection (contacts, food, overseas travel, recent antibiotic treatment, nosocomial).

Within the Royal Children's Hospital all specimens of faeces from patients with diarrhoea should be sent to the bacteriology laboratory initially, where microscopy and tests for rotavirus and adenovirus, when indicated, will be performed. Further tests including bacterial culture and test for other viruses will depend on the clinical information provided. Specimens of normal faeces or rectal swabs received from inpatients without clinical information will be assumed to be for surveillance purposes and will be cultured for MRSA only.

A sample of approximately 5 g of faeces (two or three spoonfuls) is suitable for a microscopic and culture examination. A rectal swab is less satisfactory than faeces and suitable for culture only; a swab that shows no faecal staining on the cotton wool is inadequate and will not be processed.

Reporting of Faecal Examination

Within the Royal Children's Hospital the results of tests for adenovirus, rotavirus and microscopy for parasites will be available within 48 h (Monday–Friday). Results of bacterial culture are usually available within 48 h. Final identification of a specific pathogen may require a further 24 h.

Threadworms

The worms lay their eggs in the perianal folds during the night. Samples should be collected in the early morning. The sticky side of the tape is pressed on to the skin near the anus. Then the tape is placed sticky side to the microscope slide, replaced into the plastic bag and returned to the laboratory. Kits are available from the bacteriology laboratory.

Amoebiasis

Infestations with *Entamoeba histolytica* is rare in Victoria, but may have been acquired overseas. It is necessary to discuss with the laboratory the arrangements for examining a fresh specimen of faeces.

***Note:* Within the Royal Children's Hospital faeces for fat globules/tryptic activity are examined in the gastroenterology laboratory. Faeces for viral culture from patients who have suspected enteroviral infection (for example) should be sent directly to the virology laboratory. (Separate specimens and request cards are necessary when tests are required from both laboratories.)**

RESPIRATORY SPECIMENS

Collection of Specimens

Nasopharyngeal aspirate (NPA)

NPA should be collected for immunofluorescence (IF) and culture for *Bordetella pertussis*, *Chlamydia trachomatis* and respiratory viruses. Within the Royal Children's Hospital they should be collected early in the morning, if possible, to arrive in Virology by 0930 h. Specimens collected outside laboratory hours should be stored in a refrigerator, 4°C (not frozen) and sent to the laboratory next morning. Results of IF examination are available on the same day. Cultures may take up to 3 weeks. A separate NPA is preferred for culture of *Mycoplasma pneumoniae*.

Sputum

Samples of sputum (not saliva) should be collected in standard universal containers. The quality of specimens will be assessed by microscopic examination and, if they are unsuitable, cultures will not be done. Microscopy and cultures for mycobacteria will be done on request only. Routine cultures will take at least 48 h and possibly 72 h for a complete report.

Gastric lavage

Early morning gastric lavage using normal saline, is used to obtain a sample for an examination for *M. tuberculosis* when the patient cannot produce sputum. Special bottles containing a caustic solution are available from the laboratory, and the lavage should be placed in this solution as soon as collected. Report on the culture for *M. tuberculosis* takes up to 6 weeks and no report can be expected before 3 weeks.

Throat swab

Throat swabs should be sent to the laboratory in transport medium. They are cultured routinely for *Streptococcus pyogenes* only. In patients with membranous tonsillitis in whom diphtheria is suspected a special request for culture of *Corynebacterium diphtheria* should be made. Check the patient's immunization status. If an NPA is not available for viral culture a throat swab should be taken and broken off into viral transport medium.

PUS

If available, a quantity of pus, transported to the laboratory as quickly as possible in a syringe or sterile container is optimal. This is suitable for immediate Gram stain, aerobic and anaerobic culture. If required, smears and cultures for mycobacteria and/or *Actinomyces israelii* should be specifically requested.

Pus swabs are often the only specimen available. 'Dry' swabs are not adequate for culture of many types of bacteria. Transport media (e.g. Amies) should be used for all swabs sent for culture. In some circumstances Gram-stained smears are a rapid and helpful way to assess the likely causes of infection. Smears made from swabs in transport media or from dry swabs are unsatisfactory and therefore, smears should be made directly when the swabs are taken.

Collection of Specimens

The following procedure is suitable for collection of swabs from any site of obvious infection, e.g. conjunctivitis (see eye swabs), cellulitis, discharging abscess, wound infection or vaginal discharge.

Using a plain cotton wool swabstick, swab the lesion or purulent discharge and make smears, to cover about the middle one-third of each of two labelled glass microscope slides. Discard the swab carefully — it is potentially infective. Replace the slides in the container and fill in the label provided. Using the Transwab provided, swab the lesion or discharge again and place the swab into the tube of transport medium immediately. Label, return to the laboratory together with slide container in a plastic bag.

EYE SWABS

A kit is available from the laboratory for collection of specimens from patients with conjunctivitis. All purulent material should be removed with an ordinary cotton swab which should be used to make smears on glass microscope slides and replaced into Amies transport medium (see above).

Swabs from neonates will be cultured routinely for *Neisseria gonorrhoea* and other bacteria. Specimens from infants less than 3 months of age with conjunctivitis should be examined for *Chlamydia trachomatis*. Swabs should be collected after swabs for bacterial smears and culture because epithelial cells, not pus, are required. A cotton tipped wire swab (available in 'eye kit') is then used to scrape the conjunctiva of the lower palpebral fissure firmly. The swab is then cut off (using ordinary scissors) into *Chlamydia* transport medium. A separate swab is used to make a smear on the slide provided for IF. The IF result will be available in about 1 h; *Chlamydia* culture requires 2–7 days.

GENITAL SWABS

A kit is available from the laboratory for collection of genital specimens. Smears from vaginal discharge should be made directly onto glass microscope slides. Swabs should be sent to the laboratory in transport medium. They will be cultured routinely on gonococcal medium.

If sexual abuse is suspected or if the girl is sexually active, examination for *C. trachomatis* should be performed as well. In pre-adolescent girls, a vaginal swab is adequate; in sexually active females, a cervical swab should be obtained. In this case all purulent cervical discharge should be removed from the cervix (and used for smears and bacterial cultures). A cotton tipped wire swab should be rotated in the cervical canal for at least 15 s and then the tip cut into *Chlamydia* transport medium. A separate swab should be used to make a smear on the glass slide provided for IF. Swabs, slides and *Chlamydia* transport media are available from the laboratory. Rectal swabs for *Chlamydia* or gonococcal culture may be indicated (boys or girls) and should be collected and transported as for genital swabs. Urethral swabs for Gram stain and culture for *N. gonorrhoeae* and *C. trachomatis* should be collected from sexually active boys with urethral discharge.

SWABS FROM OTHER MUCOUS MEMBRANES

For example nose, throat, rectal (faeces is usually preferable) or uninfected skin (e.g. for detection of MRSA carriers). Smears are generally not helpful in this situation but swabs should be collected, as above, and placed in transport medium.

Note: When swabs are taken outside laboratory hours, transport medium should be stored at room temperature, not in a refrigerator.

STERILE ASPIRATES (PLEURAL, PERITONEAL, JOINT)

It is recommended that the specimen be collected into a sterile heparinized bottle (available from bacteriology) so that a cell count can be performed.

TISSUE

Biopsies for bacteriological culture must not be placed in formalin. They should be submitted in a universal container. *The laboratory should be notified as soon as possible after a decision is made to perform tissue biopsy, so that appropriate specimens, transport media and culture media can be discussed.* Where possible such specimens should arrive in the laboratory during normal laboratory hours.

CEREBROSPINAL FLUID (CSF)

See also Bacterial Meningitis p. 19. CSF is examined in the following manner at the Royal Children's Hospital. Procedural details may differ at other centres.

Culture

All specimens of CSF are cultured for bacteria and for virus when cell counts are consistent with viral meningitis. Microscopy and culture for other CNS pathogens are not performed routinely and patients in whom such infections are suspected should be discussed with the microbiologist.

Test for Bacterial Antigens

Latex agglutination for antigens of *Haemophilus influenzae* type b, *Streptococcus pneumoniae*, *Neisseria meningitidis* will be done immediately on abnormal CSF.

CSF Reports

Abnormal CSF microscopy results (suggesting infection) will be phoned immediately to the requesting doctor. Microscopy reports and the 24 h culture report are returned within 24 h from the time the specimen is received at the laboratory (Monday–Friday). A further report is returned after the culture has been incubated for 48 h.

BLOOD CULTURES

Collection Of Blood Cultures

See Paediatric Procedures pp. 178–80.

Blood culture reports

Blood cultures are examined twice daily and reported at the end of the first 2 days, and reported finally after 7 days. If endocarditis or brucellosis are suspected the blood cultures are incubated for longer. Positive blood cultures are reported by phone immediately to the requesting doctor.

Blood culture for viruses

Unclotted blood in a heparinized or sequestrene tube should be sent for isolation of viruses.

FUNGAL EXAMINATION

Collection of skin, nails and hair — see Paediatric Procedures pp. 178–80.

VIROLOGICAL EXAMINATION AND SEROLOGY

Virus Isolation

Tissue culture isolation for adeno-, cytomegalo- (CMV), entero-, herpes simplex (HSV), myxo-, paramyxo-, rhino-, rubella and varicella zoster (VZV) viruses.

Antigen Detection

- IF for respiratory viruses, HSV, CMV, *Chlamydia trachomatis, Bordetella pertussis* and VZV.
- Enzyme immunoassay (EIA) for hepatitis B surface antigen (HBsAg)
- Electron microscopy for herpes group, viruses causing diarrhoea and others as required

Serology

IgG and IgM for antibodies against: CMV, Epstein-Barr virus (EBV), HSV, measles, mumps, *Mycoplasma pneumoniae*, rubella, VZV, *Toxoplasma gondii*, hepatitis B and *Bordetella pertussis*.

Other serological tests are: Antistreptolysin O titre (ASOT), antiDNAse B, screening test for syphilis — rapid plasma reagin (RPR) test.

Tests are continually being developed and evaluated according to need so that the above list may alter from time to time. Tests other than the above can be arranged with other centres.

Specimens

- *CNS infections* (aseptic meningitis, encephalitis, polio, polyneuritis): throat swab, urine, faeces, CSF, clotted blood for serology
- *Congenital infections:* throat swab, urine, clotted blood
- *Conjunctivitis:* conjunctival swab (see bacteriology notes), throat swab, faeces
- *Exanthemata:* measles—NPA, urine, clotted blood; rubella—throat swab, urine, clotted blood

- *Gastroenteritis:* faeces (see bacteriology notes)
- *Hepatitis:* blood
- *Infectious mononucleosis syndrome:* unclotted blood for culture, throat, urine
- *Myocarditis/Pericarditis:* throat swab, faeces, urine, clotted blood
- *Parotitis:* throat swab, urine, faeces
- *Pleurodynia:* throat swab, urine, faeces
- *Puo:* throat swab, urine, faeces
- *Respiratory infections:* NPA — same day rapid diagnosis available if specimen received by 0930 h.
- *Vesicular lesions:* hand, foot and mouth — throat swab (or NPA), faeces, vesicle swab; herpangina — throat swab (or NPA), faeces, vesicle swab; herpes simplex — vesicle (rapid diagnoses by IF or electron microscopy also available — contact laboratory); varicella zoster — vesicular fluid for culture — contact laboratory for rapid diagnosis

IMMUNIZATION

HAEMOPHILUS INFLUENZAE TYPE b VACCINE

Vaccines for the immunization of children against *Haemophilus influenzae* type b (HIB) are now becoming available in Australia. Children under the age of 5 years are of greatest risk. At the time of going to press (August 1992) one vaccine, PRP-D (ProHibit) is licensed for used for children 18 months–5 years. All such children should be vaccinated. Newer vaccines effective for children younger than 18 months are likely to become available in the coming months and will supersede the PRP-D vaccine.

SCHEDULES

Immunization schedules differ from state to state in Australia. Readers are advised to check with local authorities.

The Health Department of Victoria recommends the following course of immunization:

Age	*Immunizations*	*Route*
2 months	Triple Antigen	Intramuscular
	Polio (Sabin)	Oral
4 months	Triple Antigen	Intramuscular
	Polio (Sabin)	Oral
6 months	Triple Antigen	Intramuscular
	Polio (Sabin)	Oral
12–15 months	Measles/mumps/rubella (MMR)	Subcutaneous
18 months	Triple Antigen	Intramuscular
5 years or prior to school entry	CDT	Intramuscular
	Polio	Oral
10–16 years (girls)*	Rubella	Subcutaneous
15–19 years or prior to leaving school	Adult diphtheria and tetanus	Intramuscular

* Preferably in last year of primary school or first year of high school.

Tetanus Immunoprophylaxis of Wounded Patients According to Immunization Status

Type of wound	*Last dose of tetanus toxoid (0.5 mL)*	*Immune*[†]		*Partly immune*[‡]		*Non-immune*[§]
		Tetanus toxoid (0.5 mL)*	*Tetanus immunoglobulin (250 units)*	*Tetanus toxoid (0.5 mL)*	*Tetanus immunoglobulin (250 units)*	
Tetanus-prone wounds**	If < 2 years ago	No	No	Yes, and ensure that the course is completed	Yes	Give 250 units of tetanus immunoglobulin and at the same time administer 0.5 mL tetanus toxoid (or CDT or ADT*), but in the opposite limb and with a separate syringe. Ensure completion of the course
	If 2–10 years ago	Yes	No			
	If 10–20 years ago	Yes	Yes			
	If 20 years ago	Yes, and additional dose 4–6 weeks later	Yes	Yes, and additional dose 4–6 weeks later		
Other wounds (i.e. not tetanus-prone)	If < 10 years ago	No	No	Yes, and ensure that the course is completed.	No	Initiate course of tetanus toxoid and ensure that the course is duly completed
	If 10–20 years ago	Yes	No			
	If 20 years ago	Yes, and additional dose 4–6 weeks later	No	Yes, and additional dose 4–6 weeks later	No	

* CDT or ADT may be substituted when simultaneous boosting of diphtheria is required.

† Individuals who have received at least three doses of tetanus toxoid.

‡ Individuals who have received only one or two doses of tetanus toxoid.

§ Includes doubtful or uncertain immunity.

** The types of wounds which favour the growth of *C. tetani* are as follows: compound fractures, penetrating wounds, wounds containing foreign bodies, especially wood splinters, wounds complicated by pyogenic infection, wounds involving extensive tissue damage and/or bruising, burns, any superficial wound obviously contaminated with soil, dust or horse manure in which there has been a delay of more than 4 h in receiving topical disinfection or surgical cleansing. ADT for adults and children 8 years of age and older. CDT for children up to 8 years.

IMMUNIZATION PRECAUTIONS

Immunization should not be carried out during the course of a significant acute illness. Mild local reactions occur frequently (up to 50%) following Triple Antigen and *do not* contraindicate further Triple Antigen vaccination. Re-analysis of the epidemiological data has failed to confirm that there is an increased risk of permanent brain damage following the Triple Antigen. Previously held contraindications are unproven. When in doubt over Triple Antigen administration an opinion from a paediatrician should be sought.

MMR and polio are all live attenuated viruses. The precautions relating to these include: vaccination should be avoided in those children receiving corticosteroid or immunosuppressive therapy including general radiation, children suffering from malignant conditions and household contacts of patients with malignancy or immunosuppression should not be given oral polio to reduce the chance of spread to the child.

Allergies to hen's egg should not be an absolute contraindication to MMR. In patients with a history of anaphylactic reactions to egg ingestion MMR vaccine should only be given after consultation with an appropriate specialist and where facilities for resuscitation are available. A general history of allergic symptoms is not a contraindication to childhood immunization.

Pregnancy is an absolute contraindication to rubella immunization, and should be avoided for two full menstrual cycles following administration.

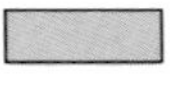

ISOLATION PRECAUTION POLICY OF THE ROYAL CHILDREN'S HOSPITAL

Within the Royal Children's Hospital patients who have a communicable disease or nosocomial (hospital acquired) infection caused by virulent pathogenic organisms, require 'isolation precautions' to prevent spread of infection.

The isolation policy should be followed as closely as possible for the protection of patients or staff. However, other arrangements may be required if an isolation room is not available, there are insufficient nursing staff available or the patient's clinical condition is such that isolation may jeopardize his/her management.

With the exception of protective isolation, any changes suggested by the Consultant should be discussed, as soon as possible, with the Infection Control Clinical Nurse specialist or if she is unavailable with the Medical Microbiologist. Once implemented, isolation procedures should not be changed without such discussion.

CONDITIONS WHICH REQUIRE ISOLATION PRECAUTION NOTICES

Protective Isolation

- **Agranulocytosis or severe neutropenia**
- **Burns and severe skin disease (extensive and non-infected)**
- **Immune deficiency**
- **Transplant recipient (recent)**

Standard Precautions

Wound and skin

- **Conjunctivitis — gonococcal (until appropriately treated for 24 h)"**

- **Exfoliating skin disease colonized with multiresistant bacteria**
- **Herpes simplex infections with extensive lesions**
- **Herpes zoster (shingles)**
- **Infected dermatitis or eczema**
- **Multi or unusually resistant bacteria (infections)**
- **Scalded skin syndrome**
- **Syphilis with skin or mucous membrane lesions**
- **Streptococcal group A infections (until appropriately treated for 24 h)**
- **Wound or burn infections which cannot be occluded**
- **Scabies (until appropriately treated for at least 24 h)**
- **Pediculosis (contact infection control for further information)**

Enteric

- **Food poisoning**
- **Gastroenteritis — bacterial and viral**
- **Giardiasis, cryptosporidiosis**
- **Hepatitis A**
- **Typhoid**

Respiratory

- **Bronchiolitis**
- **Croup**
- **Diphtheria**
- **Hand, foot and mouth disease**
- **Influenza**
- **Meningococcal meningitis (until treated for 24 h)**
- **Mumps**
- **Measles**
- **Pertussis**
- **Pneumocystis**
- **Pneumonia due to multiresistant bacteria**
- **Rubella**
- **Scarlet fever**
- **Tuberculosis — open pulmonary or discharging wound**
- **Varicella (chicken pox)**

Blood precautions: Strict or limited

All patients who are bleeding externally, when the bleeding cannot be contained.

HIV INFECTION AND AIDS

The human immunodeficiency virus (HIV) is the causative agent of the acquired immunodeficiency syndrome (AIDS). It is important to distinguish between infection with HIV, which may be asymptomatic during a variable latent period, and the progressive immunological derangement which leads to AIDS.

PAEDIATRIC RISK GROUP

Adolescents (Same as for Adults)

- Homosexual or bisexual males

- Intravenous drug users
- Sexual contacts of persons with HIV or from groups with increased risk for infection
- Transfusion recipients, particularly patients with congenital bleeding disorders, who received blood products before 1985

Younger Children

- Infants of mothers who are known to be HIV positive or who are members of a high risk group
- Children receiving blood or blood products before 1985

CLINICAL FEATURES

Clinical presentations consistent with paediatric HIV infection include: prolonged fever, failure to thrive or weight loss more than 10%, generalized lymphadenopathy, hepatosplenomegaly, parotitis, chronic or recurrent diarrhoea and chronic thrush. Laboratory tests may show lymphopenia, abnormal T-cell subsets and hypergammaglobulinaemia.

The most recent Communicable Diseases Centre case definition of paediatric AIDS includes progressive neurological disease, lymphoid interstitial pneumonia, opportunistic infection (e.g. *Pneumocystis carinii* pneumonia), recurrent episodes of serious bacterial infections and secondary malignancy.

DIAGNOSIS

Patients who are recognized as belonging to one of the high risk groups require counselling and informed consent before testing for HIV antibodies. Specific antibody detection is a sensitive indicator of HIV infection in adults and children, but it is not diagnostic in infants because passively transferred maternal antibody may persist for up to 15 months. The presence of HIV glycoproteins or proviral DNA sequences confirms the presence of HIV infection.

The testing for HIV infection should be undertaken on a confidential basis.

Subsequent management of paediatric HIV is generally by a group of physicians, nurses and allied health professionals who have a special interest in the needs of these patients. **Within the Royal Children's Hospital the clinical nurse consultant for paediatric AIDS co-ordinates clinic services that the families may require.**

Management of blood spills and needle stick injuries are discussed in the following section.

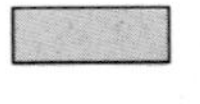

UNIVERSAL PRECAUTIONS FOR PREVENTION OF BLOOD-BORNE VIRUS INFECTION

The following is the Universal Precautions policy of the Royal Children's Hospital.

AVOID PENETRATING INJURY WITH POTENTIALLY CONTAMINATED SHARP OBJECTS

1 All sharp objects — needles, scalpel blades, glass, etc. should be disposed of immediately in sharps containers (large yellow plastic jars with the 'Biohazard' label).

2 Sharps containers should be located in or close to treatment areas; they should not be more than two-thirds full and the lid should be replaced immediately after use.
3 Needles should not be recapped or removed from syringes manually; needle guards are available for this purpose if removal of the needle is necessary.

AVOID CONTACT WITH BLOOD OR OTHER POTENTIALLY INFECTED BODY FLUIDS BY USE OF PROTECTIVE BARRIERS IF CONTACT IS LIKELY AND BY IMMEDIATELY CLEANING UP ACCIDENTAL SPILLS

1 All blood, body fluids containing visible blood and objects contaminated with blood should be regarded as potentially infectious.
2 In general, it is recommended that gloves be worn when undertaking or assisting invasive procedures including venepuncture, insertion of intravenous lines or aspiration of body fluids including lumbar puncture. The risk of contamination of the hands with blood is low in some circumstances and experienced personnel may choose not to use gloves routinely. However, they should always be used by operator and assistant (if applicable).
   a If the person taking blood or assisting has cuts, scratches or dermatitis on her/his hands.
   b If the patient is uncooperative.
   c When collecting blood from infants by heelprick.
   d In an emergency situation especially if the patient is bleeding.
   e If the blood-collector is inexperienced.
3 Gloves should be worn when attending to patients who are bleeding externally from accidental or surgical wounds, epistaxis, haematemesis, etc; this includes patients who are menstruating if they require assistance with changing sanitary napkins.
4 Goggles, mask and a disposable impervious apron should be worn, in addition, when attending to patients who are bleeding in such a way that splashing of blood is likely to occur.
5 All blood spills should be cleaned up immediately using rubber gloves, disposable cloths and sodium hypochlorite 0.5% (5000 parts/10^6 available chlorine). All surfaces in hospitals which are likely to be exposed to blood spills should be able to be thoroughly cleaned or laundered. Disinfectant should be in contact for at least 30 min. For spills, it is often difficult to leave hypochlorite in place for 30 min. An alternative method is to place some 0.5% hypochlorite solution on a wad of paper towels, wipe the spill with this wad, then discard the contaminated paper towels into an infectious wastebag. It may then be necessary to wipe the area again with hypochlorite, then clean the area with commercial detergent.
6 Blood-stained linen should be treated as potentially infectious and discarded into yellow 'infectious' meltaway bags and then yellow nylon drawstring linen bags.
7 Blood-stained dressings, paper towels, sanitary napkins and other disposable items should be discarded into yellow 'infectious' waste bags which should be placed into a second yellow waste bag for disposal when no more than two-thirds full.

ANY ACCIDENT INVOLVING SIGNIFICANT EXPOSURE TO BLOOD OR BODY FLUIDS, CONTAMINATED NEEDLESTICK INJURY OR SIGNIFICANT EXPOSURE TO MUCOUS MEMBRANES OR NON-INTACT SKIN SHOULD BE REPORTED IMMEDIATELY (SEE EXECUTIVE MEMORANDUM NO. 89/57).

PROCEDURE TO BE ADOPTED IN THE CASE OF STAFF MEMBERS EXPOSED TO PATIENT'S BLOOD: BY NEEDLESTICK INJURY, EYE SPLASH OR HEAVY SKIN CONTAMINATION

General Comments

1. Blood should be washed off skin with soap and water or from eyes with water, immediately.
2. An incident form should be filled in immediately.
3. Staff should report to Staff Clinic, usually within 24 h. If the incident occurs on Friday afternoon or at the weekend she/he should report to the Admitting Officer at once and should report to Staff Clinic on Monday morning.

Within the Royal Children's Hospital, if the patient whose blood was involved is known to be infected or at risk of infection with human immunodeficiency virus (HIV), Staff Clinic or the Clinical Nurse Consultant in Paediatric AIDS should be contacted immediately. After hours contact the Infectious Disease Specialist on call (see below).

NOTE: NEEDLESTICK INJURY OR OTHER SIGNIFICANT EXPOSURE TO BLOOD OR BODY FLUIDS SHOULD BE REPORTED IMMEDIATELY. BASELINE SERUM *MUST* BE AVAILABLE FOR SUCH AN INCIDENT TO BE IMPLICATED AS THE CAUSE OF BLOOD-BORNE VIRUS INFECTION IN A STAFF MEMBER.

Known High Risk Patient

1. If the patient whose blood was involved is a high risk patient for hepatitis B.
   - **a** Check current hepatitis B surface antigen (HBsAg) status of patient (this will usually be in the patient record).
   - **b** Check immunization status of staff member.
     - If fully immunized and known to have seroconverted (i.e. antiHBs positive) no further action is required.
     - If immunized but the antiHBs status is not known, *and* the patient is HBsAg positive, blood should be taken from the staff member and hepatitis B immune globulin (available from Red Cross Blood Bank) given within 48 h or preferably 24 h of the accident. AntiHBs will be tested as soon as possible; if negative the course of vaccination should be repeated and antibody status tested again 6 weeks after the last dose.
     - If not immunized and the patient is HBsAg positive, blood should be taken immediately, and hepatitis B immune globulin given as soon as possible.
2. A course of hepatitis B vaccine should be started immediately if necessary, that is, if the staff member has not seroconverted or has not been immunized. The importance of a full course of immunization should be explained to the staff member and if he/she chooses not to have vaccine, this fact should be recorded on his/her Staff Clinic record.
3. It is not necessary to test the staff member's blood for HBsAg before hepatitis B immune globulin is given, but blood should be collected. Blood from the staff member will be stored for future testing for HIV antibody if necessary.

Blood test for HIV will not be done without the staff member's informed consent and only after discussion with the staff doctor who will ensure confidentiality.

4 **Within the Royal Children's Hospital, if the patient is believed to be infected with HIV the Clinical Nurse Consultant in Paediatric AIDS should be contacted immediately to discuss the need for prophylaxis with zidovudine.**

This depends on the patient's HIV status and the degree of exposure. After hours the Infectious Disease Specialist on call should be contacted. If necessary zidovudine treatment will be arranged by the Infectious Disease Unit, appropriate follow-up will be arranged and strict confidentiality maintained.

Low or Unknown Risk Patient

1 If the patient whose blood was involved is not known to be a high risk patient, his/her blood should be tested for HBsAg as soon as possible if the staff member has not been fully immunized against hepatitis B. The urgency with which this is done and whether the patient should be tested for HIV antibody will be determined by the patient's underlying condition and whether there are any risk factors for HBsAg or HIV carriage. This should be discussed with the Infectious Disease Specialist on call.

2 The procedure outlined above should be followed if the patient proves to be an HBsAg carrier.

3 If the staff member has been immunized, his/her antiHBs status should be determined if this has not already been done.

Other Considerations

1 If the source of the blood is unknown, e.g. a needlestick injury has involved a needle which has been incorrectly discarded, the risk should be assessed according to whether there are, or have recently been, any high risk patients in the ward or department.

2 If the risk is considered to be high and the staff member is not known to be immune, a request for hepatitis B immune globulin may be successful. If not, a course of vaccine should be started immediately. Post-exposure immunization is quite effective even without the use of hepatitis B immune globulin.

NOTIFIABLE DISEASES IN VICTORIA

Notifiable diseases vary from state to state. Readers are advised to consult local authorities for information on local regulations.

Notifiable infectious diseases in Victoria are divided into four groups on the basis of the method of notification and the information required. Special notification forms are used and these are available from:

- **Medical Records Department (Royal Children's Hospital)**
- **Department of Health — Phone (03) 616 7145**

Completed forms are taken to the discharge clerk in Medical Records who will send them to:
THE CHIEF HEALTH OFFICER
Statewide Services
Health Department Victoria
PO Box 4003
Melbourne Victoria 3001

Details should also be entered on the back of the yellow case divider.

Numbers for notification of disease:

Phone number	(03) 616 7482
	(03) 616 7132
	(03) 616 7127
or	(008) 034 280
Fax number	(03) 616 7147 (Attention: Chief Health Officer)

After hours, contact the Duty Medical Officer. Ring the paging service on (03) 614 4600 and give pager no. 46870.

GROUP A DISEASES

- Australian arbo encephalitis
- Anthrax
- Botulism
- Cholera
- Food-borne and water-borne illness (two or more related cases)
- Legionellosis
- Measles
- Meningitis or epiglottitis due to *Haemophilus influenzae*
- Meningococcal infection (meningitis or meningococcaemia)
- Plague
- Poliomyelitis
- Primary amoebic meningo-encephalitis
- Rabies
- Typhoid and paratyphoid fevers
- Typhus
- Viral haemorrhagic fevers
- Yellow fever

A case of any of these diseases should be notified to the Health Department Victoria by telephone or fax upon initial diagnosis (presumptive or confirmed) with written notification to follow within 7 days.

GROUP B DISEASES

- Amoebiasis
- Arbovirus infections (except for Australian arbo encephalitis)
- Brucellosis
- *Campylobacter* infection
- Giardiasis
- Hepatitis, viral — all forms including: hepatitis A, B, C and non-A non-B, hepatitis (viral, unspecified)
- Hydatid disease
- Leprosy
- Leptospirosis
- Listeriosis
- Malaria
- Mumps
- Pertussis
- Psittacosis (ornithosis)
- Q fever
- Rubella (including congenital rubella)

- Salmonellosis
- Shigellosis
- Taeniasis (tapeworm infections)
- Tetanus
- Tuberculosis
- Yersiniosis

For these, written notification only is sufficient, within 7 days of confirmation of diagnosis.

GROUP C DISEASES

- Chancroid
- Donovanosis
- Gonorrhoea (all forms)
- Lymphogranuloma venereum
- Other chlamydial infections
- Syphilis (all forms)

These sexually transmitted diseases should be notified using the same notification form, but, to preclude identification of the patient, only the first two letters of the given name and surname of the patient are required.

GROUP D DISEASES

AIDS

Written notification is required within 7 days of confirmation of diagnosis. A separate form is used for this purpose due to the need to have national uniformity in collection of data. To preclude identification of the patient, only the first two letters of the given name and surname of the patient are required.

Cancer

Does not include any type of skin cancer other than melanoma. Notifications are to be made by hospitals and pathology laboratories only, direct to the:

ANTI-CANCER COUNCIL OF VICTORIA
1 Rathdowne Street
Carlton South 3052
Phone: 662 3300

Congenital Malformations

Within Victoria notification of all major and minor congenital malformations is encouraged. Notification procedures differ from state to state.

Within the Royal Children's Hospital forms are available in wards and outpatient areas. One copy remains with the Unit Record, the other is to be forwarded to the Perinatal Statistics Unit or the Department of Genetics. Notifying doctors are requested to signify the notification by marking the appropriate box on the white disease notification forms in the Unit Record. Enquiries are to be directed to the Department of Genetics.

CHAPTER 10

RESPIRATORY CONDITIONS

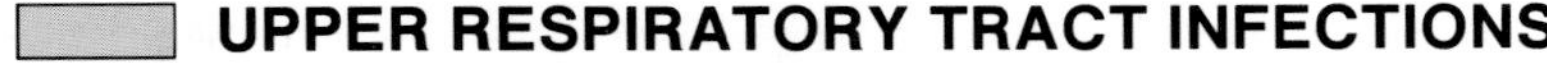

UPPER RESPIRATORY TRACT INFECTIONS

AETIOLOGY

Viruses are responsible for at least 90% of upper respiratory tract infections. The only common important bacterial pathogen, β-haemolytic streptococcus, is uncommon under the age of 4 years. The presence of fever, tender cervical lymph nodes and tonsillar exudate are suggestive of β-haemolytic streptococcal infection.

TREATMENT

Viral

Symptomatic if necessary. Paracetamol if fever is above 39°C or distressing. Ephedrine nose drops for nasal obstruction (maximum duration of therapy is 48 h).

Probable Streptococcus

Penicillin: a total course for 10 days is given. If the child is very sick, initial therapy may be by injection. Paracetamol if fever is above 39°C or distressing.

Beware of the child with signs of a mild upper respiratory tract infection but who has severe constitutional symptoms. Look for another diagnosis such as meningitis.

ACUTE OTITIS MEDIA

AETIOLOGY

Bacterial pathogens include:

- *Streptococcus pneumoniae*
- *Haemophilus influenzae* species
- *Moraxella catarrhalis*

Respiratory viruses are also common pathogens in mild otitis media and should be suspected especially when associated with coryzal illness.

TREATMENT

Paracetamol for relief of pain or if fever above 39°C. Antibiotics — amoxycillin is used for a total course of 7–10 days. Amoxycillin–clavulenate is an alternative. Failure to respond within 48–72 h signals the need for an ENT opinion but myringotomy is rarely indicated. Review after 4–6 weeks to check hearing.

COUGH IN CHILDHOOD

Cough is a common symptom of respiratory illness in children. Viral respiratory tract infection and asthma are by far the commonest cause of cough, which is usually of short duration in these conditions; in respiratory tract infection rarely longer than 2 weeks and in asthma 4–6 weeks. Repeated episodes with symptom-free periods in between are characteristic. A cough of some weeks to a couple of months duration is suggestive of whooping cough, mycoplasma infection, inhaled foreign body or an area of segmental or lobar collapse following a respiratory infection. A chest X-ray is generallly warranted in a child with a cough of this duration. A chronic cough of months duration indicates suppurative lung disease such as cystic fibrosis or other forms of bronchiectasis or chronic inhalation of milk or other foods. In these children the cough may clear with a course of antibiotics but it rapidly recurs once the antibiotics are ceased. A careful clinical history of the pattern of cough together with a chest X-ray usually determines the cause of a cough in children with repeated episodes, or a subacute or chronic cough. A specialist opinion may be indicated in such cases.

LARYNGOTRACHEOBRONCHITIS (CROUP)

Characterized by initial viral upper respiratory tract infection, harsh cough, hoarse voice and stridor. Children with laryngotracheitis must be admitted to hospital if they have sternal or suprasternal retraction at rest. Persistent stridor at rest without retraction indicates less severe obstruction but children with this sign usually warrant admission. The child with laryngotracheitis is likely to deteriorate late at night; therefore the child should rarely be sent home at night, especially if presenting in the Emergency Department after 2200 h.

TREATMENT

Minimal handling. Nurse in a warm, humid environment. Mist is an unproven form of treatment. Careful observation. Important signs of hypoxia are restlessness, increasing pulse and respiratory rate and cyanosis. Exhaustion may be manifested by decreasing respiratory effort. Adequate fluid intake. Oral fluids should be given frequently and in small amounts. Fluids given by gavage or intravenously are usually contraindicated because of the restraint involved. Sedation is contraindicated.

Antibiotics have no place in the management of acute laryngotracheobronchitis. They may be indicated if there is associated infection such as otitis media.

Nebulized adrenaline may be used to obtain temporary relief of obstruction. Dose: 1 in 1000 (0.1%) 0.05% mL/kg per dose (maximum 5 mL) by inhalation. Circumstances that may justify its use include: immediately prior to transfer from a metropolitan district hospital to the Royal Children's Hospital, while awaiting intubation to be organized, or if deterioration occurs late in the course of the illness when recovery would normally be expected. Repeated doses may occasionally be used in a child in whom it is desired to avoid intubation, e.g. established subglottic stenosis. It should not be used as definitive treatment and after its use the child must be observed very closely as rebound obstruction frequently occurs. Mechanical relief of obstruction if hypoxia develops, see p. 9, Paediatric Emergencies.

Administration of oxygen is difficult because of age of the child. It should be used if the child is hypoxic while arrangements are being made for intubation.

BRONCHIOLITIS

This is an acute viral illness in children usually between 2 weeks and 9 months of age, manifested by cough, wheezy breathing, hyperinflated chest, widespread fine crackles and frequent expiratory wheezes on auscultation.

Admission indication: increasing respiratory distress manifested by difficulty in feeding.

TREATMENT

- *Minimal handling.* Careful observation of colour, pulse, respiration and measurement of oxygen saturation by pulse oximetry.
- *Oxygen* is the most important agent in the treatment of moderate to severe bronchiolitis. Inspired oxygen percentage should be sufficient to maintain oxygen saturation above 90%. Continuous positive airways pressure or artificial ventilation in the occasional infant who develops respiratory failure.
- *Fluids.* If the baby is unable to feed orally, fluids are given intravenously at about 40% maintenance once any dehydration has been corrected.
- *Antibiotics* are indicated only in the rare situation of established secondary bacterial infection when penicillin is used, or in very severe disease when flucloxacillin and cefotaxime should be given intravenously, while awaiting culture results.

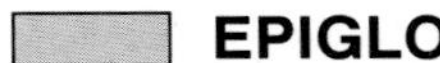

EPIGLOTTITIS

DIAGNOSIS

This differs from laryngotracheitis in the following ways:

- The child appears sick because of associated septicaemia.
- The onset is with fever and lethargy, and symptoms of respiratory obstruction develop after 2–6 h. There may be a history of a preceding upper respiratory tract infection.
- The stridor is soft, and the expiratory element is often dominant with a snoring or gurgling quality. Cough is not a prominent feature.
- Difficulty in swallowing and excess salivation with drooling are common.

All children with suspected epiglottitis require urgent admission to hospital. In Victoria consultation with PETS is recommended for patients seen outside the Royal Children's Hospital. Readers in other states should contact major paediatric centres for regional recommendations. (See p. 9.)

TREATMENT

- *Do not lie the patient flat.* Do not examine the larynx unless anaesthetist is present and able to intubate.
- *Chloramphenicol:* initial dose 40 mg/kg, i.v. or i.m. continuing therapy 25 mg/kg 8 hourly, i.v. (75 mg/kg per day) and then orally for a total duration of 4–5 days. Rifampicin prophylaxis for patients at the end of therapy and for contacts as per *H. influenzae* meningitis (see p. 21).
- *Adequate fluids.* If the patient has an intravenous line fluids can be given intravenously. Do not give more than 40%–60% of maintenance requirements.
- *General care:* see p. 79 Laryngotracheobronchitis.

- *Mechanical relief of obstruction:* see p. 9 Paediatric Emergencies. At least 80% will require intubation.

PNEUMONIA

The child with pneumonia usually has tachypnoea, and often has an expiratory grunt and there are focal signs in the chest. The latter may be difficult to detect. A diagnosis of pneumonia, especially in younger children, can usually only be made with radiological confirmation. Viruses, especially respiratory syncytial and parainfluenzae type 3, are the most common cause in young infants. *Mycoplasma pneumoniae* is a common pathogen in children in the over 5 year age group but does also cause pneumonia in younger children.

Streptococcus pneumoniae is by far the commonest bacterial pathogen in all age groups. The next is *Staphylococcus aureus* followed by *H. influenzae*. Many older children can be satisfactorily managed at home, but almost all under 24 months should be admitted to hospital.

Attempts should always be made to achieve an aetiological diagnosis. Throat swabs and sputum are of no value for bacterial culture. Postnasal mucus (nasopharyngeal aspirate) is useful for virological culture. Blood culture should be done before antibiotics are administered and urine should be examined for bacterial antigens. If pleural fluid is present this should always be aspirated for diagnosis before antibiotics are commenced. Thoracic medical or surgical consultation is indicated before the chest is needled irrespective of the hour. If the effusion is large, thoracic consultation about drainage is always indicated.

TREATMENT

Antibiotics

Because of the inability to make an aetiological diagnosis on clinical grounds, antibiotics are indicated in all cases. In children under 24 months of age, penicillin, initially intravenously or intramuscularly, is used in mild and moderate cases, while in severe cases when *S. aureus* is thought likely, flucloxacillin and gentamicin are used. Flucloxacillin and cefotaxime are alternatives especially if *H. influenzae* infection is likely. In children over 2 years of age, penicillin or erythromycin (particularly in children over the age of 5) is used.

If *S. pneumoniae* is thought to be the likely pathogen, marked clinical improvement with resolution of fever should occur within 24–36 h of commencing adequate doses of penicillin. If this is not the response, the infection is highly unlikely to be due to *S. pneumoniae*. In these circumstances further investigations to make an aetiological diagnosis should be undertaken rather than simply change antibiotics. Referral for thoracic medical advice is usually indicated in these circumstances. Response in patients with *M. pneumoniae* infection is often much slower. *H. influenzae* pneumonia frequently responds to penicillin.

General Management

Minimal handling, careful observation of colour, pulse and respirations, measurement of oxygen saturation by pulse oximetry, increased inspired oxygen concentration and an adequate, but not excessive fluid intake are all important. If fluids are given intravenously, the rate should be 40% maintenance once any dehydration is corrected.

ASTHMA

EMERGENCY ROOM TREATMENT

The treatment will be modified by the past experience with this particular patient and the medications given in the last 6 h and the response to them. Reassurance of parents and child is important in all cases. The need for and appropriateness of interval therapy should be reviewed in all children presenting in the emergency room with an acute episode of asthma.

Mild Attack

This should settle with a single dose of inhaled sympathomimetic. This can be delivered as 1 mL of salbutamol for children over 5 years and 0.5 mL for those younger, diluted to 4 mL with saline in a nebulizer driven by oxygen at 8 L/min for 10 min. Alternatively, four puffs from a metered aerosol in a spacer rebreathed for 30 s can be used. Bronchodilator therapy should be continued for 24–48 h after cessation of wheeze and again is best given by inhalation: metered aerosol in children over the age of 8; a metered aerosol plus spacer in younger children. In young children under the age of 3 or 4 with mild episodes of asthma, an oral sympathomimetic can be used, but this is less effective than the drug by inhalation and has more side effects.

Moderate Attack

This should be treated for the first hour with three doses of salbutamol (1 mL diluted to 4 mL with saline), each given for 10 min by a nebulizer driven by oxygen at 8 L/min. A child with a moderate attack, who improves completely with this regimen, can be sent home to continue inhaled bronchodilators for 48 h as described for a mild attack. A short course of oral corticosteroids should be considered for children being sent home in the following circumstances: a moderate attack that improves but does not clear completely with three doses of inhaled sympathomimetic, a child on maintenance inhaled corticosteroids, a second attendance within 12–24 h of an episode persisting for 2–3 days despite regular bronchodilators. An initial dose of 1 mg/kg prednisolone up to 40 mg is reasonable. This should be repeated after 8–12 h. A daily dose of 1 mg/kg up to 20 mg could be continued for the next 2–3 days or the dose tapered over this period depending on response. A child on maintenance inhaled steroids may require oral steroids for 7–10 days.

Children with moderate episodes who do not improve substantially with three doses of nebulized salbutamol will require hospital admission.

Severe Attack

Almost all patients will require admission. Emergency treatment, while admission is being arranged, may include:

- Oxygen
- Salbutamol 1 mL diluted to 4 mL with saline by nebulizer driven by oxygen 8 L/min given continuously.
- Corticosteroids. Most patients with a severe episode of asthma will need a short course of corticosteroids. This may be initiated in the emergency room. They can be given orally or should an intravenous infusion be required because of the patient's inability to swallow or concern about the state of hydration, they may be given intravenously.

INPATIENT MANAGEMENT

Mild and Moderate Episodes

If the patient has settled by the time he/she reaches the ward, or does so after a further one to two doses of salbutamol, therapy other than inhaled salbutamol 3–4 hourly usually will not be required. If there are still signs of significant airways obstruction, the salbutamol should be continued at least 3–4 hourly and a short course of oral corticosteroids commenced.

Severe Attack

- Oxygen
- Salbutamol by inhalation (1 mL in 3 mL saline, 10 min by nebulizer driven by oxygen at 8 L/min). This may be repeated 1–4 hourly depending on the severity of the asthma. When given more frequently than every 3–4 hours, repeated medical assessment is essential. If needed more frequently than every hour, nursing in the Intensive Care Unit is normally indicated. In the Intensive Care Unit the nebulized salbutamol may be given continuously.
- Corticosteroids should be commenced if not initiated in the Emergency Department. It should normally be given orally with an initial dose of about 1 mg/kg prednisolone to a maximum of 40 mg. The dose should be repeated after 8–12 h. A similar dose can be given daily for the next 1–3 days.
- If intravenous fluids are required (e.g. the attack is very severe), intravenous steroids should be used. During the first 24 h these should be given as 1 mg/kg methyl prednisolone 6 hourly. During the second 24 h the dose should be reduced to 1 mg/kg 12 hourly. Most patients will not require intravenous fluids for longer than 48 h. Intravenous fluids should be given at no more than 40% maintenance once any dehydration has been corrected.
- Aminophylline: 10 mg/kg loading dose followed by 5 mg/kg added to intravenous 6 hourly may be used in patients not responding to frequent nebulized salbutamol and intravenous corticosteroids. Aminophylline would normally be used only in patients likely to need management in Intensive Care and serum levels monitored. Patients on maintenance theophylline therapy should have the drug continued either orally or intravenously.
- Ipratropium bromide. Nebulized ipratropium 1 mL 4–6 hourly may be added to the salbutamol for severely distressed patients not responding to the above therapy. More frequent doses should not be used because of the risk of atropinization.
- Antibiotics are rarely indicated, and should not be used unless there is good evidence of coexistent bacterial infection. Chest X-rays are rarely necessary unless there is clinical evidence of a pneumothorax. This is exceedingly uncommon in childhood asthma. Blood gases are indicated in severe episodes not responding promptly to therapy.
- Good nursing care, careful observation and reassurance to patient and parents are essential.
- Monitoring of peak expiratory flow pre- and post-bronchodilator in children over 6 years to assess recovery.

After care of the acute episode

- Salbutamol continued by inhalation: nebulizer, metered aerosol or metered aerosol plus spacer.
- Prednisolone is given orally following removal of intravenous line. This can be given

either as a daily dose of 1 mg/kg (maximum 40 mg) for 2–3 days or in a reducing dose as below:

Day 1	30 mg/day
Day 2	15 mg/day
Day 3	5 mg/day or maintenance dose
Day 4	Cease

A patient on maintenance inhaled steroids may need a longer course of oral steroids.

LONG-TERM MANAGEMENT

This requires close personal relationship between doctor, parents and child. Parents must be fully informed about the natural history and prognosis, and reassured.

All parents and older children should be given a crisis plan for the management of a sudden severe episode that does not respond immediately to the usual bronchodilators. This will normally be the calling of an ambulance and continuous use of an inhaled bronchodilator, irrespective of dose, until professional assistance arrives.

Episodic Asthma

An inhaled sympathomimetic is required for the acute episode. If the attacks are more frequent than every 4–6 weeks, sodium cromoglycate should be considered as prophylaxis. If this is not adequate, the next stage would be to substitute inhaled steroids for the sodium cromoglycate and continue inhaled sympathomimetic as necessary. It is important in children with presumed episodic asthma to ensure that there is no persisting airways obstruction between episodes by measuring lung function, preferably ventilatory capacity and forced expiratory volume in 1s (FEV_1), when the child is well. Children with episodic asthma do not normally require a peak flow meter at home.

If there is no effective response to sodium cromoglycate after 6–8 weeks, further continuation of this therapy is not warranted.

Chronic Airways Obstruction

This is present in the child who wheezes many days or nights, who may have chest deformity and who has wheezes in his/her chest when examined. Lung function tests will show airways obstruction. There are four levels of therapy:

- *Stage 1.* Regular inhaled sodium cromoglycate plus inhaled sympathomimetic as necessary.
- *Stage 2.* Regular inhaled beclomethasone dipropionate (to 800 μg/day) or inhaled budesonide plus inhaled sympathomimetic as necessary.
- *Stage 3.* Regular inhaled beclomethasone dipropionate 800 μg/day or inhaled budesonide plus slow release theophylline plus inhaled sympathomimetic as necessary.
- *Stage 4.* Regular inhaled beclomethasone dipropionate (in excess of 800 μg/day) or inhaled budesonide plus slow release theophylline plus if necessary regular oral steroids plus inhaled sympathomimetic as necessary.

Progression from one stage of therapy to the next should be because of failure to control symptoms or achieve acceptable airways function. Nights disturbed by asthma, tightness in chest on awakening in the morning, exercise limitation, or excessive use of extra inhaled sympathomimetics indicate inadequate control. Lung function should be normal or near normal and this is assessed by measuring peak expiratory flow (PEFR) and FEV_1

when the patient is symptomatically well. Diurnal variation in PEFR of greater than 20% indicates poor control. Once asthma is well-controlled, PEFR need be measured only occasionally and during exacerbations. If during an exacerbation PEFR is less than 50% at best and does not increase to near normal levels with a dose of inhaled sympathomimetic, a short course of oral corticosteroids may be indicated. Children requiring stage 4 therapy should normally be under the care of a paediatric thoracic physician as the risk of side effects from the disease and its treatment are substantial. These children are at risk of sudden death.

The most efficient way to deliver an inhaled drug is by use of a metered aerosol and spacer. This results in the least pharyngeal deposition. This mode of administration should always be used for doses of inhaled steroids in excess of 800 μg/day. A turbohaler is 50% more efficient and results in a little less pharyngeal deposition than metered aerosol alone. This may be a compromise for a patient on a low to moderate dose of inhaled steroids who will not use a spacer device.

Nebulized budesonide has a very limited role in the management of asthma. It should be limited to those infants too young to use a spacer (with mask) with very troublesome persistent asthma. Nebulized steroid will be deposited on the face and in the eyes unless specific precautions are taken.

General Considerations

Comprehensive education of parent and patient about asthma is essential for proper care:

- To achieve good compliance with medication
- To avoid unnecessary restrictions
- To overcome misconceptions about asthma and its management
- To ensure that patient and family enjoy as normal a life-style as possible

FOREIGN BODY IN THE BRONCHIAL TREE

SYMPTOMS

- Coughing or choking episodes while eating nuts or other solid food or while sucking a small plastic toy or similar object. This story should never be dismissed.
- Persistent coughing and wheezing. Remember 'all that wheezes is not asthma' and beware of the sudden onset of a first wheezing episode in a child in the toddler age group in whom there is no history of allergy, especially if it follows a choking episode or if the breath sounds are diminished over one lung. Parents may not volunteer the history of possible inhalation. One out of every eight episodes of foreign body inhalation is not witnessed.

SIGNS

- Diminished breath sounds over whole or part of one lung
- Wheeze

INVESTIGATIONS

Chest X-ray is take in full inspiration and full expiration to exclude obstructive hyperinflation or an area of collapse. Normal X-rays do not absolutely exclude a foreign body.

MANAGEMENT

Admission is indicated for all patients with suspected inhaled foreign body. If there is any doubt, consult the thoracic physician on call.

Bronchoscopy

As radiological examination may be normal, bronchoscopy is necessary in almost every child in whom there is a story strongly suggestive of an inhaled foreign body. Bronchoscopy in children is difficult and it requires an expert paediatric endoscopist teamed with an experienced paediatric anaesthetist. It should only be done in a major children's hospital. Once a foreign body has passed through the larynx, it is very rare for there to be an immediate threat to life, and referral to the nearest children's hospital is usually quite safe.

CHAPTER 11

CARDIOVASCULAR CONDITIONS

WHEN TO INVESTIGATE A MURMUR

Approximately 50% of normal school children and 70% of infants have soft heart murmurs. In an asymptomatic child such murmurs most often have the characteristics of a 'vibratory murmur' (Still's murmur), a 'venous hum', a 'pulmonary flow murmur', or a 'carotid bruit'. Such murmurs are fairly easy to identify on the basis of their characteristic timing, pitch, and behaviour with changes in posture. However, some practice is required to become confident in identifying these common innocent murmurs.

Where doubt exists about the nature of a murmur it is appropriate to arrange an ECG and chest X-ray. If the patient has any symptoms which suggest a possible structural cardiac problem, or if the X-ray or ECG are in any way suspicious, a specialist consultation, with a view to a possible echocardiogram, should be arranged.

It should be noted that distinction between organic and innocent murmurs can be particularly difficult in the first 3 months of life. If in doubt, the auscultation should be repeated at 3–6 months of age, by which time it is usually easier to achieve a firm diagnosis either way.

HEART FAILURE

RECOGNITION

The main symptoms in infants are dyspnoea on feeding or at rest, poor feeding and failure to thrive. Physical signs include tachycardia, tachypnoea, intercostal and subcostal recession, Harrison's sulci and hepatomegaly.

Cardiomegaly is almost always present (best seen on X-ray).

A previously well child presenting with recent manifestations of cardiac failure requires urgent echocardiography to exclude pericardial effusion and/or tamponade.

MANAGEMENT

- *Diuretics.* Frusemide (1 mg/kg once or twice daily). This should be accompanied by a potassium sparing diuretic (e.g. spironolactone) or potassium supplements.
- *Digoxin.* It is not necessary to formally digitalize patients with heart failure [except those with supraventricular tachycardia (SVT) or atrial fibrillation]. Maintenance digoxin should be given in a dose of 5 μg/kg/12 hourly. If digitalization is necessary a total loading dose over 24 h of 40 μg/kg may be given (in premature infants 20 μg/kg). The first dose should be one-half of the total digitalizing dose. Further doses (25% of total digitalizing dose) should be given after 6 and 12 h. Serum digoxin levels are useful in assessing adequacy of digitalization. The

therapeutic range is 1.5–2.5 ng/mL. Infants tolerate higher levels (up to 3.5 ng/mL).

- *Vasodilators* such as captopril, may be helpful. They should be introduced with the patient in hospital so that blood pressure may be monitored.

OTHER MEASURES

- *Prostaglandin E_1*. Prostaglandin should be considered in neonates with cardiac failure, if it is probable on clinical grounds, that they have a ductus-dependent defect, in which part, or all, of the systemic circulation is compromised as a result of a cardiac defect (e.g. hypoplastic left heart syndrome, critical aortic stenosis, aortic interruption, coarctation syndrome).
- *Oxygen*. Should be administered if hypoxia is thought to be related to pulmonary congestion or respiratory infection.
- *Inotropic drugs* (e.g. dopamine, dobutamine). May be infused if severe cardiac failure is accompanied by poor peripheral perfusion. (Dose — initially 5 μg/kg per min by intravenous infusion; dobutamine may be given into a peripheral line, dopamine into a central line.)
- *Positive pressure ventilation*. Should be considered if the infant is progressing to cardiorespiratory failure.
- *Sodium bicarbonate*. Correction of acidosis may be required in severe situations.
- *Antibiotics*. These should be given if superimposed infection is present or suspected, especially in the sick neonate.

NEONATAL CYANOSIS

Rapidly progressive cyanosis in the early newborn period may be related to the presence of a ductus-dependent cyanotic defect (e.g. pulmonary atresia). It may also be due to transposition (which is also partly duct dependent as patency of the ductus allows improved mixing).

INITIAL ASSESSMENT

Should include:

- Chest X-ray
- ECG
- Blood gases
- Hyperoxic test
- Blood group and cross match.

Hyperoxic Test

Arterial Po_2 should be measured after administration of 100% oxygen by face mask, head box or endotracheal tube for 10 min. The sample should be taken from the right radial artery if possible. Right to left shunting of blood through the ductus in the newborn period can give misleadingly low Po_2 values in samples taken elsewhere.

An arterial Po_2 rising to 150 mmHg makes structural cyanotic heart disease unlikely, in which case cyanosis is probably related to lung disease. Most major cyanotic defects (e.g. transposition, pulmonary atresia) presenting in the newborn period will show arterial Po_2 levels in the range of 50–70 mmHg, or lower, after 100% oxygen.

MANAGEMENT

Initial management includes infusion of prostaglandin E_1 (10–20 ng/kg per min) and if necessary correction of acidosis. Prostaglandin E_1 may cause apnoea, so intubation for transport should be considered. Oxygen may be administered, usually in a concentration of 30%.

Diagnosis can usually be achieved by echocardiography.

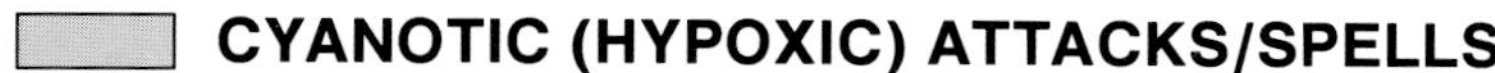

CYANOTIC (HYPOXIC) ATTACKS/SPELLS

Severe cyanotic attacks, sometimes leading to loss of consciousness, are a characteristic feature of Fallot's tetralogy, but may occasionally occur with other cyanotic lesions. Episodes may be spontaneous, but are often precipitated by exertion, feeding or crying. Intercurrent infection and dehydration may play a part.

Attacks are manifested by increasing cyanosis and/or pallor, shortness of breath, distress, out of proportion to the precipitating situation. Possible loss of consciousness in severe attacks. Episodes frequently occur first thing in the morning.

MANAGEMENT

- *First aid.* The first aid treatment of an attack is to quieten the child and try to stop him crying. The child should be picked up, cradled and soothed, and nursed in the knee–chest position over parent's shoulder. Morphine 0.2 mg/kg, i.m. may be helpful in severe cases.
- *Oxygen.* Administration of oxygen is of *limited* benefit, but should be given provided it does not provoke further distress to the child.
- *Bicarbonate.* Severe acidosis may develop and require correction, but in milder cases which resolve spontaneously the acidosis will correct itself and does not necessarily require bicarbonate administration.

In extreme cases the infant may require intravenous fluid replacement, correction of acidosis, intubation and a positive pressure ventilation, etc.

β-Blocking Drugs (propranolol)

This may be used prophylactically to prevent spells in a child who has started to have attacks. Dose 0.5–1.0 mg/kg 8 hourly. This should only be used as a temporary measure while further investigation and surgery are planned.

SUPRAVENTRICULAR TACHYCARDIA

Pallor, dyspnoea and development of cardiac failure are the usual manifestations of an episode of SVT in infancy (rate usually between 180 and 300 beats/min). Pulse is very rapid, of small volume and regular.

DIAGNOSIS

The ECG shows a regular narrow complex tachycardia. If P waves can be seen these should be present with each complex. In many cases P waves are not readily seen as they are hidden on the T waves.

MANAGEMENT

Early consultation is advised. The diving reflex may be utilized with placement of polythene bag containing cold water with ice cubes over the forehead, eyes and nose for 15–20 s. This may lead to reversion. If the infant's condition is stable and cardiac failure is absent the next line of treatment is digitalization. Digoxin should be given intravenously. The tachycardia will usually not revert for several hours with digoxin alone. If the infant is severely symptomatic, or has evidence of congestive failure, DC cardioversion should be considered (1 J/kg shock — synchronized).

Verapamil may be given in children over the age of 1 year. The initial dose should be 0.1 mg/kg given slowly intravenously (over 5–10 min), under continuous ECG monitoring and this may be repeated after 15–20 min, if no response. Intravenous calcium should be available if hypotension occurs. Verapamil is contraindicated if the complexes are broad and/or if the rhythm is irregular.

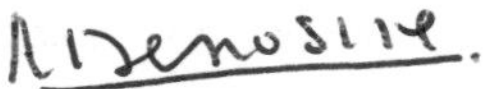

CHAPTER 12

GASTROINTESTINAL CONDITIONS

ACUTE INFECTIOUS DIARRHOEA

DIFFERENTIAL DIAGNOSIS

Never accept an admitting diagnosis of gastroenteritis just because the child is in the gastroenteritis ward. Always ask whether the symptoms could be caused by another medical problem or an acute surgical problem such as:

- Appendicitis
- Intussusception
- Malrotation
- Urinary tract infection
- Otitis media
- Meningitis

ASSESSMENT

The most important complication of acute infectious diarrhoea is water and electrolyte depletion.

The most accurate indication of the degree of fluid depletion is a recent change in bodyweight. Starvation produces no more than 1% of bodyweight loss per day. Any change in excess of this is due to water loss. For assessment of the degree of dehydration see p. 43.

MANAGEMENT

The management of gastroenteritis has changed over the last 5 years. Whereas we used to starve children, recommend clear fluids such as flat lemonade until the diarrhoea settled, and put intravenous lines into moderately dehydrated children, we now:

- Continue breast feeding
- Use oral rehydration
- Feed hungry children
- Avoid drugs

Treatment is aimed at restoring and maintaining water and electrolyte balance and restoring normal nutrition.

Oral Rehydration

A solution of 2% glucose and 50–90 mmol/L sodium will greatly enhance absorption of water from the small bowel and can be used to rehydrate children with even moderately severe dehydration provided they are not shocked.

Vomiting is not a contraindication to oral rehydration. It is best to give small amounts frequently, especially if there is a history of vomiting. Oral rehydration encourages early return of appetite.

Solutions

Sachets containing glucose and electrolyte powder can be bought at chemist shops and added to water as required, e.g. Gastrolyte. They contain glucose, sodium, potassium, chloride and citrate and should be used to correct dehydration. Solutions of sugar in water (without salt) can be used for maintenance of hydration in mild or moderate diarrhoea without dehydration.

- Sucrose (table sugar): 1 heaped teaspoon in 200 mL water
- Cordials: 1 part to 6 parts water
- Lemonade: 1 part to 4 parts water
- Fruit juice: 1 part to 4 parts water

Parent Education

The most important message is that children with diarrhoea need to drink more fluid more often (because water loss is the main cause of morbidity and mortality). Some parents mistakenly believe that fluid in at the top end is the cause of fluid out at the bottom end.

Home-made solutions and reconstitution of packets of oral rehydration powder must be accurate. Parents sometimes believe that if a small amount of sugar or salt is good, then a large amount must be better. They should be warned of the dangers of making up solutions incorrectly.

Indications for Admission

- Severe illness
- Moderate or severe dehydration
- Family unable to cope
- Very young babies (< 6 months old)
- Diagnosis in doubt
- Associated problem, e.g. ileostomy

Treatment Guidelines

No dehydration

Children with no clinical features of dehydration can usually be managed as outpatients. Breast feeding should be continued on demand, and formula-fed infants should be given their normal feeds with extra water. Vomiting babies will tolerate half-strength feeds better than full strength. Children with mild to moderate diarrhoea can continue on their normal diet with extra water. This can be given as water, cordial, diluted fruit juice or diluted lemonade (see text). Food can be stopped for up to 24 h, but starvation beyond this may delay recovery.

Mild dehydration

Children with severe diarrhoea or mild dehydration should be given large quantities of fluid, e.g. 200 mL/kg per 24 h or 8 mL/kg per h. This amount should be translated into an easily understood message, such as 50 mL every 30 min. Ideally, an oral rehydration solution such as Gastrolyte should be given. It is not usually necessary to admit these children.

Moderate dehydration

Moderate to severely dehydrated children should be admitted and given oral rehydration. Most can be rehydrated orally, even if they are vomiting, and all children who are not shocked should be given a trial of oral rehydration, i.e. adequate volumes of a physiologically balanced fluid by mouth or via a nasogastric tube. The aim is to rehydrate them quickly using a glucose–electrolyte solution. The deficit is calculated and one and a half times this volume is given over 6 h. Example:

10 kg child, 8% dehydrated
Deficit = 800 mL
Replacement volume = 1200 mL
= 200 mL/h for 6 h or until rehydrated

Thereafter, give maintenance fluids at 4 mL/kg per h or as desired. Breast feeding should be continued as soon as oral rehydration is complete, or before if this takes longer than 6 h.

If a child is tired or cannot keep up with losses, a nasogastric tube should be inserted. Small amounts of fluid should be given frequently, especially if there is vomiting. Re-assess after 4–6 h, and if the child is still clinically dehydrated and has not gained weight, give fluids intravenously.

Severe dehydration with shock

Children who are shocked need immediate resuscitation with intravenous fluids.

Intravenous Therapy

Indications:

- Failed oral rehydration
- Severe dehydration with shock
- Gastroenteritis complicated by another problem, e.g. ileostomy or cyanotic congenital heart disease

Resuscitation fluid

Normal saline is usually used, but any isotonic fluid will do. Plasma expanders are not necessary unless hypoproteinaemia is suspected. Give 20 mL/kg of stable plasma protein solution (or equivalent) as quickly as possible to treat circulatory failure. This should be repeated if there are still signs of shock.

Replacement and maintenance fluid

Isotonic saline (1/2) in 4% dextrose to which 20 mmol/L of potassium chloride is added. Sodium bicarbonate is added if there is persistent acidosis (normally acidosis will correct itself as the patient is rehydrated). Aim to replace the deficit over 24 h if the serum sodium is normal. The maintenance requirement is 4 mL/kg per hour up to 10 kg. Example:

10 kg child 10% dehydrated
Deficit 1000 mL = 40 mL/h for 24 h
Maintenance 4 mL/kg per hour = 40 mL/h
Total 80 mL/h for first 24 h, then 40 mL/h

Oral rehydration solution and breast milk should be offered once the circulation has been restored; it may be possible to remove the drip after a few hours. Appetite is restored more quickly in children given oral fluids.

Biochemical Investigations

Electrolyte and acid–base studies are not required routinely. However, they are indicated if there is prolonged diarrhoea with severe dehydration, disturbance of the conscious state or convulsions. Electrolyte and acid–base measurements should be done in any child requiring intravenous fluid, and they should be done more readily in any child less than 3 months old.

Special Circumstances

Hypernatraemic dehydration

These children may be more dehydrated than they appear. They must be rehydrated very slowly. Twenty to 40 mL/kg should be given quickly to restore the circulation if the child is shocked, but the remainder of the deficit should be replaced over not less than 48 h if intravenous fluid is used. As long as rehydration is done slowly, the intravenous fluid used does not need to have a high sodium concentration; a suitable solution is 1/2 isotonic saline in 4% dextrose with 20 mmol/L of potassium chloride and 10 ml/L 10% calcium gluconate. Oral replacement should be over at least 24 h. Severe hypernatraemia causing fitting or coma requires consultation with intensive care.

Hyponatraemic dehydration

Severe hyponatraemia causing fitting or coma requires consultation with intensive care.

Malnutrition

Malnourished children may appear more dehydrated than they actually are. Initial resuscitation may include a protein solution (stable plasma protein solution) if peripheral circulatory failure is present. Such infants are depleted of magnesium and potassium. Obese infants may be more dehydrated than the clinical signs indicate.

Drug Therapy

Antidiarrhoeal agents and antiemetics are not recommended for children with gastroenteritis. They can have dangerous side effects. Antibiotics have a limited role; they are occasionally required in neonates, severely ill infants with toxic symptoms that may be related to septicaemia or in severe shigellosis.

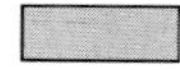

SUGAR INTOLERANCE

LACTOSE INTOLERANCE

After infectious diarrhoea, infants may have temporary lactose intolerance. Approximately 50% of formula-fed babies less than 6 months old with infectious diarrhoea requiring admission to hospital are unable to tolerate normal amounts of lactose for at least a week. Occasionally lactose intolerance may persist for some months.

Clinical features of sugar intolerance are:

- Persistently fluid stools
- Excessive flatus
- Excoriation of the buttocks

Diagnosis

Collect the stool fluid in napkins lined with plastic. Dilute 1 part of stool fluid with 2 parts water. React 15 drops of the resultant mixture with a Clinitest tablet. A colour reaction corresponding to 3 or 4% or more reducing substances indicates that sugar intolerance is present and probably the main cause of continuing diarrhoea.

Management

Breast-fed babies rarely have clinically significant lactose intolerance and breast feeding should be continued unless diarrhoea is persistent and the baby is failing to thrive. Formula-fed babies should have their feed changed to a full strength lactose-free formula such as Delact or Digestelac. After 3–4 weeks the usual formula may be reintroduced by substituting for the lactose-free milk in increasing proportions over 2–3 days.

Note. Response to soy formula does not mean that milk allergy is present. The problem is more likely to be post-infectious lactose intolerance responding to elimination of lactose.

MONOSACCHARIDE INTOLERANCE

Much less commonly, infants may be unable to absorb normal amounts of monosaccharide. Diarrhoea will continue even with a lactose-free formula. Monosaccharide intolerance requires specialist consultation.

GASTRO-OESOPHAGEAL REFLUX

This is a common cause of vomiting in infancy. The vomiting is related to posture and often occurs when the infant is laid down. This vomiting may commence in the first few days of life. It does not generally cause failure to thrive, but may do so in severe cases. Chest complications are sometimes seen. Symptoms of inhalation pneumonia, recurrent or persistent cough and wheeze may be present and can occur without vomiting. Peptic oesophagitis with anaemia and blood flecked vomitus may also occur.

TREATMENT

Nurse the child prone, and prop up head of the cot with bricks or boards. Thicken the feeds with Carobel, infant Gaviscon or cornflour.

CONSTIPATION

There is usually no organic basis to constipation. It is uncommon in the early months of life, and when it occurs is often the result of poor fluid intake. Older children may become constipated because they suppress the desire to defecate when distracted by other activities. Children past the toddler age with severe constipation may develop faecal soiling as a result (see p. 27). Apparently painful defecation or blood on the surface of the stools suggests the presence of an anal fissure.

Hirschsprung's disease is a rare cause of constipation and exclusion of this disorder by rectal biopsy is unnecessary unless the onset of symptoms dates back to early infancy or there is some other clinical indication such as considerable abdominal distension or failure to thrive.

Abdominal palpation and rectal examination will usually reveal abnormal amounts of firm faeces. However, faecal retention above the rectum may occur and is not always obvious on clinical examination. The tone of the anal sphincter and the presence of anal stenosis should be assessed. The anus should be inspected for a fissure.

MANAGEMENT

The aim of treatment is to empty the colon and to prevent re-accumulation of abnormal amounts of faeces using either laxatives or enemas. In babies, ensuring an adequate fluid intake and including fruits such as prunes and high residue cereals and vegetables may suffice. If not, dioctylsodium sulfosuccinate drops (Coloxyl) are usually effective and safe. In older children, laxatives such as lactulose or standardized senna are useful. The development and maintenance of a regular toileting routine is also important.

In general the dose of laxative needed is the one that is effective in achieving the passage of at least one soft but formed stool each day. This dose should be gradually reduced with the aim of eventually weaning the patient off laxatives. The longer constipation has been a problem, the longer it takes to achieve this aim. Parents should be told that months of treatment are likely to be required. A common mistake is to give intermittent short courses of treatment which do not allow readjustment of colonic size and sensation to occur adequately. When an anal fissure is present local anaesthetic ointments may be applied whenever the child shows a desire to defecate, until healing of the fissure is achieved.

TODDLER DIARRHOEA

This is a clinical syndrome characterized by chronic diarrhoea often with undigested food in the stools of a child who is otherwise well, gaining weight and growing satisfactorily. Stools may contain mucus and are passed between three and six times a day, often looser toward the end of the day. Its onset is usually between 8 and 20 months of age. There is often a family history of functional bowel disease. Treatment is usually reassurance and explanation. No specific drug or dietary therapy has been shown to be of value.

COW'S MILK PROTEIN INTOLERANCE (CMPI)

Symptoms related to ingestion of food or milk may be induced by any one of several components. These may be due to immune or non-immune effects. Allergic responses to cow's milk protein may result in rapid or delayed onset of symptoms. Rapid onset responses are less common, often characterized by the sudden onset of vomiting, and rarely by acute anaphylaxis. Delayed onset responses may be more difficult to diagnose, and present with diarrhoea, malabsorption or failure to thrive, and occasionally intestinal loss of protein or blood.

CMPI can only be diagnosed with a complete and thorough history, and with unequivocal reproducible reactions to elimination and challenge. Laboratory tests may help but are not substitutes for clinical assessment. After a definitive diagnosis is established, cow's milk protein should be removed from the diet and replaced with either soy or a hydrolysed formula. Most food allergies in infants improve or resolve with increasing age.

CHAPTER 13

RENAL TRACT CONDITIONS

ACUTE RENAL FAILURE

ACUTE OLIGURIA AND ANURIA

The definition of severe oliguria is a urine output of less than 250 mL/m^2 per day (approximately 8–10 mL/kg per day).

Three clinical situations occur:

1. Urinary obstruction should be suspected in the presence of sudden complete anuria provided the catheter is placed correctly and not blocked. Ultrasound will help reveal the cause.
2. Renal hypoperfusion causing oliguria should be suspected in the presence of clinical dehydration or septicaemia leading to hypotension. Blood volume expansion is necessary.
3. Renal tissue injury, e.g. acute post-streptococcal glomerulonephritis or secondary to hypoperfusion or nephrotoxin. Frusemide 4 mg/kg should be given intravenously and, if there is no response initiate treatment for continuing anuria.

CONTINUING ANURIA

- Fluid intake is restricted to the previous 24 h losses from stools, urine and other losses. Less than this will be given if fluid overloaded or hypertensive. Fluid of approximately 250 mL/kg^2 per day must be given also to account for net insensible water loss.
- Electrolytes are not required during this phase, but need to be given during the recovery of diuretic phase.
- Calories as carbohydrate are given for energy to spare tissue protein from catabolism, which accentuates the rise in blood urea. Ten to 20% glucose, oral Caloreen or Polyjoule are suitable.
- Peritoneal dialysis will be required for hyperkalaemia, severe uraemia (blood urea > 50 mmol/L), acidosis or water overload leading to hyponatraemia, oedema, or hypertension and should always be considered if anuria persists for more than 24 h. If urine output does not increase after intravenous frusemide, any degree of hyperkalaemia requires immediate dialysis.

HYPERKALAEMIA

Hyperkalaemia is an indication for dialysis if urine is not formed after intravenous frusemide (see above). A serum potassium of above 6 mmol/L is accepted as the indication for this management. Higher values not requiring treatment may be found in the neonatal period.

If cardiac arrhythmias are present, rapid but temporary benefit may be achieved by:

- Sodium bicarbonate 2 mmol/kg, i.v.
- Insulin short acting 0.1 units/kg with 2 mL 50% dextrose/kg
- Calcium gluconate 10% given intravenously slowly (0.5 mL/kg)

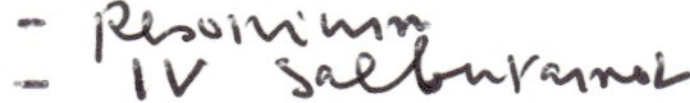

CHRONIC RENAL FAILURE

The commonest causes in children are: reflux nephropathy/hypoplasia, obstructive uropathy, chronic glomerulonephritis/glomerulosclerosis and medullary cystic disease.

Clinical features which occur when the glomerular filtration rate falls below 20 mL/min per 1.73 m^2 (i.e. when the serum creatinine > 0.25 mmol/L) include:

- Anaemia which is hypoplastic in origin
- Osteodystrophy/rickets and hyperparathyroidism
- Short stature
- Hypertension, acidosis or polyuria

Management should be undertaken by a paediatric nephrologist who may perform a renal ultrasound and biopsy. If the serum creatinine is below 0.25 mmol/L then usually no treatment is required except for continued follow-up by the nephrologist. When the creatinine is above 0.25 mmol/L the child may need phosphate and protein restriction, blood transfusions, calcium carbonate and calcitriol.

End Stage Renal Failure

Is defined as serum creatinine above 0.8–1.0 mmol/L and is usually accompanied by severe lethargy. Management includes continuous ambulatory peritoneal dialysis or haemodialysis with a view to transplantation.

HYPERTENSION

ACUTE SEVERE HYPERTENSION

Indications for Urgent Treatment

- Diastolic BP of 110 mmHg or more
- Any hypertension associated with cardiac failure or encephalopathy (e.g. convulsions or impaired conscious state)

Drugs

Initial treatment for acute hypertensive emergencies will be either sublingual nifedipene or intravenous diazoxide with intravenous frusemide if there is associated salt and water overload (e.g. acute nephritis). Nifedipine is given sublingually by placing the contents of a 10 mg capsule under the tongue. BP falls within 30 min. The dose may be repeated four to six times a day. Diazoxide 5 mg/kg is given rapidly intravenously in not more than 15 s. This dose may be repeated if a satisfactory drop in BP is not immediately achieved. A dose of 5 mg/kg may be given up to four times in 24 h if necessary. As repeated administration leads to sodium retention, frusemide (0.5 mg/kg) is recommended if more than two doses of diazoxide are given. After the first dose of nifedipine or diazoxide, oral drugs are started as soon as possible. Clonidine, hydralazine and phenoxbenzamine may be required occasionally.

Dialysis

Severe hypertension in acute renal failure not responding to the above therapy is likely to need dialysis to control BP.

CHRONIC HYPERTENSION

The aim of therapy is to reduce BP to the upper limits of normal (generally < 140/90) the following drugs are used:

- Propanolol 1 mg/kg, t.d.s. and increase every 2–3 days up to 5 mg/kg daily, may be used to commence treatment, atenolol 25–100 mg once a day is an alternative
- If response is unsatisfactory (diastolic BP > 100) add a vasodilator (hydralazine 0.5–1 mg/kg, t.d.s., or prazosin 0.25–0.5 mg, t.d.s. initially, or nifedipine 10–20 mg, b.d.)
- Occasionally a diuretic (chlorothiazide, frusemide) or a converting enzyme inhibitor (captopril, enalapril) will be required

CHAPTER 14

HAEMATOLOGICAL CONDITIONS

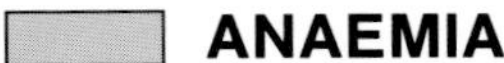

ANAEMIA

It is important to remember that there is a variation in the lower limit of normal haemoglobin at different ages. The initial investigation required is a haemoglobin and blood film. Any further investigations will be determined by the blood film appearance. Where possible, treatment should be deferred until a definitive diagnosis is made. Transfusion should be avoided in nutritional anaemias if possible. (See The Pale Infant and Child on pp. 22–24. For normal values see table on p. 199.)

THALASSAEMIA MAJOR

Transfusion

This is now performed for most patients on an outpatient basis in the Day Medical Unit (3 North) at the Royal Children's Hospital. The patient is transfused to a high normal haemoglobin level using packed cells, frequently depleted of white cells, to maintain the haemoglobin above 10 g/dL.

Desferrioxamine

This is usually given with each unit of blood transfused. A dose of 0.5 g is used. Subcutaneous infusions administered by a constant infusion pump are given overnight for 5–6 days/week.

Penicillin prophylaxis is given to all patients who have had a splenectomy.

SICKLE CELL DISEASE

Patients may present with a crisis which may be haemolytic, infarctive, aplastic or splenic sequestration. Splenic sequestration is a medical emergency, the child presenting with hypovolaemic shock, anaemia and acute splenic enlargement. Most patients in crisis require admission. Consultation with the clinical haematologist on duty is essential in the management of these patients.

DRUG-INDUCED HAEMOLYSIS

Drugs known or thought to have produced a haemolytic anaemia when taken orally by subjects with a deficiency of erythrocyte glucose-6-phosphate dehydrogenase or with haemoglobin H disease:

- *Antimalarials:* chloroquine; Pamaquine; Pentaquine (mepacrine); Primaquine; Quinacrine (Atabrine); Quinine
- *Antipyretics and analgesics:* acetanilide; acetylsalicylic acid; aminopyrine (Pyramidon); phenacetin (Acetophenetidin); quinidine

- *Nitrofurans:* nitrofurantoin (Furadantin); nitrofurazone (Furacin); acetylphenylhydrazine
- *Sulfones:* diaminodiphenylsulfone (DDS); sulfoxone (Diasone); thiazosulfone (Promizole)
- *Other drugs:* aminosalicylic acid; chloramphenicol; dimercaprol (BAL); methylene blue; naphthalene; phenylhydrazine; probenecid (Benemid); trinitrotoluene; Vitamin K (water soluble analogues; Synkavit)
- Fava beans (broad bean) may also produce haemolysis in patients with this deficiency.

COAGULATION DISORDERS

HAEMOPHILIA (FACTOR VIII DEFICIENCY)

Desired Levels of Factor VIII for Control of Haemorrhage

Most bleeding can be controlled with a single dose calculated to increase the Factor VIII level to 30–50%. Remember a minor head injury can become serious, the Factor VIII level should be raised to 100% and the patient admitted.

Dose

These levels are achieved by infusion of Factor VIII; concentrate (CSL). In general, 1 unit of Factor VIII/kg raises Factor VIII levels by 2%. Thus 15 units/kg will increase Factor VIII to 30% and 25 units/kg to 50%.

Mouth Bleeding

Use Cyclokapron tablets. For children less than 4 years old 0.5 g, q.i.d.; for children older than 4 years 1 g, q.i.d.

General Measures

These are applicable to all congenital bleeding disorders.

- **Analgesia**. Do not give aspirin. Avoid narcotic analgesics.
- **Do not give intramuscular injections**. Splinting of limbs reduces pain.

Consult with the haematologist on duty on the need for joint aspiration. Beware of risk of Volkmann's ischaemic contracture in forearm bleeds and of femoral nerve palsies with retroperitoneal bleeds tracking underneath the inguinal ligament.

VON WILLEBRAND DISEASE

This responds to cryoprecipitate, or less predictably, to Factor VIII concentrates. The half-life of Von Willebrand's factor is approximately 4 h, but Factor VIII levels continue to be increased for 48–72 h after infusion of cryoprecipitate. Further doses are given if bleeding recurs.

CHRISTMAS DISEASE (FACTOR IX DEFICIENCY)

This is treated with Prothrombinex (prothrombin concentrate). (Each 10 mL of Prothrombinex contains approximately 200 units of Factor IX.)

- *Requirements*. As in haemophilia.

- *Dose.* In general 1 unit Factor IX/kg increases the Factor IX level by 1.6%.
- *Frequency.* Injections at 24 h intervals (half-life for Factor IX = 24 h).

RARE BLEEDING DISORDERS

When the diagnosis of the disorder is in doubt, treatment with fresh frozen plasma (20 mL/kg) until the precise defect is known.

EMERGENCIES IN ACUTE LEUKAEMIA

Complications of acute leukaemia are the immediate cause of most early deaths rather than the leukaemia itself. It is important that they be recognized early and treated vigorously to ensure the patient's survival.

The most likely complications are infection, haemorrhage, toxic drug reactions, hyperuricaemia and other metabolic disturbances. Cultures and appropriate broad-spectrum intravenous antibiotics are used to treat infection. Platelets and blood transfusions are used to treat haemorrhage. Adequate hydration, allopurinol, biochemical monitoring and attention to fluid balance are used to treat hyperuricaemia.

USE OF BLOOD COMPONENTS

Many forms of anaemia do not require transfusion, which may on occasions be hazardous to the patient. Removal of the cause of the anaemia and replacement of the deficiency will frequently produce a rapid rise in the haemoglobin and avoid the need for transfusion.

WHOLE BLOOD

Used to maintain the blood volume during acute blood loss and for transfusion of patients with sickle cell anaemia in crisis.

PACKED RED CELLS

Used in preference to whole blood in the treatment of anaemia, except when blood loss is sufficient to produce hypovolaemic shock. Packed cells are especially indicated for cardiac failure, renal disease, liver disease and autoimmune haemolytic anaemia.

LEUCOCYTE DEPLETED AND/OR WASHED CELLS

For patients with demonstrated leucocyte or platelet antibodies.

FRESH BLOOD

Fresh blood (less than 3 days of age) is used in neonates.

Formulae For Calculation Of Volume Required

This assumes a haematocrit of 33% for whole blood and 66% for packed cells.

- Whole blood (mL) = wt (kg) × g% Hb rise required × 6
- Packed cells (mL) = wt (kg) × g% Hb rise required × 3

PLATELETS

Indicated for bleeding associated with thrombocytopenia, especially in leukaemia and aplastic anaemia.

Dose: 6 units/m^2

The normal lifespan for platelets is 10 days, but the effective lifespan of transfused platelets may be greatly shortened if the patient is bleeding or in the presence of infection. Transfusion may be required every 1 or 2 days for control of bleeding or more frequently if there are clinical indications. Platelets should not be refrigerated and should not be infused through a filtration set. They must be stored on a rocker.

COAGULATION FACTORS

- Factor VIII concentrate
- Cryoprecipitate
- Prothrombinex

see coagulation disorders

FRESH FROZEN PLASMA

Each pack contains approximately 300 mL. Dose 10–20 mL/kg. Indications:

- Emergency therapy of congenital bleeding disorders
- Congenital bleeding disorders not responsive to cryoprecipitate or Prothrombinex
- Post-extracorporeal circulation

STABLE PLASMA PROTEIN SOLUTION (SPPS)

Contents:

- 86% albumin and 14% globulin as a 5% solution i.e. 5 g plasma protein in 100 mL
- Sodium: 130–150 mmol/L
- Potassium: 4–6 mmol/L
- Calcium: 1.5–2.5 mmol/L

Used to expand blood volume in shock.

ALBUMIN

Contents:

- 20% albumin in 10 or 50 mL of buffered solution
- Sodium: 60 mmol/L

This solution is stable under refrigeration for as long as 4 years. Use is restricted to hypoproteinaemia and raised intracranial pressure. The solution has an osmotic equivalent of up to four times that of SPPS. Hence, if isotonicity is required, the administration of an appropriate volume of fluid should follow.

IMMUNOGLOBULINS (Ig)

Normal γ-globulin

This is obtained from pooled serum. Indications:

- Hypogammaglobulinaemia. Loading dose of 400–600 mg/kg is given. This may be repeated if IgG levels remain low. Maintenance doses are given every 4 weeks to maintain IgG levels above the 5th percentile. Dose adjustment should be made in consultation with the immunologists. Major reactions to pH modified intravenous globulin are not common. Consult with the immunologists if these occur, and with the protocol in the day transfusion centre.
- Infectious hepatitis contacts 0.2 mL/kg, i.m. (maximum 5 mL).
- Measles contacts 0.2 mL/kg, i.m. daily in children less than 12 months and

0.5 mL/kg, i.m. for immunocompromised children (maximum 15 mL; split dose and give in two separate sites).

Hyperimmune γ-globulins

Varieties currently available are:

- Anti-Rh (D) for prophylaxis of Rh haemolytic disease in the newborn.
- Tetanus for both prophylaxis and therapy (see p. 69).
- Varicella (zoster immune globulin) for prevention of chicken pox when it may be life threatening, e.g. in immune deficiency states. Must be given within 72 h of exposure. Dose: 2 mL (0–5 years), 4 mL (6–12 years), 6 mL (adult).

These products are available from either the Red Cross Blood Transfusion Services — anti-Rh(D) and zoster immune globulin — or from the Commonwealth Serum Laboratories.

BLOOD TRANSFUSION REACTIONS

Type	*Symptoms and signs*	*Treatment*	*Prevention*
Pyrogenic	Pyrexia, rigors, anxiety and restlessness	Slow rate of flow Antihistamines	If not better in 30 min, discontinue transfusion
Allergic	Usually pyrexia and rigors, urticaria facial and laryngeal oedema, dyspnoea Cyanosis and peripheral collapse	Discontinue transfusion Adrenaline Antihistamines. Hydrocortisone, i.v.	Prophylactic antihistamines Use appropriate leucocyte poor or washed cells
Haemolytic	Pyrexia, rigors, lumbar pain, pain in vein, jaundice, haemoglobinuria, haemoglobinaemia, oliguria later	Obtain expert advice Check all labels Take blood samples Save urine Discontinue transfusion	Careful grouping and cross-matching Care in storing blood Check labels prior to transfusion
Infected blood	Pyrexia, pain in limbs and chest, pallor, dyspnoea, headache, shock	Discontinue transfusion Save donor blood Treat shock Antibiotics	Care in collecting Storage of blood at correct temp. Observation of expiry time
Circulatory overload	Pulmonary oedema, dyspnoea, headache, venous distension, heaviness in limbs Maybe pyrexia and rigors	Slow rate of flow Diuretic frusemide Digoxin Venesection if extreme	Use of packed cells Give all fluids very slowly If in doubt, give frusemide

ONCOLOGY

The management of paediatric cancers is a specialized field within the discipline of paediatrics and is best undertaken under the supervision of a fully trained specialist in a tertiary referral centre.

In Victoria the Department of Haematology and Oncology provides consultation on children with a malignancy who require medical attention. The therapeutic effects of modern chemotherapy involve multiple systems and are complex. The Department is ready to provide liaison both within the hospital and outside. This can be obtained during office hours on (03) 345 5652 or 345 5656 and after hours through the specialty registrar on call at the hospital.

While recognizing the broad spectrum of situations that a child undergoing treatment for a malignancy may encounter, some general guidelines are set out. Any child receiving chemotherapy who has a fever must be considered likely to be neutropenic and should have white cell count performed. If the child's total neutrophil count is less than 500 then appropriate cultures should be taken and broad spectrum intravenous antibiotics should be given to prevent overwhelming septicaemia.

CHAPTER 15

NEUROLOGICAL CONDITIONS

EPILEPTIC SEIZURES

FEBRILE CONVULSIONS

The term febrile convulsion (FC) is used when no other cause for a convulsion is found in a febrile child over 6 months and under 5 years of age. Criteria for diagnosis are:

- Temperature > 38 °C
- No evidence of an inflammatory process directly involving intracranial structures, e.g. meningitis, encephalitis
- No past history of afebrile seizures

Simple FC are brief, non-focal, tonic or tonic–clonic seizures. Although simple FC are not thought to be harmful, prolonged and focal FC may result in cerebral injury and possibly the development of subsequent epilepsy (recurrent afebrile seizures). Epilepsy occurs in 2–4% of children who have had a simple FC.

Management of a FC consists of termination of a continuing convulsion with rectal diazepam, paracetamol and general temperature lowering measures, and a search for the cause of the fever. Unless a definite cause is present, and the child is otherwise well, CSF should be examined to exclude meningitis.

Occasionally FC are recurrent, despite general measures to control fever. Rectal diazepam 0.4 mg/kg with fever can be used as FC prophylaxis, although it is better used to terminate potentially prolonged FC. If particularly troublesome, consultation with a paediatrician is advised. There is no evidence that prophylaxis of simple FC prevents later epilepsy.

PRIMARY GENERALIZED EPILEPSY

This term describes the group of childhood epilepsies characterized by recurrent generalized tonic–clonic seizures and/or absence seizures of unknown (presumed genetic) aetiology. First seizure is usually between 4–16 years age, in an otherwise normal child. Prognosis is generally good for seizure control and remission in later childhood or adulthood.

PARTIAL (FOCAL) SEIZURES

Partial seizures arise from a localized area of cortex in one cerebral hemisphere and are often due to underlying structural pathology. Metabolic disturbances, e.g. hypoglycaemia and hypocalcaemia may also produce partial seizures. Two common forms of partial epilepsy are temporal lobe epilepsy and benign focal epilepsy of childhood.

Breath holding attacks: see p. 25.

Status epilepticus: see Paediatric Emergencies p. 10.

INDICATIONS FOR COMMENCING ANTICONVULSANTS

The decision to investigate and treat a child following a seizure depends on many factors. Many children have only a single convulsion and treatment would not normally be commenced unless there are clinical features to suggest an increased risk of recurrence. These include:

- The seizure was prolonged (more than 10 min)
- The seizure was partial
- There is evidence suggesting organic cerebral damage, such as developmental delay, a history of birth injury, head injury or previous meningitis

If seizures are recurrent, maintenance anticonvulsants are generally indicated.

Principles of Anticonvulsant Therapy

Most patients can be controlled as well on one anticonvulsant as with two or more, and polypharmacy should be avoided if possible. Introduce or change one anticonvulsant at a time, except in emergency situations. Anticonvulsants should be given an adequate trial before withdrawal.

Start low and go slow to avoid side effects during introduction.

Individuals vary greatly in dosage requirements and tolerance, with young children and infants typically requiring relatively large doses. If seizure control is inadequate or non-compliance or clinical toxicity is suspected, check anticonvulsant blood levels.

Avoid sudden withdrawal of anticonvulsants.

Depending on the type of epilepsy, several years free of seizures are generally required before anticonvulsants are withdrawn. EEG is generally not a good predictor of convulsion recurrence following anticonvulsant withdrawal. Withdrawal is done gradually over several months. Sudden withdrawal may precipitate status epilepticus in some patients.

See table of guidelines for use of the common anticonvulsants at the end of this chapter.

WEAKNESS OF ACUTE ONSET

The acute onset of symmetrical limb weakness usually has a peripheral neuromuscular or spinal cord origin. Toxins (e.g. snake or tick bite), metabolic disturbance, systemic illness and psychogenic causes have to be considered under appropriate circumstances. Two key questions require urgent consideration:

- Is there a treatable cause?
- Is there respiratory or pharyngeal dysfunction of sufficient degree to warrant, irrespective of the cause, management in an intensive care unit?

Myasthenia gravis should be considered in any child with relatively acute onset limb weakness particularly if accompanied by ptosis, eye movement disorder, pharyngeal or respiratory insufficiency. A diagnostic/therapeutic trial of parenteral anticholinesterase is warranted if myasthenia is a possibility.

Guillain-Barré syndrome is often not recognized in its early stages when there may only be an 'ataxic' gait. The child should be transferred to a tertiary referral centre at the time of diagnosis as respiratory weakness may occur rapidly and plasma exchange (and possibly γ-globulin) need to be commenced early if they are to be effective. Similarly, the child with suspected infant botulism should be transferred urgently to a centre capable of undertaking long-term ventilation.

Confirmation or exclusion of spinal cord compression (trauma, tumour, abscess, haematoma, skeletal anomaly) is an urgent priority. Brisk deep tendon reflexes or extensor plantar responses may not be prominent early and a sensory level is often the most important clue to a myelopathy. Spinal imaging is required when acute 'transverse' myelopathy is suspected.

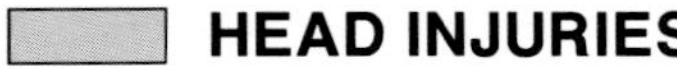

HEAD INJURIES

ASSESSMENT

History

It is essential to determine the nature of the injury, its severity, the time of occurrence and the clinical course prior to consultation.

General and Neurological Examination

These findings will provide a baseline for further assessment and must be carefully recorded. Cervical spine injury must also be diagnosed or excluded as it may occur in association with head injury.

Radiological Examination

Skull X-ray is indicated when the force of impact producing the head injury is considered significant. If the child is unwell enough to warrant a skull X-ray then the child should be in hospital under observation.

Within the Royal Children's Hospital skull X-rays may only be ordered for children with head injuries by the neurosurery registrar or neurosurgery consultant if the child has been or is to be admitted. Children may present to the Emergency Department with skull X-rays performed outside the hospital that show fractures; therefore the following management guidelines mention skull fractures.

There is no place for a skull X-ray 'just in case'.

Cervical spine X-ray is necessary when there is a suggestion that the spine has been damaged and as a routine in all patients with severe head injuries.

A CT scan is indicated in all patients with significant head injury particularly if there is the possibility of an intracranial haematoma.

BLUNT HEAD INJURY

This form of injury is due to an impact on a flat surface which produces an acceleration–deceleration type of injury.

Effects

- *Scalp haematomas are common.* In the infant or young child it may be responsible for a significant reduction in the circulating blood volume.
- *Skull fracture.* Significant injuries may not necessarily have a skull fracture, but the majority do. Conversely, a skull fracture may not be associated with significant brain injury. The fracture is usually linear and it may extend to the skull base. Involvement of the nasal, paranasal or middle ear spaces implies that the injury is compound, with the risk of infection. Check for CSF rhinorrhoea or otorrhoea.

- *Concussion.* The duration of unconsciousness is an indicator of the severity of the concussion.
- *Localized brain damage.* This is due to local deformity at impact which is not generally an important factor except for some injuries in infancy, or surface laceration of the brain due to brain movement within the skull.
- *Intracranial haemorrhage.* Subarachnoid and subdural haemorrhages are usually due to surface laceration of the brain. In extradural haemorrhage, a dural vessel is torn by distortion at or near the point of impact, especially if on the lateral aspect of the head.

Clinical Course

Most patients rapidly recover from the effects of concussion in 12–24 h. Delay or reversal of recovery suggests haemorrhage, brain swelling, infection or an extracranial complication — most commonly an impairment of ventilation.

Management of Blunt Head Injuries

Mild

A brief loss of consciousness (< 5 min) suggests a mild injury, and these patients can be sent home after an initial 4 h observation in emergency. Adequate explanation must be given to the parents and they must be given a head injury form. The patient should be reviewed the following day, either by the LMO or in emergency.

Mild blows on the side of the head are potentially serious, and these patients should be admitted.

Serious

The potential seriousness is indicated by:

- Longer period of unconsciousness
- Deterioration in conscious state, behaviour or vital signs
- Neurological defects
- Bleeding or CSF leak from nose or ear
- Severe bleeding from scalp wound
- Superficial haematoma on the side of the head may be associated with an extradural haematoma even if no fracture is seen on X-ray

Children with these signs will require admission and must be observed carefully for at least 48 h.

Delayed Presentation

These are in four categories:

1. Symptoms and signs as described for potentially serious head injuries. These patients should be admitted.
2. Patients with a wide linear fracture and a large scalp haematoma over the fracture need admission.
3. A linear fracture in otherwise well patients with no haematoma should be seen by the neurosurgical registrar who will also arrange for the patient to attend outpatients in 5–7 days time.
4. An apparently well patient should be sent home after appropriate advice, with instructions to return immediately if any worries develop.

LOCALIZED HEAD INJURY

Injuries of this type are relatively more common in children than in adults.

Effects

- Simple or compound depressed fracture are common
- Infection may occur with compound injuries
- Focal contusion or laceration of the brain may be present to a varying size or depth and may produce neurological signs or seizures
- Concussion may be absent

Management

X-rays are always required, and should be performed as part of the admission including, where indicated, tangential views. CT is helpful. Admission for neurosurgical assessment is required in most cases.

Prevention of infection: all compound injuries should be placed on antibiotics immediately and the wound covered by a head dressing.

CARE OF THE UNCONSCIOUS PATIENT

- Maintain airways
- Observation for vital and basal neurological signs
- Temperature regulation
- Fluid and electrolyte balance
- Nasogastric aspiration to avoid inhalation of gastric contents

Anticipation of Complications

Early evaluation of the patient to assess the development of complications such as compression and infection is essential. Observation for the complications associated with extracranial injury is also important. The patient whose clinical features are not improving should be referred to the neurosurgeon.

Head Injury Instruction to Parents

For the next 24 h keep a careful watch over the patient who should be roused at least every 2 h. The child must be brought back to emergency department immediately if you notice any of the following:

- The child becomes unconscious or more difficult to rouse
- The child becomes confused, irrational or delirious
- Convulsions, or spasms of the face and limbs occur
- The child complains of persistent headache or neck stiffness occurs
- Vomiting occurs frequently
- Bleeding from the ear or recurrent watery discharge from the ear or nose

A head injury information sheet is available in emergency for issue to parents.

CSF SHUNTING PROCEDURES

SUBACUTE SHUNT OBSTRUCTIONS

Aetiology

- *Upper end block*. The tube is too long or blocked by the choroid plexus.
- *Lower end block*. The tube is too short or blocked by abdominal tissues.
- *Disconnection*.

Symptoms

- Headache
- Drowsiness
- Vomiting
- Fits
- The same as a previous episode

Signs

- Fontanelle tension
- Cranial percussion note
- Focal neurological signs
- Change in vital signs
- Deterioration in conscious state
- Recent increase in head circumference in infants

Specific Signs

- *Upper end block*. The pump depresses but does not refill.
- *Lower end block*. The pump is difficult to depress. An X-ray of the chest or abdomen will give an indication of the length of the tube.
- *Disconnection*. The signs depend on the site of the disconnection. Ventricular tube disconnection is unusual and has the same signs as upper end block. Pump disconnection produces local swelling. Disconnection along the course of the tubing may produce local swelling. X-rays may demonstrate a disconnection.

Assessment

The neurosurgeon will want to know:

- The symptoms and signs including the state of the pump and shunt tubing
- The findings on plain X-ray, CT head scan or ultrasound
- The type of shunt: Pudenz or Holter, atrial or peritoneal

SHUNT INFECTION

This should be suspected in any child with a shunt who has recurring obstruction, fevers, anaemia, general malaise, splenomegaly.

TABLE OF GUIDELINES FOR USE OF THE COMMON ANTICONVULSANTS

Drug	*Status epileptïcus*	*Generalized tonic–clonic seizures*	*Partial simple or complex*	*Typical absence (petit mal)*	*Myoclonic/ tonic/atypical absence*	*Prominent side effects*	*Oral dosage*
Carbamazepine (Tegretol)	–	+ + +	+ + +	–	–	Drowsiness, irritability, GIT	10–15 mg/kg per day
Sodium valproate (Epilim)	+	+ + +	+	+ + +	+ + +	Hepatotoxicity, nausea, anorexia vomiting see text	20–50 mg/kg per day
Clobazam (Frisium)	–	+ +	+	+ +	+ + +	Drowsiness, irritability	5–30 mg/day
Clonazepam (Rivotril)	+ + +	+ +	+ +	+ +	+ + +	Irritability and behaviour disorder	0.1–0.25 mg/kg per day
Phenytoin sodium (Dilantin, DPH)	+ +	+ + +	+ + +	–	–	Gum hyperplasia, ataxia, nystagmus, serum-sickness like illness, cognitive	5–8 mg/kg per day
Phenobarbitone	+ +	+ + +	+ +	–	–	Cognitive, irritability overactivity or drowsiness	3–5 mg/kg per day
Ethosuximide (Zarotin)	–	–	–	+ + +	+	Gastrointestinal disturbance, thrombocytopenia	20–40 mg/kg per day
Nitrazepam (Mogadon)	–	–	–	–	+ +	Drowsiness, increased bronchial secretions	Work-up slowly from 1.25 mg/day
Diazepam (Valium)	+ + +	–	–	–	+ + + (i.v. only)	Drowsiness	Intravenous 0.1–0.2 mg/kg slowly

Sodium valproate should be used with caution in children under 3 years of age, particularly where multiple anticonvulsants are being used and underlying cerebral pathology is present.
Cognitive side effects are common to all anticonvulsants, particularly benzodiazepines, barbiturates and phenytoin.

CHAPTER 16

DEVELOPMENTAL DELAY AND DISABILITY

ASSESSMENT OF CHILD DEVELOPMENT

An integral part of paediatrics is the monitoring of children's development. Developmental screening is not definitive. Screening is designed to sort out children who probably do have developmental delay from those who probably do not. Screening may include, but is not limited to the administration of formal developmental screening tests, such as the Denver II. Children who fail developmental screening should be referred for standardized developmental assessment – either to a paediatrician or to a multidisciplinary assessment team.

Developmental screening tests, such as Denver II, need to be formally administered, and are not merely history check-lists. Please refer to the Denver Manual for details.

GUIDE TO DEVELOPMENTAL MILESTONES

The following table is included to give a guide to developmental milestones. It cannot be used as a screening tool. The ages set out are those when at least 90% of a normal group of children will achieve the test, and the figures in brackets represent the range from 25th to 90th centiles for achievement.
(Abbreviations: W = weeks, M = months, Y = years)

Age	*Gross motor*	*Fine motor adaptive*	*Language*	*Personal–social*
1 M	Lifts head momentarily while prone (0–3 W)	Visual following to mid-line (0–5 W)		Watches face (0–4 W)
2 M	Lifts head momentarily to erect position when sitting	Hands predominantly open	Vocalizes (0–7 W)	Smiles responsively (0–7 W)
3 M	Lifts head to 90° while prone (0–10 W)	Visual following past mid-line (0–10 W)	Laughs (6–10 W)	
4 M	Head steady when held erect (6–17 W)	Plays with hands together (6–15 W)	Goos and gurgles	Excited by approach of food
5 M	No head lag when pulled to sitting (3–6 M) Rolls over	Grasps rattle (10–18 W) Reaches for object with palmar grasp (3–5$\frac{1}{2}$ M)	Squeals (6–18 W)	Smiles spontaneously (6 W–5 M)

(Continued over)

Guide to developmental milestones (continued)

Age	*Gross motor*	*Fine motor* *Adaptive*	*Language*	*Personal–social*
6 M	Lifts head forward when pulled to sit (9–19 W)	Passes block hand to hand ($4\frac{1}{2}$–$7\frac{1}{2}$ M)	Turns to voice ($3\frac{1}{2}$–$8\frac{1}{2}$ M)	Friendly to allcomers
8 M	Maintains sitting position without support		Repetition of syllables, e.g. ba ba, Dada	Feeds self biscuit (5–8 M) Tries to get toy out of reach (5–9 M)
10 M	Stands holding on (5–10 M)	Index finger approach	'Mum' 'Dad' without meaning (6–10 M)	
12 M	Walks holding on to furniture ($7\frac{1}{2}$–$12\frac{1}{2}$ M)	Crude finger–thumb grasp (7–11 M)	Imitates speech sounds (6–11 M)	Gives up toy
15 M	Walks alone ($11\frac{1}{2}$–15 M)	Neat pincer grasp of pellet (9–15 M)	'Mum' and 'Dad' with meaning (9–15 M)	Indicates wants ($10\frac{1}{2}$–$14\frac{1}{2}$ M)
$1\frac{1}{2}$ Y	Walks well ($11\frac{1}{2}$–18 M)	Tower of two blocks (12–20 M)	Three words other than 'Mum', 'Dad' (12–20 M)	Drinks from cup (10–17 M)
2 Y	Walks up steps without help (14–22 M)	Scribbles (12–24 M)	Points to one named body part (14–23 M)	Feeds self with spoon (12–24 M)
$2\frac{1}{2}$ Y	Throws ball (15–32 M)	Builds tower of four blocks (15–26 M)	Combines two words (14–27 M)	Helps in house — simple tasks (15–24 M)
3 Y	Pedals tricycle (21 M–3 Y)	Imitates vertical line (18 M–3 Y) Copies circle ($2\frac{1}{2}$–$3\frac{1}{2}$ Y)	Uses three word sentences	Puts on clothes (2–3 Y)
4 Y	Balances on one foot 5 s ($2\frac{3}{4}$–$4\frac{1}{2}$ Y)	Copies square	Gives first and last name (2–4 Y)	Dresses with supervision ($2\frac{1}{4}$–$3\frac{1}{2}$ Y)
5 Y	Hops on one foot (3–5 Y)	Draws man in three parts (3–$5\frac{1}{2}$ Y)	Knows some colours (3–5 Y) knows age	Dresses without supervision ($2\frac{1}{2}$–5 Y)

DEVELOPMENTAL DELAY AND DISABILITY

All children with a disability have a potential for further development and the principles of normal development apply. Specific disabilities in one area of development frequently cause secondary disabilities in other areas. The needs of children with developmental disabilities are the same as those of non-disabled children.

Once suspicion regarding a child's development has been raised a full paediatric consultation is required. The history should include full details of the family, obstetric, neonatal and developmental history. Observation of how the child looks, hears, moves, explores, plays and communicates is essential prior to formal examination. Understandably, parents will be anxious about a child with a disability. A sensitive approach is therefore essential at all times.

Developmental assessment may be ongoing and provides the family with an understanding of a child's development, and outlines goals which may reduce his or her disability and reduce any handicapping effects. Assessment and management may include physiotherapists, speech pathologists, educationalists, occupational therapists, psychologists and social workers.

PRINCIPLES OF ASSESSMENT

- The utilization of play as a fundamental assessment tool
- The promotion of optimal performance of the child
- The gearing of the assessment towards remediation rather than merely producing a profile
- The involvement of the parents in the assessment process
- Close linking of the assessment services with offering help and support

Policies regarding education differ from state to state. Local availability of early intervention and family support services should be sought from local authorities. The following section provides more specific information for Victorian readers.

EARLY INTERVENTION

Early intervention services in the community have developed over the last 10 years and are available through Community Services Victoria Early Childhood teams; (listed at the conclusion of the chapter), some hospitals and Yooralla and Spastic Societies. The overriding philosophy is now of normalization with integration of children into normal generic services. Details about specific early intervention programmes and local support services can be obtained from these organizations.

EDUCATION

In Victoria, the policy of the Ministry of Education is to encourage integration of children with disabilities into regular schools. The special schools still have an important role for many children where the disability is severe or if there are inadequate supports within the regular school system.

FAMILY SUPPORTS

Parents need to be aware of the facilities that are available to them, to assist in the care of their disabled child. Supports available include the Child Disability Allowance, council home help and Noah's Ark.

Respite care in the form of special home help is available from local councils. Overnight respite care can be obtained from Interchange, mothers and babies hospitals, nursing homes, community residential units and usually with generic foster care agencies.

Institutional care for children is no longer an option. Consumer organisations can provide information, parent support and advocacy. The main groups in Victoria are:

DOWN SYNDROME ASSOCIATION OF VICTORIA (DSAV)
55 Victoria Parade
Collingwood 3066
Phone: 419 1653

STAR, VICTORIAN ACTION ON INTELLECTUAL DISABILITY INFORMATION AND RESOURCE UNIT
247–251 Ross House
Flinders Lane
Melbourne 3000
Phone: 650 2730

ACTION GROUP FOR DISABLED CHILDREN
1st Floor
55 Victoria Parade
Collingwood 3066
Phone: 419 3119

INTELLECTUAL DISABILITY

Intellectual disability is defined as a significantly subaverage general intellectual functioning existing concurrently with deficits in adaptive behaviour and manifested during the developmental period. Up to 2.5% of children have an intellectual disability (0.5% moderate, severe or profound, 2% mild). Although the cause is often not known, the single most common cause of moderate intellectual disability is trisomy 21.

PRESENTATION

- At birth with known syndromes or malformations
- With marked delay in major milestones
- Delay in specific milestones
- Secondary handicaps, e.g. behavioural problems

INVESTIGATIONS

Routine investigations include:

- Skull X-ray
- TORCH screening in neonates
- Chromosomes
- Urine metabolic screen
- Creatine phosphokinase
- Thyroid function studies

Other investigations may include:

- CT scan
- Mucopolysaccharide screen

MANAGEMENT

Regular vision and hearing assessment is required for all children with major handicaps. Investigation of known associated anomalies should be carried out, for example, cardiac status in children with trisomy 21. Referral to a geneticist may be appropriate to exclude single gene disorders and provide parents with recurrence risks.

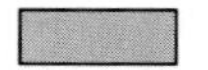

CEREBRAL PALSY

Cerebral palsy is a persistent but not unchanging disorder of movement and posture due to a defect or lesion of the immature brain. It occurs in about 2 per 1000 live births.

AETIOLOGY

Cerebral palsy is not a single entity but a term used for a diverse group of disorders, whose cause may relate to events in the prenatal, perinatal or postnatal periods. Fewer than 1 in 10 cases results from perinatal hypoxia. In the vast majority of children the cause is unknown.

CLASSIFICATION

- The type of motor disorder, e.g. spasticity, athetosis
- The distribution, e.g. hemiplegia, diplegia
- The severity of the motor disorder

ASSOCIATED DISORDERS

- Visual problems
- Hearing deficits
- Epilepsy
- Intellectual disability
- Perceptual problems

Some children have only a motor disorder.

MANAGEMENT

Management of the child with cerebral palsy involves:

1 Accurate diagnosis with genetic counselling.

2 Assessment of the child's capabilities and referral to appropriate services for the child and family. Liaison with kindergarten and school is important.

3 Management of the associated disabilities and health problems.

- **a** All children require a hearing and visual assessment.
- **b** Careful assessment and management of epilepsy.
- **c** Dietary guidance, as obesity and undernutrition are common problems.
- **d** Advice regarding constipation, which is a frequent occurrence.
- **e** Management of drooling with techniques employed by speech pathologists, by the use of medication or surgery in a small group of children.
- **f** Orthopaedic management. Any operative procedure requires consultation with a physiotherapist who will be essential in the postoperative rehabilitation phase. Surgery is mainly confined to the lower limb.
    - *The hip.* Non-walkers and those only partially ambulant are prone to hip subluxation and eventual dislocation. Early detection is important. Hip X-rays should be performed at yearly intervals. Dislocation, which may cause pain and difficulty with perineal hygiene, is difficult to treat once it occurs.
    - *The knee.* Hamstring surgery may be necessary to improve gait pattern.
    - *The ankle.* Equinus deformity is commonly corrected.

4 Referral to, and ongoing liaison with allied health professionals is essential to enable children to achieve their optimal, physical potential and independence. The physiotherapist provides advice regarding methods to encourage movement, and about footwear, splints and walking aids, and may also give individual treatment. The occupational therapist helps parents to develop their child's upper limb and self-care skills, and is also involved in suggesting suitable toys, and equipment for home care. The speech pathologist provides guidance with communication and severe feeding problems. Other professionals that may be helpful include the medical social workers, the psychologist, the special education teacher and the community nurse.

VICTORIAN STATE-WIDE SERVICES FOR DISABLED CHILDREN

NOAH'S ARK
28 The Avenue
Windsor 3181
Phone: 529 1241

ROYAL VICTORIAN INSTITUTE FOR THE BLIND
Burwood Highway
Burwood 3125
Phone: 288 6081

SPASTIC SOCIETY OF VICTORIA
135 Inkerman Street
St Kilda 3182
Phone: 537 2611

YOORALLA SOCIETY OF VICTORIA
52 Thistlethwaite Street
South Melbourne 3205
Phone: 698 5222

VICTORIAN EARLY CHILDHOOD TEAMS: COMMUNITY SERVICES VICTORIA

Early Childhood teams provide services and liaison with other agencies for children with developmental disabilities, including intellectual disability.

EARLY CHILDHOOD SERVICES
Box 760
Geelong 3220
Phone: (052) 26 4540

EARLY CHILDHOOD SERVICES/
EARLY INTERVENTION
PO Box 334
Traralgon 3844
Phone: (051) 74 0755

CHILD & FAMILY SUPPORT SERVICES
LODDON/CAMPASPE REGION
PO Box 5133
Bendigo 3550
Phone: (054) 43 2411

CHILD & FAMILY HEALTH SERVICES
142 Lime Avenue
Mildura 3500
Phone: (050) 23 7866

PLAYHOUSE EARLY INTERVENTION
PO Box 566
Ballarat 3353
Phone: (053) 31 7633

EARLY CHILDHOOD SERVICES/
EARLY INTERVENTION
PO Box 1060
Shepparton 3630
Phone: (058) 21 4644

NORTHERN MALLEE (SUBREGION)
CHILD & FAMILY HEALTH SERVICES
45 Campbell Street
Swan Hill 3585
Phone: (050) 32 1811

EARLY CHILDHOOD SERVICES
PO Box 2
Box Hill 3128
Phone: 890 9311

EARLY CHILDHOOD SERVICES
PO Box 2234
St Kilda West 3182
Phone: 536 1777

EARLY CHILDHOOD TEAM
PO Box 630
Ringwood 3134
Phone: 870 9077

SENIOR EARLY INTERVENTION WORKER
PO Box 1223
Wodonga 3690
Phone: (060) 55 7777

EARLY INTERVENTION
& FAMILY SERVICES
67 Henna Street
Warrnambool 3280
Phone: (055) 61 9444

CHILD & FAMILY SERVICES
Mount Street
Heidelberg 3084
Phone: 457 9111

EARLY CHILDHOOD SERVICES
11 Chesterville Road
Cheltenham 3192
Phone: 581 2222

STEP AHEAD PROGRAM
Suite 4/5 Robinson Street
Dandenong 3175
Phone: 794 0600

EARLY CHILDHOOD SERVICES
PO 200 Sydney Road
Locked Bag No. 7
Brunswick 3056
Phone: 389 2700

WORKERPLAYMATE EARLY CHILDREN'S INTERVENTION
PO Box 633
Horsham 3400
Phone: (053) 81 9555

EARLY CHILDHOOD SERVICES
273 Barkly Street
Footscray 3011
Phone: 689 6500

SPINA BIFIDA

GENERAL

Spina bifida is the commonest severe congenital malformation of the nervous system. The degree of impairment from the spinal cord pathology varies. Most children have some element of lower limb dysfunction, sensory loss and a neurogenic bladder and bowel. Eighty per cent have progressive hydrocephalus requiring surgery.

Management requires collaboration between health education and welfare professionals and the child and family. Most children attend regular schools. Families require a great deal of support.

INITIAL MANAGEMENT

Neurosurgical and paediatric assessment of the newborn infant is undertaken to determine if early surgery to close the spinal defect should be recommended. Clinical and ultrasound observation to detect and monitor the presence of hydrocephalus is important. Ventriculoperitoneal shunts are inserted in 80% of cases. Orthopaedic and urological consultations and investigations are undertaken in the neonatal period to provide baseline information for subsequent management. A small number of infants require early management of talipes or a high pressure neurogenic bladder.

The families must be fully informed about the diagnosis, the natural history, prognosis and reassured that assistance is available.

LONG-TERM MANAGEMENT

Goals

- The maintenance of good health
- The promotion of the development of the child's functional capacities to the maximum possible extent
- The promotion of satisfactory family functioning
- The development of independence and self-care skills in the growing child and the transfer of responsibility from professionals to family and patient

Specific Professional Goals

Orthopaedic

Independent mobility is the primary goal of the orthopaedic surgeon and physiotherapist. Almost all children learn to walk during childhood. The degree of assistance required in the form of surgery, bracing, crutches, etc. varies with the level of the lesion. Those with high lesions often choose in adolescence to use a wheelchair as their primary method of mobility.

Urology

The primary goals of the urologist are the development of continence at a developmentally appropriate age and the maintenance of satisfactory renal functioning. In the past an ileal conduit was constructed early in infancy. Several hundred patients with ileal conduit attend the Royal Children's Hospital. Clean intermittent catheterization is now the preferred first method of treatment. Not all children respond to this and additional support may be necessary in the form of condom drainage or wearing protective clothing. Surgical bladder augmentation or the insertion of artificial urinary sphincters may be required.

Neurosurgery

Depending upon the form of neonatal management undertaken after discussion between neurosurgeon, paediatrician and family the neural tube defect is closed early or late. If hydrocephalus becomes established a ventriculoperitoneal shunt is inserted. In those infants for whom conservative early treatment is undertaken a shunting procedure may precede excision of the lesion and careful observation of the head circumference should be undertaken in all individuals surviving the perinatal period.

Paediatric

Within Victoria the staff of the Spina Bifida Services (physicians in the Department of Child Development and Rehabilitation, social workers, physiotherapists, occupational therapists and stomal therapists and neuropsychologists) provide a co-ordinated and comprehensive care structure for children and families. Strong links exist between this service and education and welfare services in the community.

Specific Acute Problems

Urinary tract infections

These occur frequently. Younger children and those with an ileal conduit present with constitutional symptoms, in particular headache, fever, irritability and vomiting. If infection is suspected a specimen is obtained as follows:

- *Bladder specimen* is obtained by catheter or suprapubic aspiration, a bag specimen may well be contaminated.
- *Conduit specimen* is obtained using a double catheter technique because of the possibility of colonization of the stoma. Interpretation of urine results of double catheter specimens can be difficult. A pure growth suggests infection but a mixed growth may need to be further evaluated. Treatment is along standard lines.

Discharge from the bladder

This occurs in a patient with ileal conduit. This is usually either an infection (pyocystis) or a seminal discharge. If an infection is suspected five daily Neomycin bladder washouts via a urethral catheter are required.

Ulceration of an ileal conduit stoma

This occurs frequently particularly if the child is not drinking adequate volumes of fluid. Referral to a stomal therapist is required.

Problems with the ventriculoperitoneal shunt

These are common. Shunt occlusion or other malfunction may present with headache, irritability, vomiting or other signs of raised intracranial pressure. These signs may also be present in individuals with a urinary tract infection or a viral illness. If in doubt, urine specimen should be obtained to eliminate significant urinary tract infection. Occasionally shunt malfunction may be an episodic phenomenon or occur over time with changes in school performance, personality and behaviour. Urgent referral to a neurosurgical service is required.

Pressure sores

These occur in all children at some time. Footwear, orthopaedic appliances and even the hospitalization of a normally mobile child may pose particular risks. Management should be supervised by a consultant clinic (plastic surgery, orthopaedic or spina bifida).

Pathological fractures

These occur infrequently and usually in those with a high lesion. Local swelling and erythema with or without deformity and usually without pain are common symptoms. Orthopaedic advice should be sought in management.

Constipation

This is a common long-term difficulty but may present as an acute impaction. Dietary advice, laxatives and enemas may be required.

Epilepsy

Some 15% of children with spina bifida have epilepsy, treatment is along the usual lines.

SPEECH AND LANGUAGE DELAY

Delayed development of speech and language is common. The delay may occur alone, or be associated with other conditions such as hearing impairment, global developmental delay or environmental deprivation.

Indicators of speech and language difficulties may include parental concern, lack of babbling/vocalization in the infant, unintelligible speech, poor language comprehension, lack of expressive speech and dysfluency. Early referral to a speech pathologist is important and should be considered as part of the paediatric assessment.

CHAPTER 17

CHILD PSYCHIATRY

CHILD PSYCHIATRY SERVICES IN VICTORIA

The organization of child psychiatry services differs from state to state. Readers are referred to local authorities for the availability of services in their region.

Victorian Child Psychiatry services are largely provided on a regional basis. The Royal Children's Hospital Department of Child and Family Psychiatry provides services to hospital inpatients and outpatients who require ongoing care; complex patients whose needs are best served in a tertiary setting. Patients who have been treated previously in the department, those from specific research populations and those from municipalities served by the Hospital department, i.e. Melbourne, Richmond, Collingwood, Fitzroy, Brunswick, Coburg, Broadmeadows, Bulla and Gisborne and also country Region 3.

Travencore Child and Family Centre (376 3211) serves the south-west zone of the State, including the rest of western region 6 and also country Regions 1 and 2. The Austin Hospital Child and Adolescent Psychiatry Department (459 8824) serves the north-east zone, including Regions 7 and 4. The South Eastern Child and Family Centre (529 8799) and the Monash Medical Centre (550 1111) serve the south-eastern zone, including Regions 8 and 5. Any of these agencies may be used to consult on other child psychiatry resources in their areas or to discuss referrals to their services.

NOTES ON INTERVIEWING FOR PSYCHIATRIC PROBLEMS IN CHILDHOOD

As well as interviewing parent(s) and child together, see each separately if possible, to get a more complete picture. Check why the family have presented at this particular time. Note that children, the less intelligent or educated, and those with language and cultural disadvantage are more likely to be misunderstood and to misunderstand questions, to be afraid or hostile and to use somatic complaints to communicate distress.

Use simple language and try to understand the predicament of the child and the family. One's own response to the child and the family is a vital aspect of the assessment.

Assess the detail of the problem behaviour, history, frequency, context and the responses of family members. Assess the meaning of the problem behaviour to the family and the ways in which they have attempted to solve the problem, including professional advice previously sought.

Inquire about: pregnancy, delivery, nursing relationship, development in early years, preschool and school life, educational progress, peer relations, interests, family structure, recent stresses, marital relationship, family supports and extended social network, intergenerational difficulties, illnesses and separations.

Observe the following:

- Affect: range, variability and form, e.g. flat, anxious etc
- Play: confidence, competence, co-ordination, activity, creativity, etc
- Thinking: content (including suicidal thoughts), concentration, organization, orientation, form of thought, dreams, wishes, etc
- Personality: behavioural style, adaptability/rigidity, openness/defensiveness, ability to engage in a relationship

FAMILY CRISIS

Children are even more dependent on their families than are adults, and their self-perception, emotional life, understanding of people and relationships and behaviours are intimately connected with the views and the behaviour of their families.

Parental responsibilities and obligations include nurturance, care and protection of children; the establishment of limits and rules; the provision of security and emotional space to play and develop; appropriate education, stimulation and involvement.

Where parental competence is undermined by illness, poverty, ignorance, stress, lack of supports and other factors, then many children show evidence of behavioural disturbance. Overactivity, aggression, self-stimulation, destructive behaviour, stealing, running away and suicidal behaviour may all be evidence of family difficulty. While these behaviours bring the predicament of the child to the attention of others, they are also often perceived by parents as 'bad' and they in turn, punish or reject the child. A cycle of unsatisfactory interactions develops where the parents feel bad and angry and the child feels bad and angry.

At various points in the crisis-filled careers of some families, children may be presented at emergency departments with the problems located inside them. They may carry such labels as 'hyperactive', 'suicidal', 'possessed', 'bad', 'out of control', etc. At such times it is helpful to focus on the difficulties of the caretakers, as well as on those of the child, and clarify the interactional cycles or habits that can organize their lives.

One should balance the disadvantages of offering crisis admission with the benefits of being able to establish appropriate responsibilities and community supports once the problem becomes clearer.

ACTION

- Social work and psychiatric consultation may be very helpful
- Crisis social work/psychiatry referrals for assessment
- Liaison and referral to appropriate community agencies

ATTEMPTED SUICIDE

This most often presents as a drug overdose in children over 9 years old, but may take more violent forms such as cutting oneself or attempted hanging. Most are an expression of long-standing difficulties between parent(s) and child where care, co-operation and communication are unsatisfactory. The suicidal act is usually associated with difficulties in control, protests and unhappiness. About one-quarter are more serious expressions of suicidal intent, often in association with depressed mood and other depressive symptoms. It is always dangerous simply to dismiss a self-injurious act as attention seeking.

Action

Do not delay necessary medical attention. Consult the duty psychiatric registrar to determine whether urgent psychiatric assessment, admission or referral for outpatient assessment is required. Interview the child alone, parent(s) alone and family together and evaluate underlying difficulties, strengths and likely responses of the family to this crisis.

ANXIETY DISORDERS

These present with high underlying levels of autonomic arousal and subjective fear or panic. It may occur in attacks or as a persisting state.

PANIC ATTACKS

Can occur following severe stress or trauma, or threats to the child's integrity or the child's family support systems. Associated with palpitations, chest pains, hyperventilation, nausea, giddiness, trembling, sweating, abdominal pain, etc. There may be separation anxiety with increased clinging to parents.

Action

After examination and understanding of the origin of the fear, explanation and planned follow-up is usually sufficient. More difficult cases should be discussed with the duty psychiatry registrar for emergency psychiatric assessment or urgent outpatient appointment.

CONVERSION REACTIONS

May be associated with paralysis, blindness, deafness, pains or other sensory changes which have no organic basis. Usually occurs in association with recent stresses, family difficulties with emotional communication and difficulties in providing emotional support.

Action

If admission for full medical and psychiatric assessment is needed, refer to the duty psychiatric registrar. Otherwise, consider elective consultation with the psychiatric registrar, or referral to medical outpatients and psychiatry.

SCHOOL REFUSAL

The child is brought with the complaint of panic and distress on being sent to school. The presenting symptom is often some somatic problem of pain. To be distinguished from truancy where the child avoids school without the accompanying anxiety symptoms and often without parents' knowledge.

Action

Full physical examination should precede psychiatric referral. Consult with duty psychiatry registrar to determine referral for urgent psychiatric assessment and management. Urgent return to school is a high priority.

DEPRESSION AND BEREAVEMENT

GRIEVING

May occur in response to loss of attention and support if parents are unavailable or are themselves grieving as well as following more obvious losses. Protest at the loss with overactivity and rage may be followed by sadness, depression and withdrawal.

Action

Parents need explanations and the children need support by adults who can understand their response to the loss. Assist family to get appropriate support and counselling.

DEPRESSION

May present with low, flat or sad mood, self-deprecation, hopelessness, social and academic withdrawal, sleep and appetite disturbance, changed activity levels, suicidal thoughts or attempts, etc. May be associated with conduct disturbances, anxiety symptoms or psychotic symptoms.

Action

As depressed children are at increased risk for suicide, consult duty psychiatric registrar. Early outpatient appointments are needed.

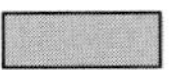

ANOREXIA NERVOSA AND BULIMIA

Obsessional pursuit of thinness involves rigid dieting, purging or vomiting and exercise in various proportions. Patients usually minimize or deny their difficulties, becoming distressed or hostile if these are pursued. Families are often distressed at times of presentation to hospital. Current treatment involves a family orientation and the decision to admit should follow both medical and psychiatric assessment, unless the patient is severely chachectic or hypotensive.

Action

Medical outpatient or adolescent services referral. Duty psychiatry registrar consultation and/or referral to psychiatry.

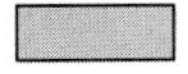

MAJOR PSYCHIATRIC DISORDERS (PSYCHOSIS)

Psychosis is a general term for states in which mental function is grossly impaired, so that reality testing and insight are lacking and delusions, hallucinations, incoherence, thought disorder and/or disorganized behaviour may be apparent. In the case of 'organic' psychoses there may also be clouding of consciousness, confusion and disorientation as well as perceptual disturbances. Short-term memory impairment is common in organic brain syndromes.

Anticholinergics, anticonvulsants, antidepressants, antimalarials and benzodiazepines have been associated with psychotic reactions in young people as have substances of abuse (amphetamines, cocaine, opiates, hallucinogens, etc.) Organic brain syndromes commonly follow even minor head injury.

Adolescents may occasionally present in an acutely psychotic state with no prior history of drug ingestion or head injury. In this case the possibility of a 'functional' psychosis, schizophrenia or manic-depressive disorder should be considered. The latter often presents with elated mood, grandiose ideas, increased energy and reduced sleep requirements.

Action

The hospital medical officer should make a clinical evaluation and call the duty psychiatric registrar. Most of these children will require admission for full psychiatric and medical work-up. Do not sedate the child unless essential, before he/she is seen by the psychiatric registrar.

SEXUAL AND EMOTIONAL ABUSE OF CHILDREN

This is an increasingly recognized phenomenon. Signs of neglect and emotional abuse are often non-specific but suspicion should be raised when infants, preschoolers or school-age children behave in the following ways:

- Persistently angry, socially avoidant, defiant, disobedient and overactive.
- Anxiously attached, watchful of their patients, having limited ability to enjoy things, intensely ambivalent to parents.
- Low self-esteem, depressed or unresponsive, developmental and emotional retardation, poor social skills and overinhibitions.
- Signs of sexual abuse are also usually non-specific, but include the above and various behavioural problems (phobias, bad dreams, eating and sleeping disorders, depression, school problems, delinquency, etc). There may be overt manifestations of sexual preoccupations including precocious and inappropriate sexual activity, promiscuity and aggressive sexual behaviours.

Action

See Child Abuse chapter, pp. 127–130. Psychiatric consultation is often useful in conjunction with involvement of the Child Protection Unit.

CHAPTER 18

CHILD ABUSE AND NEGLECT

Child abuse occurs when a child experiences some physical, emotional or mental damage, occasioned other than through accident by the behaviour of one or more individuals. Child abuse may be divided into four main types although it is important to recognize that there is considerable overlap between them.

- *Neglect* is the failure of parents to adequately safeguard the health, safety and well-being of the child
- *Emotional abuse* is the distortion of the parent–child relationship that deprives children of the consistent nurturing of body and mind that would enable them to develop fully.
- *Physical abuse* includes inflicted physical violence directed against children such as bruises, burns, head injuries, fractures, abdominal injuries, suffocation, drowning and includes intentional poisoning with drugs or other substances and the syndrome known as Munchausen's by proxy
- *Sexual abuse* is the involvement of dependent, developmentally immature children and adolescents in sexual activities that they do not fully comprehend and to which they are unable to give informed consent

INDICATORS OF ABUSE

There are certain indicators or signs which may be used to alert someone to the possibility that a child is being abused. Some of these indicators are more clear-cut than others, for example, unexplained bruising or burn marks, or certain physical signs of sexual abuse. Behavioural indicators are more difficult to assess but they are often just as important as the more obvious physical signs. Many of these indicators are common to all forms of abuse and may include repeated unfounded complaints of physical illness, frequent accidents (the apparently 'accident prone') child, previous injury or concern of siblings, if injuries are not consistent with the child's stated cause or the child's developmental level.

Indicators of sexual abuse may include inappropriate sexual activity, prepubescent venereal disease, genital or rectal trauma or pregnancy.

IN ALL CASES OF SUSPECTED CHILD ABUSE, CONSULT THE CHILD PROTECTION UNIT

THE CHILD PROTECTION UNIT AT THE ROYAL CHILDREN'S HOSPITAL

The Child Protection Unit is a multidisciplinary team within the hospital that provides a 24-h, 7-day-a-week service for child abuse. It is available for advice on the assessment and management of all cases of suspected and

recognized child abuse for both inpatients and outpatients, within the Royal Children's Hospital:

Location: 5th Floor, South East Building
Phone: 345 6391
After hours via switchboard for on-call social worker

The Unit does not have legal power to investigate cases of suspected or recognized child abuse but has established links with the statutory child protection agencies, i.e. Community Services Victoria and the Community Policing Squad.

GUIDELINES FOR MANAGEMENT OF CHILD ABUSE

The following protocol represents Royal Children's Hospital policy in relation to child abuse in all its forms and is applicable to all health professionals within the hospital.

It should be noted that at all times the well-being and safety of the child is of paramount importance although help for the parents and the family is an integral part of the management.

Note: Owing to the complexities involved in child sexual abuse, a different approach is required. The guidelines for management for child sexual assault are therefore differentiated from other forms of abuse.

CHILD ABUSE (EXCEPT CHILD SEXUAL ABUSE)

All children need appropriate referral for thorough assessment.

Within the Royal Children's Hospital the child should be seen without delay by the Admitting Officer or the Emergency Registrar. The Ambulatory Paediatric Social Worker (after hours the on-call Child Protection Unit Social Worker) should be notified without delay.

Clinical Evaluation

A thorough clinical evaluation of the child and family is mandatory. Physical, emotional, psychological and social aspects must be documented clearly.

- Detailed description of injuries with diagrams and photographs are required. To detect bone injuries, X-rays are most useful in the acute phase (up to 72 h post-injury) with bone scans indicated after this. To detect skull fractures, a skull X-ray is the most sensitive investigation.
- Developmental evaluation is required.
- Psychiatric assessment of the child and family must be considered.
- Information from community sources may be sought from maternal and child health nurses, general practitioners, other hospitals and agencies.

SEXUAL ABUSE

Children should be referred to the local health authority. Hospital admission may be required. Local regulations will govern the need for requiring the involvement of police or statutory authorities. The information below relates to the management of sexual abuse in Victoria and within the Royal Children's Hospital. Although the details may differ in other regions the principles will be of use to the reader.

Acute

If rape or sexual abuse has occurred within the previous 72 h. Collection of forensic evidence assumes great significance but the medical needs of the child are first priority.

Within the Royal Children's Hospital consult the Child Protection Unit Social Worker who will be responsible for counselling or referral for ongoing counselling. Consult the Child Protection physician or Ambulatory Consultant. The Police Surgeon is to be called in all such cases of recent sexual assault and may be assisted by the Child Protection physician or Ambulatory Consultant/Registrar. Record in the Medical Record the date the child was examined and by whom.

Sexually transmitted disease screening is usually deferred until first follow-up visit. Consider pregnancy prophylaxis. Medications are held in the pharmacy and in the after-hours drug cupboard. Consider other treatment as required.

Follow-up by the Child Protection Unit medical staff to be organized for 1–2 weeks from the first visit.

Chronic or Late Sexual Contact Greater Than 72 h

Immediate examination is rarely necessary. Forensic evidence gathering is less relevant. Focus of assessment is on the health of the child. If appropriate perform general examination. After obtaining consent of guardian and child, inspect the genitalia. Medical screening tests if appropriate. Document findings carefully. Treat if necessary.

Within the Royal Children's Hospital consult with the Child Protection Unit Social Worker regarding a joint assessment of the case, the need to consult or refer to Community Services Victoria/Community Policing Squad and to arrange for medical and social work assessments. Consult with on-call Ambulatory Paediatrics Consultant before proceeding further.

Arrange follow-up by Child Protection Unit medical staff (it may be more appropriate for the physical examination to be deferred until the child can be seen in the Child Protection Unit).

Ambulatory Paediatrics, Outpatients and Inpatients

If child abuse is suspected the social worker attached to that Unit should be contacted without delay. If there is no allocated Social Worker contact the duty social worker or, after hours, the on-call Child Protection Unit Social Worker.

Telephone Calls Regarding Child Abuse

These may be for advice in child abuse and/or for medical examinations. The caller should be referred to the Child Protection Unit duty Social Worker, or after hours, the on-call Child Protection Unit Social Worker.

Issues That May Arise

These may include parents refusing admission of the child, threat of removal of child from hospital; and access to child on Safe Custody Order.

Case Conference

Following the collection of detailed information, a case conference will be held. This should include the relevant medical and nursing staff and other involved allied health professionals such as Play Therapist, Psychologists, etc. Outside agencies involved with the child and family such as Community Services Victoria, the Police and other relevant professionals may also be asked to attend.

The following points are essential:

- There is a Chairperson who will clearly set out the aims of the Conference
- The conference is minuted and circulated to all invited participants
- That clear decisions are reached and that minority opinions (if any) are recorded
- Allocation of tasks and case responsibility is defined clearly
- A process for review is established

COURT APPEARANCES

Where medical evidence is required in court, the senior medical person involved with the child is the most appropriate person to give such evidence. It is also the responsibility of this person to prepare the medical report according to medicolegal procedures. In some cases, junior medical staff may be subpoenaed to give evidence.

The Child Protection Unit medical staff are available for consultation regarding the preparation of reports and court appearances.

Note: **Remember**

SUSPECT CHILD ABUSE, RECOGNIZE CHILD ABUSE, CONSULT THE CHILD PROTECTION UNIT

CHAPTER 19

ENDOCRINE CONDITIONS

SHORT STATURE

DEFINITION

Height below 3rd height centile. Refer to growth charts in Appendix 3.

AETIOLOGY

Physiological (commonest)

- Constitutional growth delay
- Familial short stature
- Combination of above

Growth velocity usually normal (5–6 cm/year mid-childhood). Constitutional growth delay occurs in patients who are 'late developers' and usually follows a familial pattern of growth and development.

Familial short stature is diagnosed in a healthy child with short parents. Parental height should be measured rather than guessed, and the parents' height centiles determined.

Pathological

- Nutritional (including psychosocial)
- Metabolic (systemic disease)
- Endocrine (i.e. hypothyroidism, growth hormone deficiency, Cushing's syndrome)
- Chromosomal (i.e. Turner's syndrome)
- Bone dysplastic disorders (i.e. achondroplasia)
- Miscellaneous — intrauterine growth retardation, iatrogenic (i.e. drugs, X-ray)

All are less common, growth velocity is always subnormal. Endocrine causes are relatively uncommon but are most important as they are treatable.

DIAGNOSIS

Height measurement using accurate equipment is important to establish the diagnosis of short stature. Plot measurements of height and weight on centile charts.

Body proportion measurements of arm span and lower segment (pubic symphysis to floor) should be made. Examine for skeletal dysplasias, hypothyroidism or various syndromes associated with short stature.

Notes:

- Span should be within a few centimetres of height at all ages.
- Lower segment should be greater than half the height beyond bone age 8 years.

- Height velocity. All patients with short stature should have growth measurements every 3 months for a minimum of 6 months to determine growth velocity.

Investigations

Investigate growth velocity less than 25th centile for the child's bone age and deviation from 3rd heights centile. The investigations aim to confirm the clinical suspicions. These include: thyroid function, urea and electrolytes, calcium, full blood examination, chromosomal analysis (girls only), a bone age X-ray and an exercise growth hormone screening test (random growth hormone values are meaningless).

Referral

Referral to the endocrine unit is appropriate if the short stature is marked or no obvious cause is determined, or an endocrine cause is apparent or suspected, or likely to be associated with significant pubertal delay (i.e. Turner's syndrome or marked constitutional delay).

Within the Royal Children's Hospital growth hormone treatment is available through the endocrine/growth clinic.

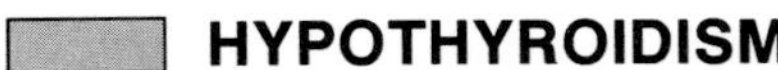

HYPOTHYROIDISM

Hypothyroidism may be congenital or acquired. Congenital hypothyroidism has an incidence of 1 : 4000 live births. Mandatory screening, conducted on the fourth day of life, detects most causes of congenital hypothyroidism.

AETIOLOGY

- Absent or ectopic thyroid glands (no goitre) are the most likely to be detected by screening
- Dyshormonogenesis (usually large goitre) is caused by a thyroid gland that cannot produce enough thyroxine and may not be detected in the neonatal period
- Acquired hypothyroidism may be caused by Hashimoto's thyroiditis, iodine deficiency or secondary to hypothalamic or pituitary disease

EXAMINATION

Clinical findings for hypothyroidism are secondary to slowed body metabolism, i.e. sluggish physical and mental activity, growth failure, coarsening of features, dry pale skin, cold intolerance and constipation.

INVESTIGATIONS

Thyroid function tests (TFT) measuring serum thyroxine (T4) and thyroid stimulating hormone (TSH) will help establish a diagnosis. Congenital hypothyroidism should be detected with a low T4 and a high TSH. Age specific ranges are quoted in the biochemistry section (pp. 189–197).

Referral to the Department of Endocrinology is important for the management of hypothyroidism.

PRECOCIOUS PUBERTY

DEFINITION

- < 8 years in girls
- < 9.5 years in boys

For pubertal staging refer to Appendix 3.

AETIOLOGY

Central Causes

Idiopathic true precocious puberty associated with elevated gonadotrophins is more common in girls than boys, where it is always associated with enlarged testes. Causes include:

- CNS abnormalities, tumours and trauma
- Inherited syndromes (e.g. neurofibromatosis and tuberous sclerosis)
- Severe hypothyroidism

Non-Central Causes

- Increased adrenal sex steroid production, particularly congenital adrenal hyperplasia in boys (testes small)
- Non-pituitary gonadotrophin e.g. β-human chorionic gonadotrophin from tumours (boys only)
- Sex steroids from ovarian or testicular tumours
- McCune-Albright syndrome
- Testotoxicosis (boys)

INVESTIGATIONS

- Oestradiol (girls); testosterone (boys)
- 24 h urinary FSH and luteinizing hormone (LH)
- TFT
- LH releasing hormone (LHRH) stimulation (not in all)

Radiology

- Bone age
- CT head scan (only if biochemistry abnormal)

TREATMENT

Referral should be made to a paediatric endocrinologist who may use medroxyprogesterone acetate, cyproterone acetate or LHRH super agonist.

CONDITIONS RESEMBLING PRECOCIOUS PUBERTY

Premature Thelarche

Isolated breast development is most common in the first 2 years of life. It usually regresses spontaneously. Breast enlargement may occur after 6 years and if there is no other sign of puberty and the oestrogen level is normal then careful observation is all that is necessary.

Premature Adrenarche (Pubarche)

This is isolated pubic hair development due to an increase in circulating adrenal androgen levels. The bone age is often slightly advanced and a careful check is needed to exclude pathological causes of excess androgen production, especially congenital adrenal hyperplasia.

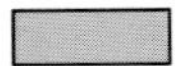

DELAYED PUBERTY

DEFINITION

Absence of pubertal changes

- > 14 years girls
- > 15 years boys

For pubertal staging refer to Appendix 3.

AETIOLOGY

Normal or Low Serum Gonadotrophins:

1. Constitutional delay most common — usually strong family history. It is often associated with poor growth velocity and delayed bone age is common.
2. Chronic illness/poor nutrition. Seen in patients with cystic fibrosis, thalassaemia and inflammatory bowel disease.
3. Endocrine causes
   - **a** Hypothyroidism
   - **b** Hypopituitarism with multiple pituitary trophic hormone deficiencies
   - **c** Isolated gonadotrophin deficiency (Kallman's syndrome)
   - **d** Prolactinoma of pituitary

Elevated Serum Gonadotrophins

Chromosomal disorders

- Turner's syndrome 45 XO (gonadal dysgenesis)
- Klinefelter's syndrome 47XXY
- Noonan's syndrome (chromosomes normal, both sexes)

Bilateral gonadal failure

Traumatic post-infectious, post-surgical, post-irradiation or chemotherapy, autoimmune or idiopathic.

INVESTIGATION

- Full blood examination and ESR
- Electrolytes and urea
- Serum proteins (exclude chronic disease)
- Thyroid function tests
- Chromosomal analysis (girls and boys suspected of having Klinefelter's)

- LH/FSH (elevated levels indicate primary gonadal failure)
- Exercise growth hormone test (if growth velocity poor)
- Serum prolactin

TREATMENT

Referral should be made to a paediatric endocrinologist who may use oxandrolone or testosterone in boys and oestrogen in girls. Androgen therapy (boys) sometimes useful if it helps to remove psychological problems.

AMBIGUOUS GENITALIA

Any child where the genitalia are not completely normal male or female should be regarded as potentially ambiguous. 'Clitoral enlargement' of any degree is abnormal. 'Hypospadias with undescended testes' is an example of ambiguity if both testes are not palpable or the 'penis' is very small.

Urgent consultation with an experienced paediatric endocrinologist or surgeon should be made on the first day of life, often by phone initially.

MANAGEMENT

In the Delivery Room

Tell the parents the baby is healthy but has a problem which prevents immediate gender assignment. Show the baby's genitalia to the parents, so they can appreciate the problem for themselves. Indicate that definite general assignment will be made within a few days, once investigations/consultation has occurred. Tell the family an expert in genital disorders will be called immediately and that a social worker will be available to assist while things are sorted out. Indicate that transfer to a tertiary referral centre may be required within the first 1–2 days. Advise parents to delay naming the baby and registering the birth until after the gender has been ascertained.

In the Neonatal Nursery

Meet with all ward staff and agree on what is to be said about the baby. No one should talk to the parents without adequate briefing. No one should give an opinion about the sex until after a proper decision is made. Keep detailed notes about communication with parents.

CHAPTER 20

DIABETES MELLITUS

For both Royal Children's Hospital and Victorian patients the Diabetes Service offers advice to patients on a 24 h basis. Parents are encouraged to ring if worried and this often avoids the need to bring the child to hospital. The specialty registrar is on call and available for phone consultations with residents and GPs at any time (03) 345 5522.

DIAGNOSIS

Diagnosis of type 1 diabetes in childhood is made on a raised blood glucose level (> 11 mmol/L) in the presence of unequivocal symptoms. There is little place for oral glucose tolerance test in diagnosis. Fasting normoglycaemia does not exclude diabetes and a raised blood glucose concentration in an ill child without symptoms is not diagnostic of diabetes.

DIABETIC KETOACIDOSIS

The management of diabetic ketoacidosis requires a team approach. Resuscitation with fluids and electrolytes carries a risk of cerebral oedema. There is some evidence that reducing the free water load while increasing sodium replacement at a constant gradual rate decreases the risk of cerebral oedema.

INITIAL MANAGEMENT

- Assess degree of dehydration. Take care not to overestimate (see pp. 43–44).
- Treat shock. Give a plasma volume expander i.v. (10 mL/kg), repeat if necessary.
- Look for treatable precipitating causes.

Intravenous Fluids

- Give calculated deficit and maintenance (see p. 43). Aim for full replacement over **48 h**.
- Use 0.9% (normal) saline.
- Add 40 mmol/L KCl if < 30 kg, 60 mmol/L if > 30 kg.
- At blood sugar level of 10 mmol/L, change to 0.45% saline in 5% dextrose, with added KCl (aim for 12 h of normal saline — may have to use 0.9% saline in 5% dextrose).

Insulin Infusion

- Start after shock has been treated.
- Use a syringe pump with a rapid-acting insulin (1 unit/mL) in 0.9% saline via a 3-way tap into a sideline.
- Dose: 0.1 units/kg per h. Reduce to 0.05 units/kg when blood sugar < 5 mmol/L and patient is metabolically improving and receiving 0.45% saline in 5% dextrose.

- Change to subcutaneous insulin when patient is alert and metabolically stable (blood sugar < 10 mmol/L, pH > 7.30 and bicarbonate > 15 mmol/L). Cease infusion 30 min after first subcutaneous injection.

Monitoring

- Nil by mouth until alert and stable. Nurse head up. Strict fluid balance.
- Clinically: Over first 24 h monitor the following hourly: glucose (glucometer), pulse, blood pressure, level of consciousness and pupils; 4 hourly temperatures.
- **Beware headache and altered behaviour** — this may indicate cerebral oedema.
- Biochemically: 2–4 hourly glucose, sodium, potassium, chloride, osmolality.
- **Beware falling sodium as glucose declines** — this may indicate cerebral oedema.

Hypoglycaemia

- Do not discontinue insulin infusion.
- Treat hypoglycaemia with i.v. 10% dextrose (2 mL/kg stat).

Cerebral Oedema (see p. 11, acutely raised intracranial pressure)

- Give mannitol 20% i.v. stat, 0.5 g/kg (repeat if necessary).
- Nurse head up.
- Restrict fluids.
- Arrange immediate transfer to ICU.

INITIAL STABILIZATION

PROTOCOL FOR INSULIN THERAPY FOR DIABETES

Assess clinically and biochemically:
(Vomiting? Acidotic? Dehydrated > 5%)

YES	NO	NO
KETOACIDOSIS	UNWELL KETONURIA MILD DEHYDRATION	NOT UNWELL NOT SIGNIFICANT KETONURIA
1 Follow ketoacidosis protocol	**1** Quick-acting insulin. 0.25 units/kg wt stat UNLESS within 2 h of a meal	**1** No insulin until next usual meal time
RESUSCITATION COMPLETE	**2** Quick-acting insulin before each meal. Dose: 0.25 units/kg at 0730 h 1130 h 1730 h	

3 Intermediate acting insulin 0.25 units/kg wt at 1730 h, but not if this is FIRST insulin dose. Then give quick-acting insulin at midnight followed by snack.

4 Order meals as carbohydrate exchanges at standard meal times: 0800 h, 1030 h, 1200 h
with snacks, 1530 h, 1800 h, 2000 h

(Continued over)

PROTOCOL FOR INSULIN THERAPY FOR DIABETES (Continued)

NEGATIVE KETONURIA AND NORMOGLYCAEMIA

5 Change insulin to twice daily mixture of short and intermediate insulins. Basis for day 1 is give total of 1 unit/kg, but modify on basis of previous day's insulin requirements.

- **a** Give one quarter of this dose as quick acting — half of this at breakfast, half at evening meal.
- **b** Of remainder (3–4 units/kg), give two-thirds at breakfast and one-third at evening meal as intermediate insulin.
  e.g. 30 kg child:one-quarter quick acting (say ACTRAPID HM) = 80.
  Give half of this twice a day, i.e. 4 units at breakfast and evening meal. Remainder as intermediate insulin (PROTAPHANE HM) = 22 units. Two-thirds of this at breakfast (15 units) and one-third at evening meal (7 units)

USUAL INSULINS USED IN CLINIC FOR NEW PATIENTS

In combinations:

1. Velosulin (quick acting) and Insulatard (intermediate) or;
2. Actrapid (quick acting) and Protaphane (intermediate) or;
3. Humulin Reg (quick acting) and Humulin NPH (intermediate).

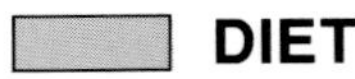

DIET

Some old patients will be on the 10 g portion system: diet should be ordered as such, and if possible changed by dietitian during admission.

APPROXIMATE TOTAL NUMBER OF EXCHANGES TO START WITH (DIETITIAN WILL ADJUST SUBSEQUENTLY)

Age	*Exc.*	*Age*	*Exc.*	*Age*	*Exc.*
1 year	8	6 years	13	11 years	17
2 years	9	7 years	14	12 years	18
3 years	10	8 years	15	13 years	19
4 years	11	9 years	16	14 years	20
5 years	12	10 years	16	15 years	20

For the 6 year old above on twice daily insulin

- 0800 h 3
- Mid-morning 1
- 12 midday 3
- Mid-afternoon 1
- 1800 h 3
- 2000 h 1

The 8 year old above would be ordered exchanges 4 : 1, 4 : 1, 4 : 1.

Toddlers are often hard to feed especially if upset; don't overfeed or it will be a battle. Older children are often ravenous, be generous and review each day.

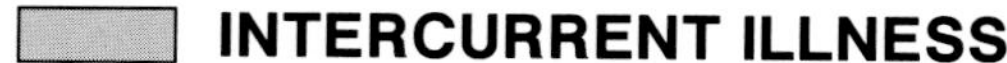

INTERCURRENT ILLNESS

Intercurrent illness usually leads to relative insulin resistance. This, together with physical inactivity leads to hyperglycaemia, and if severe, ketonaemia. On the other hand, and particularly if there is anorexia or vomiting, diminished food intake may lead to actual or potential hypoglycaemia.

INSULIN SHOULD BE MAINTAINED

Whatever the circumstances, insulin injection should not be omitted. There is a mandatory need for insulin to suppress excessive endogenous glucose production and ketonaemia even in the absence of oral carbohydrate intake.

The intercurrent illness should be treated on its own merit and not differently to a child without diabetes.

MAINTAIN CARBOHYDRATE INTAKE

A child who is anorexic and vomiting can omit the protein and fat foods but maintain carbohydrate intake largely as simple sugar-containing food or fluids. It is not necessary then to give carbohydrates in precise amounts, but they can be spaced during the day in smaller amounts at more frequent intervals.

INCREASE INSULIN IN HYPERGLYCAEMIA

A child who is hyperglycaemic during intercurrent illness should have an increase in insulin dosage, the increase depending on the degree of hyperglycaemia, but would be about 10% above normal levels. Rapid reduction of dose after the illness has cleared is usually essential to prevent hypoglycaemia.

GIVE SUPPLEMENTS OF QUICK-ACTING INSULIN IF KETONURIA

If child has hyperglycaemia and ketonuria, in addition to the 10% increase in the intermediate acting insulin, he/she will need an increase or supplementary dose of quick-acting insulin. The increase should be 10–20% of the total morning dose of combined insulins, given as unmodified insulin. This may be repeated 2–4 hourly until ketones clear and normoglycaemia is restored.

VOMITING

A diabetic child who is vomiting must have blood glucose and urine ketones estimated before an appropriate decision on insulin can be made. If vomiting persists, it is essential to check hydration and exclude ketosis.

Administration of antiemetic medication may be appropriate for vomiting during intercurrent illness but is contraindicated in the presence of ketosis or severe hypo- or hyperglycaemia when it will be ineffective and may mask signs of CNS depression.

The following clinical situations may arise in a vomiting child:

- *Normal blood glucose and no ketonuria.* Maintain insulin dose and substitute sugar-containing fluids (soft drink, cordial or fruit juice which are all approximately 10% sugar) or other easily tolerated simple carbohydrates for usual meals. Check blood glucose levels 2–4 hourly and if necessary give small supplements of quick-acting insulin for hyperglycaemia.

- *Low blood glucose values.* Reduce the insulin dose to half to two-thirds of usual dose (sufficient to suppress ketosis, but reduced to prevent hypoglycaemia). Administer fluids as above and check blood glucose hourly until blood glucose levels rise. Be prepared to administer extra quick-acting insulin during the day if blood glucose values rise.
- *Hyperglycaemia but no ketonuria.* Increase the insulin dose by 10%. Give supplements of quick-acting insulin in the dose of 10–20% of the usual total daily dose of long- and short-acting insulin. Measure blood glucose and urine ketone levels 2–4 hourly and repeat quick-acting supplements until normoglycaemia and clearing of ketonuria has been achieved.

Maintain fluids as sugar-containing fluids, the amount not being critical except to maintain hydration. If vomiting persists, or if the parents are concerned, or if you are unsure of the parents' ability to assess their child, or if vomiting extends into the night, it is essential to examine the child for ketosis.

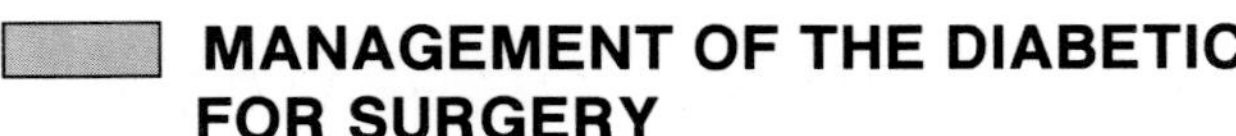

MANAGEMENT OF THE DIABETIC FOR SURGERY

The major aims are to prevent hypoglycaemia during and after surgery and ketoacidosis after surgery. Surgery should not be cancelled on the basis of the diabetic state without consultation with the diabetic team.

ISSUES TO CONSIDER

- Time of surgery
- Length of surgery
- Urgency of surgery

IF ELECTIVE AND OF A MINOR NATURE

Usually aim for morning surgery and for the diabetic to be first on the list. It is usually preferable to have child admitted the day before surgery. Child given normal food and insulin requirements until midnight prior to surgery. Ten per cent dextrose, i.v. commenced at maintenance rates 1 h before surgery. One-sixth of normal total morning insulin requirement given as unmodified insulin before surgery (i.e. if morning dose is 24 units Protophane 4 units Actrapid give 5 units Actrapid). This can be adjusted to individual patient needs. There should be regular blood glucose estimations including one just before leaving the ward.

After surgery, measure blood glucose 2–4 hourly and give extra short-acting insulin (0.25 units/kg) 6 hourly to keep glucose between 5–10 mmol/L. When tolerating oral fluids intravenous infusion can cease, blood glucose monitoring should continue 4–6 hourly and usual evening insulin given before evening meal.

IF SURGERY IS IN AFTERNOON

One-sixth of total morning insulin should be given as short-acting insulin as above and an extra dose of short-acting insulin of same dose given at 1200 h. A light breakfast consisting of the usual number of carbohydrate exchanges is given after the early morning insulin. Intravenous 5% dextrose also started at 1000 h and extra insulin given pre-operatively and postoperatively 4 hourly as required to keep blood glucose levels between 5–10 mmol/L.

SHORT ANAESTHETIC

Intravenous dextrose may not be necessary providing oral intake can be resumed soon after surgery and providing the pre-operative blood glucose concentration is not less than 8 mmol/L. If in doubt about patient's likely postoperative state then it is safer to follow regimen outlined above.

EMERGENCY AND MAJOR SURGERY

In preparing for emergency surgery, the child should first be assessed clinically and biochemically. If ketoacidosis or dehydration is present, urgent correction is required, using intravenous fluid and insulin infusion. The child should have intravenous dextrose/saline infusion and continuous insulin intravenous infusion before, during and after surgery. The initial rate will be between 0.05 and 0.1 units/kg per h according to hourly blood glucose concentration. This should continue until oral feeding is resumed.

TYPES OF INSULIN COMMONLY USED AND TIME OF ACTION IN HOURS AFTER INJECTION

Insulin	*Type*		*Start of effect (h)*	*Maximum effect (peak action; h)*	*End of effect (h)*
*Actrapid HM	Quick, clear		0.5	1–4	Up to 8
*Velosulin Human	Quick, clear		0.5	1–4	Up to 8
Humulin R	Quick, clear		0.5	1–4	Up to 8
*Protaphane HM	Moderately slow, cloudy		1.5	4–12	Up to 24
*Insulatard Human	Moderately slow, cloudy		1.5	4–12	Up to 24
Humulin N.P.H.	Moderately slow, cloudy		1.5	4–12	Up to 24
*Actraphane HM	Mixture	30% Actrapid 70% Protaphane	0.5	3–15	Up to 24
*Mixtard Human 30 : 70	Mixture	30% Velosulin 70% Insulatard	0.5	4–15	Up to 24
*Initard Human Mixtard Human 50 : 50	Mixture	50% Velosulin 50% Insulatard	0.5	4–8	Up to 24
*Mixtard 15 : 85	Mixture	15% Velosulin 85% Insulatard	0.5	4–15	Up to 24
Monotard HM	Moderately slow		3	6–18	Up to 24
Humulin L	Moderately slow		3	6–18	Up to 24
Ultratard HM	Slow		4	8–24	Up to 30
Humulin UL	Slow		4	8–24	Up to 30

*Available also in cartridge form for use in pen.

CHAPTER 21

METABOLIC CONDITIONS

INBORN ERRORS OF METABOLISM

An inborn error of metabolism should be considered in any child presenting with impaired consciousness, seizures, vomiting, hypoglycaemia (see below) or severe acidosis. The majority of presentations are in the neonatal period or during infancy.

Children with suspected or proven inborn errors of metabolism may rapidly deteriorate and die. In all cases, management should be discussed immediately with a metabolic consultant.

INITIAL MANAGEMENT

Investigations

In suspected cases, and especially in emergencies when a consultant may not be immediately available, collect and document the following:

- *Blood:* acid–base, electrolytes, liver function tests; ammonia; amino acids; lactate, ketones, fatty acids (BLF tube); glucose; save 10 mL of heparinized blood for further analysis (freeze the plasma)
- *Urine:* smell; ward test for reducing substances and ketones; save at least 20 mL for a metabolic screen
- *CSF:* if LP done for any reason, freeze 0.5–1.0 mL of CSF immediately (use dry ice if possible) for later metabolic analysis

A provisional metabolic diagnosis can be made by attention to these biochemical results.

TREATMENT

High Dose Dextrose Therapy

This provides sufficient energy to minimize protein catabolism. A higher energy intake is possible if carbohydrate is given orally in the following manner:

Age	*cal/kg per day*	*Polyjoule strength (%)*	*Dose (mL/kg per h)*
0–6 months	123	15	9
6–12 months	100	15	7
1–3 years	90	20	5
4–6 years	85	20	4.5
6–12 years	85	30	3
12–15 years	70	30	2.5
> 15 years	60	30	2.2

Carbohydrate is given as frequent small sips in the nauseated child. Otherwise it is administered 2 hourly in children under 5, and 4 hourly in children over 5 years of age. The minimal acceptable intake is 75% of the prescribed fluid orders over every two consecutive feeds, and 85% of the prescribed intake over 12 h. If this is not achieved, nasogastric or intravenous therapy is initiated.

Small infants may suffer from polyjoule-induced sugar intolerance.

Mineral Supplements are Given Routinely as:

- KCl 2.5 mmol/kg per day in four divided doses
- $NaHCO_3$ 2.5 mmol/kg per day in four divided doses

Blood electrolyte and acid–base disturbances are corrected as necessary by additional mineral supplementation.

Intravenous Therapy is Indicated for:

- Excessive vomiting
- Coma
- Diarrhoea in children with methyl malmonicaciduria or polyjoule sugar intolerance
- Not tolerating oral feeds

Commence 15 or 20% dextrose, by a peripheral or central line, respectively, and run at a rate of maintenance requirements + 20%. Monitor blood glucose strips 2 hourly and aim to achieve levels of between 10 and 20 mmol/L.

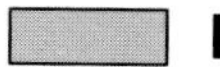

HYPOGLYCAEMIA

Hypoglycaemia frequently presents with a disturbed conscious state and/or seizures. Pallor and sweating may be absent. Hypoglycaemia is defined as a blood glucose less than 2.5 mmol/L. Causes to consider are a range of inborn errors of metabolism, drug ingestion and endocrine disorders which, on presentation in the older child, may mimic ketotic hypoglycaemia.

All children presenting with hypoglycaemia require immediate investigation and treatment.

MANAGEMENT

1 When hypoglycaemia is suspected, perform strip glucose measurement. If low, immediately collect the following specimens using the 'Hypoglycaemia kit' which is found in the Emergency Department or in the Biochemistry Department.

  a At least 5 mL (preferably 8–10 mL) of blood are required and distributed as follows:

  - Fluoride/oxalate tube: 0.5 mL for blood glucose (fill to mark)
  - BLF tube: 1.0 mL collected on to ice, and sent to the laboratory immediately for lactate, ketones and free fatty acids
  - Plain tube: 2–4 mL for insulin, cortisol growth hormone
  - Heparinized tube: 1–2.5 mL for amino acids electrolytes, Ca, Mg
  - Capillary sample: acid-base can be collected after glucose administration

  b Collect approximately 20 mL of urine for a 'metabolic and drug screen'. Ward test for ketones. Urine may be collected after administration of glucose, but delay should be minimal. Bladder tap or catheterization may be necessary.

2 Immediately correct hypoglycaemia by administration of 1–2 mL/kg of 50% dextrose, i.v. Document recovery time. If consciousness remains impaired (common in children with fat oxidation defects), continue intravenous glucose as 15% dextrose at a rate of maintenance + 20%.

3 Remember to document period of fasting, intercurrent illness, drug ingestion (especially alcohol), hepatomegaly and afterwards, muscle bulk, power and tone.

BIOCHEMICAL CHARACTERISTICS OF MAJOR INBORN ERRORS OF METABOLISM

Classification	*Metabolic acidosis*	*Ketosis*	*Lactic acidosis*	*Hyper-ammonaemia*	*Hypo-glycaemia*	*Most common diagnosis*
Aminoacidopathies	–	+ + +	–	–	±	MSUD
Organic acidopathies	+ + +	+ + +	+	+ +	–	MMA, PA, IVA
Primary lactic acidosis	+ + +	+ + +	+ + +	–	±	PDH, PC, RC
Urea cycle defects	–	–	–	+ + +	–	OTC, citrullinaemia, arginosuccinic aciduria
Unusual defects	–	–	–	–	–	Peroxisomopathies sulfite oxidase deficiency, RC, NKH
Hepatic involvement (hepatomegaly/abnormal LFT/hypoglycaemia)	+ + +	+ + +	+ + +	+ / –	+ + +	Galactosaemia tyrosinaemia gluconeogeneis defects, GSD, FAO

MSUD, maple syrup urine disease, MMA, methylmalonic acidaemia; PA, propionic acidaemia; PDH, pyruvate dehydrogenase deficiency; PC, pyruvate carboxylase deficiency; RC, respiratory chain defects; OTC, ornithine transcarbamylase deficiency; NKH, non-ketotic hyperglycinaemia; GSD, glycogen storage diseases; FAO, fatty acid oxidative defects.

CHAPTER 22

IMMUNOLOGY

GUIDELINES FOR INVESTIGATION OF IMMUNODEFICIENCY

If immunodeficiency is present there should be unequivocal evidence of infections (discharging ears, production of purulent sputum) for antibody deficiency, or severe viral infections for T-cell deficiency. A history of recurrent viral respiratory tract secretions in an apparently well child does not suggest significant immunodeficiency even if the infections are very common. Infants with chronic diarrhoea and failure to thrive should have immunoglobulins checked to exclude severe combined immunodeficiency.

Remember that measurement of IgG, A and M and a full blood count is a good screen for most treatable immunodeficiencies. Specific defects of neutrophil function are very rare. If present the patient will almost certainly have gingivitis. Look at the mouth before ordering neutrophil function tests.

Immunoglobulin subclass measurements should only be considered when there is evidence of upper and/or lower respiratory tract suppuration and hypogammaglobulinaemia has been excluded. When considering whether to measure immunoglobulin subclasses you should ask yourself does this clinical condition require regular gammaglobulin therapy if a subclass deficiency is found? If you wish to measure immunoglobulin subclasses in someone who is not IgA deficient and has a normal total IgG level discussion with a clinical immunologist will probably be required.

Measurement of T cell numbers and T cell function by mitogenic stimulation is predominantly of use in the first 6 months of life to help in the diagnosis of severe combined immunodeficiency and Di George syndrome (absent thymus, hypocalcaemia and cardiovascular anomalies). It is less likely to provide useful information thereafter. If in doubt whether immunological function testing is indicated or what test should be ordered consult with a clinical immunologist before ordering expensive and time consuming tests.

CHAPTER 23

DERMATOLOGICAL CONDITIONS

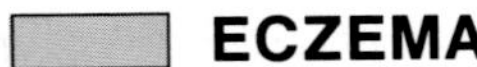

ECZEMA

NATURAL HISTORY

An itching rash appears on the face and sometimes also on the trunk and limbs, usually beginning in the first year of life. Sites of predilection in children over 2 years are the elbow and knee flexures. Spontaneous clearing occurs in most between 3 and 5 years of age.

TREATMENT

1. Avoid dryness by moisturising with simple emollients, Sorbolene + 10% glycerine, aqueous cream, paraffin.
2. Avoid heat over skin. Cool environment and apply cool/tepid compress with soft cotton material to use for itchy and warm areas frequently.
3. Avoid roughness of clothing and extra pressure on skin; use soft materials (e.g. satin).
4. Treat infection early, use topical mupirocin or oral antibiotics (e.g. flucloxacillin).
5. Anti-inflammatory creams/ointments.
   - **a** Steroid creams/ointments:
     - Hydrocortisone cream 0.5–1% applied sparingly to the affected areas twice daily for 2 days on and off is the safest topical steroid.
     - Betamethasone cream 0.01% or 0.02% or other fluorinated steroid creams, of standard strength, are indicated if the response to hydrocortisone cream is inadequate. They should not be applied to the face or nappy area. Use twice daily as above.
     - In young infants skin atrophy and adrenal suppression can occur with continuous use of standard strengths of fluorinated steroid ointments. Systemic steroid administration is not indicated.
   - **b** Zinc and tar ointment: For the management of mild eczema, modified zinc and coal tar ointment is available over the counter as Hamilton's Eczema (Tar) Cream and Ego Cream.
6. Emphasis on treating itch by cool compress early and bandaging or splinting.
7. Diet. The normal diet for the age of the child is indicated. Allergic sensitivity to food is not the only cause of infantile eczema. Urticarial reactions to some foods such as egg occur occasionally; these are sudden reactions. Discontinuation of that particular food is then necessary.
8. Sedation with trimeprazine tartrate, promethazine hydrochloride or chloral hydrate may be indicated.

SEBORRHOEIC DERMATITIS

CLINICAL FEATURES

The onset is normally in early infancy frequently at 6 weeks of life. It is a non-itchy rash characterized by erythema and scaling of the scalp (cradle cap), forehead, eyebrows, retroauricular folds, neck, axillae, groins and gluteal cleft, with patches on the trunk are typical. Napkin area is often involved giving the bipolar appearance scalp/bottom. It usually clears within the first 12 months.

TREATMENT

- Dilute salicylic (1%) and sulfur ointment (1%). This is applied twice daily for a maximum of 2 weeks for the mild rash.
- Hydrocortisone cream at a concentration of 0.5–1% is applied three times a day for the more severe or extensive rash.
- Antidandruff shampoo used once or twice weekly.

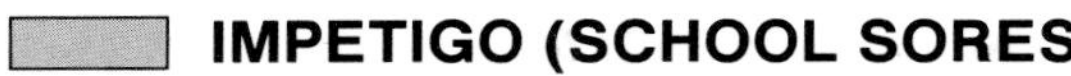

IMPETIGO (SCHOOL SORES)

CLINICAL FEATURES

This is a contagious skin infection caused by both *Staphylococcus aureus* and *Streptococcus pyogenes*. It is characterized by rounded oozing and crusted areas. It may be primary or secondary to some other condition such as eczema, scabies or papular urticaria.

TREATMENT

Bathe off crusts as often as they form with cetrimide 0.1% lotion, saline or soap and water. The topical antibiotic, mupirocin, applied three times a day may be used. Alternatively, systemic antibiotic treatments with oral flucloxacillin or cephalexin may be prescribed especially when lesions are extensive. The patient should be kept away from school until the lesions have been treated.

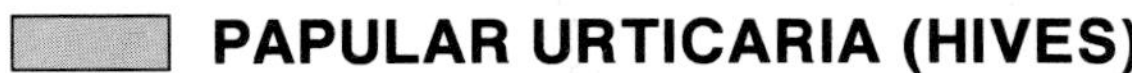

PAPULAR URTICARIA (HIVES)

CLINICAL FEATURES

This is caused by allergic sensitivity to insect bites. Groups of lesions occur most commonly in the warmer weather. There is marked itching and scratching. The lesions are papules 1–5 mm in diameter, with a transient urticarial element, surmounted by a scale, crust, vesicle or pustule.

TREATMENT

Prevention of insect bites is achieved by insecticidal spraying in the home, the use of insect repellants and treatment of pets for insects. An antipruritic lotion such as Liquor Picis Carb. 2% in Calamine lotion may be applied three times daily, or fluorinated steroids may be used. Antihistamines such as promethazine or diphenhydramine are of value. Sedation with chloral hydrate may be added if the antihistamines are inadequate in producing sedation. Secondary infection such as impetigo or pustules should be treated appropriately.

NAPPY RASH (IRRITANT DERMATITIS)

It is usually caused by prolonged contact with urine or faeces. Occasionally soaps and detergents not rinsed from the napkin may contribute.

TREATMENT

Keep the area dry by adequate changing during both day and night. A non-wettable Orlon undernapkin can be helpful. Leaving the napkin off for as long as possible during the day may aid healing. Plastic pants should not be used at night if the rash is severe. Remove faecal material from the skin without delay. Clean the area adequately with warm water.

Napkins should be thoroughly washed and rinsed to remove soap, detergent or disinfectant. At times boiling may be necessary. Zinc cream is used for mild eruptions. Hydrocortisone cream 0.5–1% is used where inflammatory change is more marked.

Note:

- Secondary candidial infection may occur and is indicated by a whitish sodden scaling at the margin of the rash. This is treated with one of the imidazole creams (clotrimazole, miconazole, econazole). Secondary bacterial infection is treated with the appropriate oral and topical antibiotic.
- Seborrhoeic dermatitis presents as a nappy rash involving the skin creases and is treated separately.

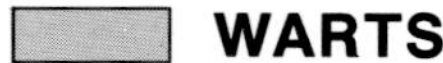

WARTS

ORDINARY WARTS

BFR paint (Royal Children's Hospital) is applied once or twice daily with a sharpened matchstick. Brilliant green, resorcinol and formalin are the constituents of the paint. Regular paring or filing every 2–3 days with pumice, razor blade or nail file will remove the surface horn. Refer to skin clinic if unduly persistent.

PLANTAR WARTS

A small pad of cotton wood soaked in 3% formalin is placed in a saucer on the floor. The area of sole involved is applied to the wool for 30 min each night. Paring every 2 or 3 days is required to remove the surface horn.

PLANE WARTS

These are usually rounded, smooth, flat or slightly elevated skin coloured or pigmented lesions. BFR paint may be applied to lesions on the hands. Refer patients with lesions of the face and elsewhere to the skin clinic.

CUMINATE WARTS

These are soft warts at the mucocutaneous junctions. All patients with this condition should be referred to skin clinic. Do not advise surgery and never use cryotherapy under the age of 10 years.

TINEA CAPITIS (RINGWORM OF THE SCALP)

This is characterized by rounded patches of hair loss with some short lustreless bent hairs a few millimetres in length. Some redness and scaling of the skin area may be present in the patch. Must be diagnosed by microscopy, culture or Wood's light.

It is usually due to *Microsporum canis* infection contracted from a cat or dog. Diagnosis is confirmed by greenish fluorescence with Wood's light. Less commonly it is due to other species of fungus such as *Trichophyton tonsurans*, which cause irregular areas of hair loss, erythema and scaling, and there is no fluorescence to Wood's light. Hairs are taken for microscopy and culture for fungus see p. 178. All children with suspected tinea capitis should be referred to skin clinic. Treatment in skin clinic usually comprises griseofulvin orally 10–15 mg/kg for 4–6 weeks or until non-fluorescent. Children may attend school providing they are being treated.

KERION (INFLAMMATORY RINGWORM)

An elevated, erythematous, tender, boggy swelling discharging pus from multiple points may develop in ringworm of the scalp. These swellings may appear to be fluctuant but incision is to be avoided. All children with suspected kerion should be referred to skin clinic. They are thought to represent an immune response to the tinea. Treatment in skin clinic is oral griseofulvin. Topical and systemic antibiotic therapy may be needed for control of secondary bacterial infection.

TINEA CORPORIS

Lesions are treated with half-strength Whitfield's ointment applied twice daily, or one of the imidazole creams (clotrimazole, miconazole, econazole). Diagnosis must be certain by above criteria.

SCABIES

This is an itchy contagious disease affecting both adults and children, due to infestation with the itch mite, *Sarcoptes scabei*. The characteristic lesion is the burrow, a linear elevation several millimetres in length, which varies in colour depending on the cleanliness of the individual, but is commonly greyish. Burrows are best seen on the hands especially between the fingers. However, in clean individuals the burrows may be very difficult to find. Papules, excoriations and secondary infection may also be present.

TREATMENT

Benzyl benzoate application (APF 1969) is used. Gammabenzene hexachloride 1% (Lorexane) may be toxic to infants. The patient and everyone in the family must carry out treatment at the same time. Paint all the skin surface from neck to toes with the lotion using a 5 cm paint brush. After drying a second coat of the lotion should be painted on to ensure that no area has been missed. The patient should not wash skin, including hands, bathe or shower during the treatment period. One 12 h period is sufficient and no further repeat treatments should be necessary unless microscopy confirms recurrence.

HEAD LICE *(PEDICULOSIS CAPITIS)*

Infestation of the scalp with the *Pediculus capitis* is associated with itching and nits are visible attached to the hairs.

TREATMENT

The agent used is Pyrifoam (pyrethrins 0.165%). Wash the hair thoroughly with soap and water. Thoroughly moisten scalp and hair and leave on overnight. Comb out with a finetoothed comb the following morning. One application should kill all the lice and prevent reinfestation for about 3 weeks. Repeat application after 1 week is usually necessary.

CHAPTER 24

OPHTHALMOLOGICAL CONDITIONS

IMPORTANT PRINCIPLES

- *Always test and record vision* as the first part of any eye examination. In infants note following and other visual behaviour, and listen to parents' impression about their child's vision.
- *A child with a squint is never too young to be seen.* Transient malalignment of the eyes is common up to 6 months of age. A child with a constant squint at any age, or any transient squint after 6 months of age, should be referred to an ophthalmologist promptly. True squints, in general, never get better by themselves.
- *Never pad a discharging eye.*
- *Always pad an eye into which local anaesthetic has been instilled* for the removal of a foreign body.
- *Do not use local steroid drops* unless corneal ulceration has been excluded by fluorescein staining. Then only use them for short periods (2 days or less) without consulting an ophthalmologist.
- *X-ray the orbit (AP and lateral) if an intraocular foreign body is suspected* from the history, even though the eye may appear normal.
- In cases of photophobia or watery eyes in the first year of life, when there is no significant discharge, *consider the possibility of congenital glaucoma.*
- All children with a *white red reflex or white masses in the retina* must be referred immediately to an ophthalmologist to exclude retinoblastoma.

TRAUMA

FOREIGN BODIES

If a foreign body or corneal ulcer is suspected instil one drop of local anaesthetic to ease the pain and facilitate examination. Suitable local anaesthetics are Ophthaine 1%, Amethocaine 0.5 or 1% or Benoxinate 0.4%. Do not use local anaesthetics for the continuing treatment of ocular pain under any circumstance.

Conjunctival

These are common and are often found on the posterior surface of the upper lid. Therefore, eversion of the lid is essential. Most foreign bodies are easily removed with a moist cotton wool swab. If they are embedded or difficult to remove, refer the patient to the duty ophthalmologist.

Corneal

If not readily removed with a moistened cotton wool swab, refer to the duty ophthalmologist. Beware of an iris nevus and iris prolapse through a perforating injury of the cornea mimicking a corneal foreign body.

Intraocular

These are generally high velocity fragments. Suspect if the history involves an explosion, striking metal on metal, or any other situation involving high speed objects (i.e. power tools, lawn mower). If the history is at all suggestive, even in the absence of local signs, X-ray of the orbit (AP and lateral) is necessary. If an intraocular foreign body is demonstrated, immediate referral to the duty ophthalmologist is mandatory.

EYELID INJURIES

All eyelid lacerations, except the most minor, should be repaired as an inpatient procedure. Suspect canalicular injury in all lacerations involving the medial aspect of the eyelids and refer to the duty ophthalmologist.

HYPHAEMA (BLOOD IN THE ANTERIOR CHAMBER)

This generally requires admission to hospital. All cases require ophthalmic referral, as there is a potential for secondary haemorrhage and loss of vision.

FRACTURE OF THE ORBITAL BONES

A blow-out fracture through the wall of the orbit is suspected if one or more of the following three cardinal signs are present:

- Restricted movement of the eye, particularly in a vertical plane, with double vision
- Infraorbital nerve anaesthesia
- Enophthalmos: this may be difficult to assess initially because of haemorrhage

Diagnosis is most often clinical. Plain X-rays and CT scan are used to demonstrate fracture of orbital wall and entrapped orbital tissue (classical sign if tear drop 'polyp' hanging from roof of the maxillary antrum). Refer to the duty ophthalmologist.

PENETRATING INJURY

It should always be considered in patients with lacerations involving the eyelids, particularly after motor car accidents. Suspect if the pupil is distorted or iris is prolapsing through the cornea or pigmented tissue is seen over the sclera. If suspected protect the eye with a cone or shield that places no pressure on the eyelids or eye and admit. Prevent vomiting with antiemetic. Refer to duty ophthalmologist immediately.

CHEMICAL BURNS

Irrigate the eye with saline or water copiously for 15 min. Instillation of local anaesthetic will facilitate this. Intravenous solution administered by a giving set is a practical method of irrigation. Refer all chemical burns to the duty ophthalmologist. Most alkali burns will require admission.

THERMAL BURNS

The ocular surface is rarely involved. Check for ulceration with fluorescein staining.

Butesin pictrate ointment is suitable for use on lid burns. Secondary lid swelling may result in corneal exposure and ocular lubricants are then required.

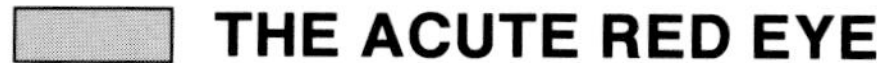

THE ACUTE RED EYE

Common causes of the acute red eye are conjunctivitis, corneal ulceration, corneal or conjunctival foreign body (see above) and iritis.

CONJUNCTIVITIS

Aetiology

- Bacterial — generally pus present
- Viral — generally watery discharge
- Allergic — history of atopy and 'itchy eyes'

Neonatal Conjunctivitis (Ophthalmia Neonatorum)

Aetiology

Neisseria gonorrhoeae: Acute severe, purulent discharge associated with marked conjunctival and lid oedema (clinical appearance is of 'pus under pressure'). Occurs within a few days of birth. This is an ocular emergency because of the risk of corneal perforation.

- Diagnosis. Urgent Gram stain for Gram negative intracellular diplococci and direct culture to appropriate culture media.
- Treatment. Admit and give intravenous penicillin or ceftriaxone. Local measures such as ocular lavage and topical antibiotics (chloramphenicol or neomycin) may be of help. Investigate and treat mother and partner.

Chlamydia: Causes about 30% of sticky eyes in the neonatal period. Fails to respond to routine topical antibiotics. Untreated there is a risk of pneumonitis.

- Diagnosis. Giemsa stain of conjunctival scraping for intranuclear inclusions. Also antibodies in tears and immunofluorescent stains of conjunctival scrapes.
- Treatment. Oral erythromycin and eye toilet. Investigate and treat mother and partner.

Other bacteria: Generally caused by *Staphylococcus*, *Streptococcus* or diphtheroids. Culture and treat with neomycin or chloramphenicol eye drops. Rapid clinical response anticipated.

Blocked nasolacrimal duct: Mucopurulent discharge with watery eye. Discharge worse upon waking and conjunctiva is not inflamed.

Chemical: Purulent discharge with lid oedema seen within 24 h of instillation of silver nitrate prophylaxis. Treatment: frequent lavage and topical neomycin.

Conjunctivitis in Older Children

Management:

Bacterial: Chloramphenicol eye drops 2 hourly by day and ointment at night.

Viral: Usually clears spontaneously. Neomycin eye drops may be given.

Herpes simplex conjunctivitis: Suspect if have lid vesicles, check for corneal ulceration and treat with 4 hourly idoxuridine ointment. Refer to the duty ophthalmologist.

Allergic: Mild cases use astringent (phenylephrine 1/8% or naphazoline 0.1%). Moderate cases use topical antihistamine (antazoline 0.5%). In severe cases refer to the duty ophthalmologist.

CORNEAL ULCERATION

Aetiology

- Trauma (with or without a foreign body)
- Herpes simplex (dendritic ulcer)

Diagnosis

Pain, photophobia, lacrimation and blepharospasm. Fluorescein stain after instillation of local anaesthetic.

Treatment

- Traumatic: chloramphenicol ointment and pad. Review in 24 h, if not healed in 48 h refer to duty ophthalmologist.
- Herpes simplex: idozuridine eye ointment and refer to next eye clinic.

IRITIS

Rare in children. Symptoms as for corneal ulcer. Pupil small and does not react well to light. Refer to the duty ophthalmologist.

PRE-SEPTAL (PERIORBITAL) AND ORBITAL CELLULITIS

Both conditions present with erythematous, swollen lids in a febrile, unwell child. In pre-septal cellulitis the lid swelling frequently prevents eye opening. The lids must be separated to exclude proptosis and limitation of eye movement (important signs of orbital cellulitis). A bent paper clip or a Desmarre's lid retractor may be used for this. Orbital cellulitis generally presents with proptosis and restriction of eye movements and is associated with sinusitis. Proptosis may be so severe that it prevents lid closure and corneal exposure may result. Bilateral orbital (or pre-septal cellulitis) may be associated with cavernous sinus thrombosis.

TREATMENT

All cases require admission (at the Royal Children's Hospital under General Paediatrics) and intravenous antibiotics. Refer all cases to ophthalmology and all cases of orbital cellulitis to ENT. Cases of orbital cellulitis require urgent CT scan to identify sinus pathology.

STRABISMUS OR SQUINT

Refer all children with squint or suspected squint to the eye clinic. This will allow amblyopia to be detected early, and perhaps prevented, and will enable any underlying pathology such as retinoblastoma to be detected. A child does not 'grow out of' a squint. However, babies in the first few months of life may have an intermittent squint, especially when feeding. If the parents report a squint the child should be referred to the eye clinic. All children with a first degree relative with a squint should have an eye examination at about $2\frac{1}{2}$ years of age.

A pseudo-strabismus (pseudo-squint) is due to a broad nasal bridge, and/or epicanthic folds. This results in the appearance of a squint, but corneal light reflexes are central and there is no movement on cover testing. Only make the diagnosis of pseudo-strabismus if absolutely certain, refer doubtful cases to the eye clinic.

BLOCKED TEAR DUCT

This is a common cause for discharge which persists after the first 2 weeks of life. It usually resolves spontaneously, due to opening of the lower end of the nasolacrimal duct. If infection is troublesome topical neomycin eye drops may be given (avoid repeated courses of chloramphenicol). Massage over the tear sac after each feed. If discharge and watering have not settled by 9 months of age refer to eye clinic for possible probing.

CONGENITAL GLAUCOMA

This is a rare condition, but early recognition is vital as prompt surgery offers a chance of cure and preservation of vision. All infants with suspected glaucoma require examination under anaesthesia to measure corneal diameter, optic disc cupping and intraocular pressure. Presenting features:

- Hazy cornea
- Enlarged cornea
- Watery eyes
- Photophobia (severe)

CONGENITAL CATARACTS

Congenital cataracts are rare, but early detection and removal with subsequent optical correction (contact lenses or spectacles), offers a good chance of visual preservation. All newborn infants should have their red reflexes examined prior to discharge from hospital. Check the red reflexes and fundi in any infant with poor visual performance (fixation and following). Nystagmus is a late sign for congenital cataracts. A child thought to have a congenital cataract must be referred urgently.

CHAPTER 25

ORTHOPAEDIC CONDITIONS

FRACTURES

If soreness persists following injury, assume it is a fracture even if the initial X-ray is normal; sprains are rare in children.

At the Royal Children's Hospital children with significant fractures are to be seen by or consulted with the orthopaedic registrar, who will advise on treatment. Plasters should be thin and padded. Plaster cylinders should be used rather than plaster slabs as the latter break easily. Except for minor greenstick fractures, plasters around the wrist and ankle should extend above the elbow or knee. If swelling is anticipated, split the plaster and padding throughout its length.

At the Royal Children's Hospital all families are to be given verbal and written plaster care instructions which emphasize the need to elevate the injured limb and the need to return to the Emergency Department if features of a tight plaster develop. All children with fractures, whether displaced or not, should be reviewed the following day at an orthopaedic clinic (weekdays) or emergency (weekend) and checked for :

- **The presence of pain**
- **The circulation and sensation of toes and fingers**
- **The integrity of the plaster**

Some children with minor fractures may be referred back to their family doctor by the orthopaedic staff. Otherwise all children are reviewed 1 week later in an orthopaedic clinic to verify that the fracture position has been maintained.

ACUTE LIMP

An acute limp may be due to injury, osteomyelitis, arthritis or spinal lesions. Local bone or joint tenderness localizes the site to be X-rayed. The following conditions need to be considered:

IRRITABLE HIP SYNDROME

An acute limp with restricted hip motion may be due to the irritable hip syndrome. If the child is generally well, afebrile, and if there is only slight restriction of movement, the child may rest at home and attend the orthopaedic outpatient clinic the following day. Otherwise the child should be admitted for further assessment and treatment.

SEPTIC ARTHRITIS

A child with an acute arthritis with limited motion and pyrexia should be admitted to hospital with suspected septic arthritis. Unless an alternative diagnosis can be established immediately, the child is managed as having an acute bacterial arthritis. Blood is collected in emergency for a full blood examination and erythrocyte sedimentation rate and for culture. Following admission, the joint is aspirated or opened under general anaesthesia and specimens are sent for culture and histology. Antibiotics that are effective against *Staphylococcus aureus* and *Haemophilus influenzae* are then given intravenously.

OSTEOMYELITIS

A child with an acute febrile illness and metaphyseal tenderness should be admitted to hospital with suspected acute osteomyelitis. In emergency, blood is collected for a full blood examination and erythrocyte sedimentation rate and for culture. An intravenous drip is inserted. The orthopaedic registrar will order antibiotics which are effective against *S. aureus*.

CHRONIC LIMP

A limp persisting for weeks or months needs careful assessment and the following conditions need to be considered:

Perthes' Disease of the Hip

This diagnosis should be suspected in young boys with a chronic limp and intermittent pain. Hip motion is restricted. An anteroposterior X-ray of the pelvis and lateral X-rays of the hips are required to confirm the diagnosis. The child should be referred to the orthopaedic outpatients.

Slipped Upper Femoral Epiphysis

This condition occurs in older children and young teenagers. The limp is often painless and hip motion is restricted. Anteroposterior and lateral X-rays of both hips will confirm the diagnosis. Urgent referral to the orthopaedic department is required. Rarely, the slip occurs acutely and requires immediate admission to hospital.

BONE TUMOURS

Chronic limp is a common presentation of malignant bone tumours, such as osteosarcoma. Careful assessment is required. If the X-rays show a likely tumour, the child requires admission to hospital for assessment and treatment.

POSTURE AND GAIT

Children at different ages have characteristic postures. It is important to give an explanation of postural development to parents.

FLAT FEET

When infants start walking they have flat feet. Arches develop over the next 4–5 years in 85% of children and most of those with persisting flat feet do not require treatment. However, advice may be given concerning footwear if there is excessive wear to the shoes.

BOW LEGS

These are very common in normal children up to the age of 2 years and very seldom require treatment. If gross bowing is present after the age of 2 years, refer for orthopaedic opinion. Rickets or skeletal dysplasias may present as severe bow legs.

KNOCK KNEES

These are also very common in normal children between $2\frac{1}{2}$ and 7 years and rarely require treatment. Obesity, if present, requires treatment.

IN-TOED GAIT

This is due to inset hips, internal tibial torsion or metatarsus adductus. Metatarsus adductus is present at birth. Internal tibial torsion is common between 1 and 3 years and is often accompanied by bow legs. Inset hips are common from 2 to 6 years. Spontaneous improvement is usual and only severe degrees require orthopaedic opinion.

OUT-TOED GAIT

An outset posture of the legs is due to an excessive range of external rotation of the hips and is a normal variant at birth. It usually corrects within the first year but may persist for 1–2 years and produce an out-toed gait. It can be expected to correct spontaneously.

CHAPTER 26

BURNS

AIMS OF TREATMENT

- Prevent and treat burn shock
- Prevent infection
- Obtain early skin cover
- Prevent hypertrophic scar formation
- Restore function and correct cosmetic defects

ASSESSMENT

AGE

The younger the child, the more likely is shock to occur for a given extent of burn.

ESTIMATION OF THE SURFACE AREA BURNED

The usual adult formula (rule of nines) is not applicable to children because the proportions contributed by the head and limbs vary at different ages. The burned areas should be plotted accurately on the body chart and the area calculated with the aid of the table (see Lund-Browder Chart p. 160). The extent of the burn only rarely is underestimated. Overestimation is common and frequently leads to excessive fluid administration.

ASSESSMENT OF THE DEPTH OF BURN

Depth of burn	*Degree*	*Cause*	*Surface/colour*	*Pain sensation*	*Treatment*
Superficial (partial loss of skin)	1st degree	Sun, flash; minor scald	Dry, minor blisters, erythema	Painful	Expose
	2nd degree	Scald	Moist whitish	Painful	Non-adherent dressing
	Deep 2nd degree	Scald, minor flame contact	Moist white slough, red mottled	Painless	Graft otherwise scarring
Deep (complete loss of skin)	3rd degree	Flame, severe scald or contact	Dry, charred whitish	Painless	Graft

In most burns, there are varying grades of injury.

LUND-BROWDER CHART

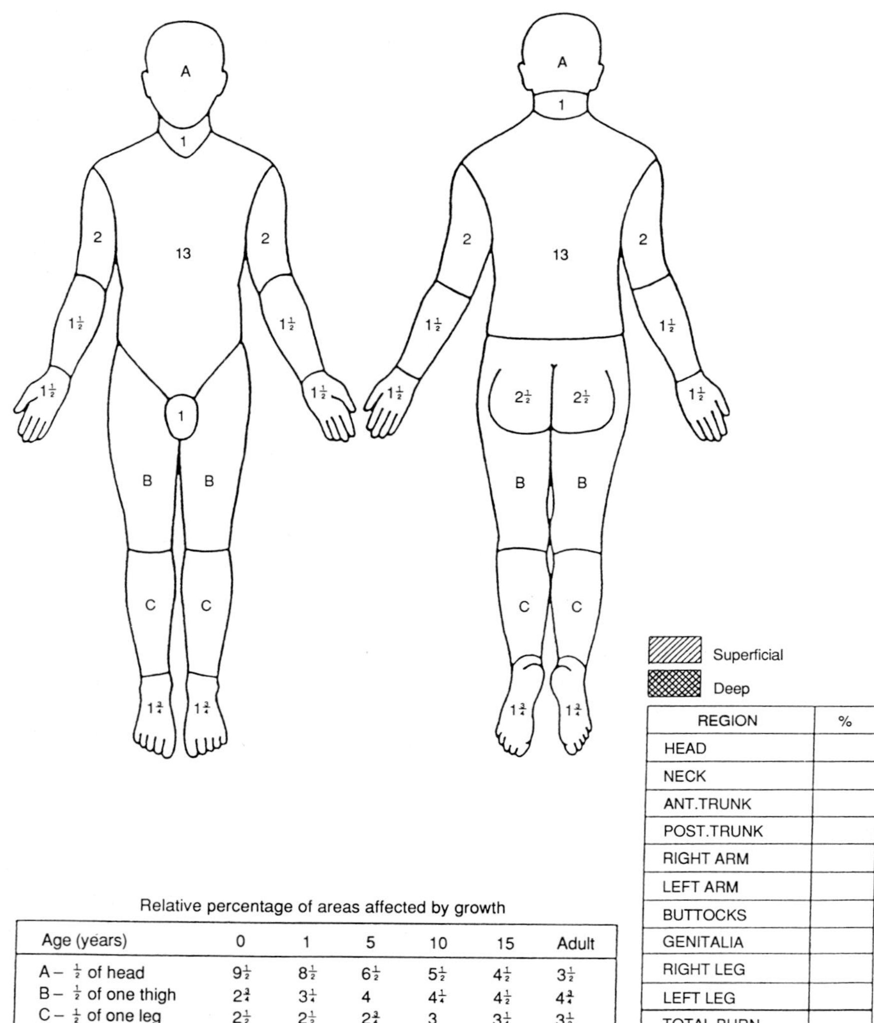

Relative percentage of areas affected by growth

Age (years)	0	1	5	10	15	Adult
A – ½ of head	9½	8½	6½	5½	4½	3½
B – ½ of one thigh	2¾	3¼	4	4¼	4½	4¾
C – ½ of one leg	2½	2½	2¾	3	3¼	3½

REGION	%
HEAD	
NECK	
ANT.TRUNK	
POST.TRUNK	
RIGHT ARM	
LEFT ARM	
BUTTOCKS	
GENITALIA	
RIGHT LEG	
LEFT LEG	
TOTAL BURN	

MANAGEMENT

FIRST AID

Instantly remove clothing or smother flame and apply cold water.

Continue cold water application in bowl or by compress for up to 60 min in minor burn and bathe for 20 min while awaiting transport to hospital, in major burn. Guard against hypothermia or cold injury.

Major burns are covered in a special foam transport dressing (if available) or a clean sheet, and blanket for warmth and given intravenous infusion, oxygen and morphine, if necessary, before admission to hospital.

BURN CONSULTATION SERVICE AT THE ROYAL CHILDREN'S HOSPITAL

Within the Royal Children's Hospital the burns surgeon on duty is available for consultation regarding the resuscitation and transfer of any child with a burn injury (03) 345 5522.

MINOR BURNS

Superficial burns of less than 8% of the body surface are suitable for outpatient treatment unless they occur on the face, neck, hands, feet or perineum. Infants under the age of 12 months are at risk and are more likely to require admission.

Treatment

Initial:

- Blisters should be left intact
- Gently cleanse, remove loose skin
- Dress with tulle gras and an absorbent dressing
- Immobilize with a first crepe bandage, plaster slab or sling if indicated

Subsequent:

- Leave the initial dressing for 5–8 days. If the dressing is soaked by exudate, redress as necessary without disturbing the adherent tulle.
- Consider grafting to the residual areas if healing is not complete by the second to third week. Graft deep 2nd degree burns by 5–10 days.
- Pain, fever and soiled or offensive dressings indicate that the dressing should be changed earlier than anticipated.

MAJOR BURNS

Superficial burns greater than 8% of the body surface area and deep burns require admission to hospital. Transfer should be considered in any child with a burn greater than 15%. Older children with more extensive superficial burns such as sunburn may be managed as outpatients. See Lund-Browder chart at the end of this chapter.

Treatment

- *Prevent and treat shock.* Intravenous therapy usually is required for burns greater than 12–15%, even though clinical shock is not evident at time of admission.
- *Prevent infection.* Careful ward management to guard against cross-infection. Antibiotics are not prescribed routinely.

Procedure

A brief history should document the time, causative agent and circumstances of the burn, the therapy already given and the child's general health. Insert intravenous line. Patients with severe burns may need a central venous line for recording central venous pressure. Draw blood for baseline laboratory studies to include haemoglobin and haematocrit, serum electrolytes and in severe burns blood grouping and cross-matching. Plan intravenous therapy (see below) and commence treatment with stable plasma protein solution (SPPS). Insert urethral catheter for hourly urine volume in all patients with burns greater than 15%. Weigh if possible, otherwise estimate weight. Extent and depth of burn is estimated carefully and charted. Analgesia or sedation as necessary using morphine intravenously or chloral orally. Morphine intravenously is given diluted as a continuous infusion, the rate of which is adjusted every 15 min until response is achieved. Morphine usually is not used in infants. Tetanus prophylaxis is given as indicated (see p. 69).

Burns care involves taking swabs of the burnt areas as well as nose, throat and rectum, to detect infection followed by limited debridement and dressings (see below). Escharotomies should be considered if the peripheral circulation to a limb is jeopardized.

Respiratory difficulties require particular attention, including possible need for intensive care or escharotomy to the trunk. Observation of general condition, pulse, respiration rate, temperature, BP and fluid balance including hourly urine output estimations are necessary.

Fluid Resuscitation

Fluid volume

Three millilitres per kilogram of bodyweight per 1% burn surface area for the first 24 h. In less severe burns 2 ml/kg bodyweight per 1% BSA may be sufficient.

Type of fluid

Colloid, SPPS or substitutes, should constitute one-quarter (in burns greater than 20%), one-third (in burns greater than 30%), one-half (in burns greater than 40%) fluid requirement depending on the depth and extent of the burn, the remainder is given as Hartmann's solution in 5% dextrose.

Fluid Maintenance

For volume of fluid (see p. 43).

Type of fluid

Use 1/2 isotonic saline in 5% dextrose to provide extra sodium.

Rate of infusion

In first 24 h:

- First 8 h one-half resuscitation fluid + one-third maintenance fluid
- Second 8 h one-quarter resuscitation fluid + one-third maintenance fluid
- Third 8 h one-quarter resuscitation fluid + one-third maintenance fluid

The 24 h period commences from the time of burning, not from the time of admission. Adjustments are made according to the hourly urine output which is the best guide to the adequacy of fluid replacement.

Expected flow is 0.75 mL/kg per h, and infusion rate is adjusted to this urine flow. In the infant and toddler a urine output of up to 1.0 mL/kg per h, is required.

Specific gravity of the urine is recorded, as is osmolality of urine and serum if poor renal function. Repeated haemoglobin, haematocrit and electrolyte estimations are made. Restlessness may indicate inadequate fluid replacement.

Second 24 h and onwards: Replacement fluid = approximately one-half volume for first 24 h. Maintenance fluid as before. Total volume is given at an even rate over 24 h, and the volume and type of fluid given are adjusted on urine flow and electrolyte estimations and decreased as shock diminishes over the succeeding days. Diuresis occurs 3–5 days post-burn.

Blood

Whole blood is required initially only in severe, deep burns, and then usually after the first 24 h post-burn when the haemoglobin concentration is falling.

Oral fluids

Gastric dilatation associated with vomiting may occur and if so a nasogastric tube should be inserted. Most children after 4–8 h tolerate small amounts of milk (30–60 mL/h). In minor burns commence oral fluids earlier. If this is tolerated, increase quantity 4 hourly. After 48 h, the majority of fluid intake is usually oral. Children who refuse to drink or who have burns to the face and mouth may require tube feeding.

Local Wound Care

Minimal debridement of loose skin is performed initially and then management continues by exposed or closed methods.

Exposure:

- Indications — for burns on face, perineum, or one surface area of the trunk.
- Treatment — allow eschar to form if superficial or apply topical silver sulfadiazine cream. Daily bath is given with warm water, mild soap and application of antibiotic cream.

Closed:

- Indications — for small children and burns on extremities. Except for face and perineum nearly all children are ultimately nursed with closed dressings.
- Treatment — an antiseptic tulle gras and gauze for superficial burns or topical silver sulfadiazine cream and Melolin for deep burns. Fingers and toes are separated with non-adherent tulle and wrapped together, not separately. Daily bath is given with warm water and mild soap, before the dressing.

Antibiotics

These usually are given only for proven infection and on the basis of sensitivity tests. On admission, swabs are taken of the burn area, nose, throat, and rectum, and the burn area is reswabbed twice weekly. If septicaemia is suspected clinically, blood culture should be performed and antibiotics such as gentamicin and flucloxacillin are commenced.

Nutrition

All children receive a high calorie diet containing adequate proteins and vitamins and iron supplements. In severe burns there is a marked increase in metabolic rate and gastric tube feeding with a complete fluid diet (e.g. Isocal, Osmolite) is instituted early over each 24 h of the day and is adjusted to hold or make a gain in bodyweight. A dietitian is involved.

Room Temperature

It is desirable that this is in the range of 22–26°C. If a child is partly exposed and nursed in a cool environment, metabolic requirements will increase.

Special Therapy

Institute physiotherapy and occupational therapy early and continue throughout the course of burn care. Splints and pressure dressings are necessary to control hypertrophic scar formation. The play therapist also has an important role.

Social rehabilitation is important as many burned children come from disadvantaged homes. Maltreated children constitute approximately 6% of admissions to the burns unit. Psychological and psychiatric consultation often is required and the hospital teacher liaises with the child's school teachers.

Follow-up

Within Victoria the District Nursing service provides care in the home, between outpatient consultations. Healed burns and grafts are kept soft with emollient. Parents and children need support and further operations are sometimes necessary to correct contractures and relieve cosmetic defects.

CHAPTER 27

EAR, NOSE AND THROAT CONDITIONS

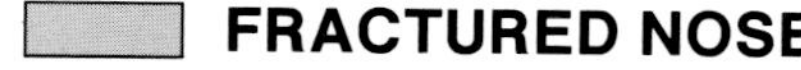

FRACTURED NOSE

There are two common types:

FRACTURE FROM A FRONTAL BLOW

This is common in toddlers and is frequently due to a fall flat on the face.

Signs

Generalized swelling. Palpable dip just below the midpoint of the nose. Thickening of the septum to a variable degree due to septal haematoma.

X-rays

A lateral X-ray may show a backward displacement of a chip of the lower margin of the nasal bone. This may be performed in the presence of soft tissue swelling.

FRACTURE FROM A LATERAL BLOW

This is more common in older children.

Signs

Nasal deformity: the nasal skeleton is pushed to one side, visibly and palpably. Septal displacement or buckling. X-rays rarely indicated.

Management

Fractures unite early. If the diagnosis is suspected refer promptly to a plastic surgeon or ENT surgeon as reduction must be arranged within a few days.

Complications

Septal haematoma: this is detected by testing the patency of the airways and examining the septum with an auriscope or nasal speculum. Urgent referral to the ENT unit is required as an untreated sizeable haematoma will progress within 24 h to septal cartilage necrosis, abscess and eventual saddle nose deformity. Admission to hospital is usually indicated, as surgical drainage is necessary.

Associated Injuries

- Orbital fracture producing enophthalmos and diplopia
- Fracture of the infraorbital margin, malar and zygoma
- Head injury with skull fracture or concussion

EPISTAXIS

MANAGEMENT OF ACUTE CASES

Digital Pressure

Pressure is applied to the nose just below nasal bones by compression of the lateral cartilages for at least 10 min, with patient upright.

Topical Local Anaesthetic and Adrenaline

Initially spray with xylocaine pressure pack. Then soak pledgets of cotton wool in a solution of cocaine 0.2% and adrenaline 1 in 20 000. Apply to the bleeding point for 15–20 min. Pressure for a longer time may cause necrosis.

Treatment of Bleeding Point

The patient should be referred if bleeding continues after removal of the cocaine and adrenaline packs because cautery by heat or chemical means may be required.

MANAGEMENT OF CHRONIC CASES

Examination must include inspection inside the nose and of the post-nasal space. The source of bleeding needs to be localized and is best achieved by use of cocaine/adrenaline packing as above. Referral to an ENT specialist is recommended. If a bleeding disorder is suspected initial management includes appropriate blood tests.

FOREIGN BODY IN THE NOSE

A patient with a long-standing foreign body in the nose presents with a foul-smelling blood-stained unilateral nasal discharge. The patient may require sedation and/or local anaesthetic for examination. Use a local anaesthetic solution of cocaine 2% and adrenaline 1 in 20 000 solution soaked in a pledget of cotton wool. This take 5–10 min to act. An auriscope is useful for nasal examination.

REMOVAL

A good light source is necessary. A hook made from a dental broach with the end 2 mm bent at the right angle is usually safe and effective for removal of a nasal foreign body. Alternatively, place the flat end of a blunt or ring probe along the floor of the nostril under the foreign body. Depress the handle of the probe so that the flat end rotates upward and forward and pushes out the foreign body. Occasionally suction may adhere to a foreign body and facilitate its removal. If difficulty is encountered referral to an ENT specialist is indicated.

FOREIGN BODY IN OESOPHAGUS

The patient may present with initial retching and vomiting, dysphagia, salivation and refusal to eat. Occasionally cough, stridor or wheeze are the only symptoms, especially in infants less than 18 months old. Retrotracheal tenderness on lateral pressure is an important sign.

REMOVAL

Removal should be performed as soon as possible since the complications of oesophageal perforation are dangerous. X-ray of the chest, abdomen and lateral of the soft tissue of the neck should be performed. If a foreign body is evident in the oesophagus on X-ray or if the X-ray is clear and the clinical features suggest an oesophageal foreign body the child should be admitted under the ENT unit or the thoracic unit.

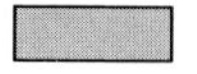

FOREIGN BODY IN THE EAR

Have one attempt at removal before calling for help. Good light is essential. This is best provided by a head worn light and viewing system.

REMOVAL

- Hook. The most commonly useful is a dental broach with the end 2 mm bent at a right angle.
- Grasping instruments: should be used only for soft non-friable foreign bodies such as cloth and paper.
- Syringing. Only use this method if the drum is intact and for friable material such as sand.
- Sucker. This is best for a tightly impacted spherical object. A large soft rubber catheter with its end cut at right angles to its axis is used.

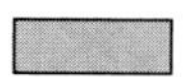

FISH BONE IN THE THROAT

In almost all cases, fish bones are caught in the base of the tongue or in a tonsil. They rarely reach the oesophagus. Fish bones are radiolucent so X-rays are unhelpful. Differential diagnosis is a scratch or infection. As complications are rare, in doubtful cases observe for 24 h.

REMOVAL

Most can be removed after application of a local anaesthetic.

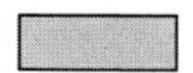

ACUTE INJURIES TO THE EAR

AETIOLOGY

- Direct trauma to the drum by a cotton bud or twig
- Indirect trauma to the drum such as a slap over the ear or a pressure wave with water
- Fracture of the petrous temporal bone following head injury

MANAGEMENT

Ruptured ear drums heal spontaneously in 80% of cases. During this time, water must be excluded from the ear canal. Blue Tac or cotton wool made greasy with Vaseline make excellent ear plugs. Uncommonly, a tympanic membrane tear forms a triangular flap with the edge rolled inwards. These cases require surgical treatment.

Oral antibiotics should be given after water-related injuries. Urgent surgical referral is indicated if the ear injury is associated with petrous temporal bone fracture. Suggestive symptoms include canal skin laceration, drum rupture, ossicular disruption, CSF leak and facial nerve damage, cochlear damage with sensorineural deafness, vestibular damage with vertigo.

SERIOUS OTITIS MEDIA

See also p. 78. Minor glue ear (e.g. brief duration, unilateral, air fluid mixture) does not require treatment as with time there is frequently improvement in middle ear ventilation. Persisting severe glue ear with significant hearing impairment may need treatment by insertion of ventilating tubes.

OTITIS EXTERNA

External ear infection is suggested by tragal tenderness and pain on movement of the pinna (e.g. chewing). Thorough cleaning of debris is essential to distinguish external from middle ear infection unless swelling and tenderness of the meatus prevent this. Extension of infection to the post-auricular lymph nodes may be difficult to distinguish from acute mastoiditis.

MANAGEMENT

Analgesia: wetting of the ear should be avoided. Thorough cleaning of the external auditory canal meatus is essential wherever possible. This particularly applies to fungal infections suggested by spores, mycelia or 'wet blotting paper' debris. Syringing of an ear with otitis externa is generally contraindicated.

Direct application of the appropriate antibiotic ointment or drops is used where the swelling is slight. If marked, pack the ear with a gauze strip impregnated with the appropriate medicament. Neomycin ointment is recommended for a furuncle. Soframycin drops are indicated if there is diffuse cellulitis. Kenacomb ointment or Sofradex or Aerocortin drops are recommended for diffuse bacterial infection (usually Gram negative) which may be primary or secondary to eczema, seborrhoea or foreign body. Locacortin Vioform drops are useful for fungal infection. Acute bullous haemorrhagic otitis, often associated with myringitis and pharyngitis, is treated symptomatically with analgesia. Local analgesia with Auralgin ear drops. Parenteral analgesia is also recommended. Systemic antibiotics are needed if pain is severe or if there is regional lymphadenopathy.

POST-TONSILLECTOMY HAEMORRHAGE

REACTIONARY HAEMORRHAGE

Restlessness and excessive swallowing may be the only early clinical indication of haemorrhage, especially in association with bleeding from the adenoidal bed. Pallor and alteration in pulse and blood pressure may also be noted.

Management

Careful repeated observations are taken. The patient is placed with the head of the bed raised if he is in good condition or lowered if in poor condition. Special measures will depend on the pharyngeal examination. Removal of a blood clot from the tonsillar fossa may be curative. The patient should be referred immediately to an ENT specialist if there is tonsillar fossa bleeding requiring treatment, continued bleeding from the adenoidal bed or if the site of bleeding is uncertain. If blood loss is significant or bleeding continues, an intravenous line is established for fluid/blood replacement.

SECONDARY HAEMORRHAGE

This occurs usually 7–10 days after operation and is generally the result of an adherent thrombus separating from tonsillar or adenoidal bed. Infection may also be an aetiological factor. Bleeding tends to be slow from numerous small vessels.

Management

Admission for careful observation and antibiotics is usually indicated. Blood transfusion is occasionally necessary.

ORBITAL CELLULITIS

Most cases of this condition follow an upper respiratory infection and most have an underlying sinusitis as the basis of transmission to the orbit. Early consultation with ENT and ophthalmology is advised. Proptosis and ophthalmoplegia are very serious signs and usually indicate an abscess. Antibiotics administered intravenously give the quickest resolution. Drainage may be necessary and X-rays of sinuses are helpful in the evaluation of the degree of sinus involvement.

CHAPTER 28

DENTAL CONDITIONS

EMERGENCIES

Within the Royal Children's Hospital the Department of Dentistry provides separate consultative services for more difficult paediatric dental problems and for major traumatic injuries. The dentist and oral surgeon 'on call' can be contacted via the switchboard. During normal hospital hours simple Emergency Department problems (such as non-urgent toothache in a normal child) should be referred to Royal Dental Hospital of Melbourne or the local dentist.

After hours emergencies:

Royal Dental Hospital of Melbourne 341 0222 (weekends 341 0427)
Weekdays: 1800–2115 h
Saturdays: 0900–2115 h
Sundays and public holidays: 0900–2115 h

or the local dentist.

TOOTHACHE AND INFECTION

Patients presenting with toothache or dental abscess and who have severe pain, elevated temperature, obvious facial swelling and/or associated lymph node involvement will require treatment with antibiotics such as penicillin (drug of first choice or erythromycin) and may need admission. A dental consultation should be made immediately for all such patients.

Children with intermittent toothache only after eating (but not the severe spontaneous pain at night which is indicative of pulpitis, peridontitis or early abscess) should be given analgesia and referred to a dentist.

LOCAL BLEEDING FROM THE MOUTH

Always wear gloves, reassure the patient and parents. Remove all blood clot with a gauze swab and identify source of bleeding such as a soft tissue laceration or bleeding from tooth socket (bone). If possible wash out patient's mouth with cold water.

SOFT TISSUE LACERATION

If bleeding is not controlled by pressure with a gauze swab, refer to the dentist on call for further management. Bleeding tooth socket usually due to extraction of a tooth with untreated infection (more rarely a haematological disorder). If possible irrigate out or remove with gauze or tweezers, any loose, broken down or excess clot. Compress alveolus between finger and thumb firmly.

If the child is co-operative, place a gauze pad over the socket, and have child bite on it for 20 min and change when soaked. If not co-operative, the parent should hold the gauze in place. Never pack anything into the socket.

Anxiety relief is frequently necessary using a tranquillizer. This should be given immediately if indicated. Antibiotics (penicillin is the drug of first choice) should be given if infection is present as indicated by history of preceding pain or abscess. If indicated this should be given immediately. Once bleeding is controlled the patient should be referred to his own dentist, or the Department of Dentistry on the following day. If bleeding continues consult the dentist on call, check hydration and admit if necessary.

TRAUMA TO TEETH AND JAWS

Treatment should be commenced as early as possible if complications such as disturbed jaw growth, malformation or malposition of permanent teeth, tooth loss, or pulp death with abscess formation are to be prevented.

SUSPECTED FRACTURES OF THE MANDIBLE AND MAXILLA

Within the Royal Children's Hospital notify the plastic surgery registrar, who will then notify the oral surgeon on call immediately on presentation and before any radiological investigations are undertaken, even if other injuries are the main problem. Tetanus prophylaxis and antibiotics should always be given immediately for a compound fracture opening into the mouth or skin. Penicillin is the drug of choice initially.

DENTO-ALVEOLAR INJURIES

Dental consultation is recommended. Tetanus prophylaxis and antibiotics are given as indicated above.

Tooth Fracture

This may involve the crown or root of the tooth without alveolar bone fracture.

Tooth Displacement

This may be palatal or labial, intrusion or total dislodgement, extrusion with fracture of the labial and/or lingual alveolar bone. Before dental consultation assess:

- Degree of fracture and/or amount of displacement
- Occlusion (whether bite is distorted)
- Mucosal lacerations

Displaced Primary Incisor Tooth (Teeth)

Compress the tooth and alveolar bone together between the finger and thumb to return the tooth to its original position. If it remains firmly in place, advise a soft diet and refer to the dentist next day. If it remains unstable, contact the dentist on call.

Displaced or Avulsed Permanent Incisor Tooth

Ideally the tooth should be replaced in its socket immediately (reimplanted). Handle tooth gently and do not touch the root surface. If not possible keep tooth moist in room temperature milk until the dentist on call arrives. If the surface is very dirty, syringe gently with body temperature isotonic saline. (Teeth which have partly dried for short periods of time may be 'conditioned' in isotonic saline for 30 min.)

The success of treatment is directly proportional to the time elapsed since injury. For the completely avulsed tooth, reimplantation after 1 h is rarely successful in the long term.

However, under certain circumstances such as a perfect caries free mouth, reimplantation may be attempted even after longer time intervals at the discretion of the dentist.

The dentist will check the position of the tooth, splint it as necessary and arrange appropriate follow-up.

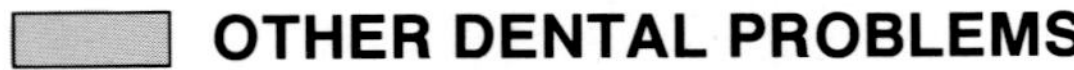

OTHER DENTAL PROBLEMS

The following problems may present as emergencies, but are generally not so. Patients presenting to the Royal Children's Hospital should be advised to ring their own dentist or the dental department (if already attending here) for an appointment at the earliest opportunity.

- Lost filling (unless associated with significant pain)
- Broken denture or orthodontic plate
- Loose band or wire of fixed orthodontic appliance. (Tuck the wire out of the way with a haemostat. Can cover sharp end with chewing gum or gutta percha from chemist.)
- Loose artificial crown
- Superficially chipped tooth

Minor laceration not requiring suturing. Give mouth rinses with warm saline and chlorhexidine gluconate 0.2% (Chlorohex, Savacol).

NORMAL DENTITION

PRIMARY OR DECIDUOUS TEETH (TOTAL 20)

	Central incisors	*Lateral incisors*	*Cuspids*	*First molars*	*Second molars*
Age in months	6–8	8–10	16–20	12–16	20–30

There is wide variation in eruption times, particularly of the deciduous teeth. At 1 year an infant has six to eight teeth, at 18 months 12 teeth and at $1\frac{1}{2}$ years, 20 teeth. Should there be no teeth erupted by 12 months, dental consultation should be sought.

PERMANENT TEETH (TOTAL 32)

	Central incisors	*Lateral incisors*	*Cuspids*	*First bicuspid*	*Second biscuspid*	*First molar*	*Second molars*	*Third molars*
Age in years	6–7	7–8	10–12	10–12	11–12	6–7	11–13	17–21

The first permanent teeth to erupt are the lower first molars and central incisors.

CHAPTER 29

ADOLESCENT HEALTH

Adolescence is a critical developmental phase covering almost a decade of physical, sexual, physiological and social change. Some health problems are almost unique to adolescence. These include the results of acting-out and risk-taking behaviour, certain habit disorders, anorexia nervosa, psychological adjustment difficulties, concerns about pubertal development and stature. Many chronic adult disorders, such as ischaemic heart disease, hypertension, alcoholism and tobacco-related disorders, have their inception at this time or are critically influenced by events during adolescence.

The developmental process may have a substantial effect on chronic disorders of childhood through maturing physiology. Of more significance in the care of chronic diseases, poor compliance may reflect a rebellious and risk-taking behaviour (a characteristic of earlier adolescence). Other young people show a responsible and self-reliant attitude to personal health (characterizing later adolescence).

There is likely to be a conflict of priorities between the social and emotional demands of adolescence and the demands on a young person to achieve good health and acceptable behaviour.

DEVELOPMENTAL TASKS OF ADOLESCENCE

- Achievement of autonomy and independence from parents
- Development of self-esteem and a sense of personal identity
- Maturity of sexual function, behaviour and identity
- Determination of a role in adult society, including a life career

HEALTH ISSUES DURING ADOLESCENCE

The Department of Adolescent Health provides a medical service both on referral and for those who attend without referral. The major categories of problems are as follows:

- School-based problems and learning difficulties (a multidisciplinary assessment programme is available)
- Concerns regarding puberty, growth and development
- Eating disorders, nutritional disorders including anorexia nervosa, obesity
- Concerns regarding sexuality, both for boys and girls, contraception, menstrual problems
- Behaviour disorders both at home and in the community
- The consequences of risk-taking behaviour: alcohol, drugs and sexual behaviour
- Affective disorders presenting with suicide attempts and gestures
- Adjustment problems for adolescents with chronic disease or disability

THE CONSULTATION

Effective consultation with an adolescent is likely to be more time-consuming than at any other age, if a doctor is to address the complex issues that are likely to be involved in health problems in adolescence. Many young people go to a doctor with a relatively minor problem, hoping for the opportunity to discuss a more sensitive or embarrassing concern. A satisfactory consultation provides the opportunity for an adolescent to develop rapport with the doctor and to discuss what seems to him/her to be important problems in his/her life. The consultation may be most helpful if the doctor:

- Recognizes that many adolescents are anxious about the consultation
- Recognizes that the parent and the adolescent may have different concerns, both of which need to be addressed
- Listens to what the adolescent has to say
- Uses appropriate and simple language in discussion
- Respects the adolescent's desire for privacy (some adolescents like a parent to be present during the examination, some do not)
- Respects the wish for confidentiality
- Respects the young person's personal judgement and decision

COMPLIANCE

Poor compliance with medical treatment is common in adolescent patients. This is important in the care of chronic disorders such as diabetes or epilepsy, and many disabled adolescents neglect hygiene and health precautions. Adherence to medical advice may be increased if:

- The consultation with the doctor has been satisfactory for the adolescent.
- The adolescent understands what the doctor has said.
- The adolescent believes that his own health concerns are being addressed, rather than just those of his parents.
- The adolescent feels he or she is not being put down but is respected.
- Treatment is simple. Increased complexity of medication dosage and schedules is linked with increased non-compliance.
- The treatment is practical. The tablet ordered before breakfast may not be taken if the teenager does not have time for breakfast. Medication at lunchtime won't often be taken at school.
- Parents are involved. Compliance increases when both parents understand the reason for treatment.

CONFIDENTIALITY AND CONSENT

Doctors respect confidentiality of adult patients including parents, but often view the confidences of children in a different light, sharing them with parents, school teachers or others who are interested in their well-being. Many adolescents resent this and may feel they have good reason to distrust the doctor who relates primarily with their parents or referring agencies.

It is wise for the doctor to discuss the confidentiality of the consultation with the adolescent, clarifying that sensitive information would only be shared with their parents with permission. It may be important for the doctor to state that he may feel it necessary to discuss some issues with a professional colleague from whom he needs help or advice. It may be wise for a student to have a copy of any report sent to his school.

Within Victoria, State law does not identify a particular age when a child's confidentiality must be respected or when a child can give consent for treatment without also securing consent of parents.

This matter is of particular concern when prescribing contraception, but may arise at other times when a teenager seeks help without parents' knowledge.

The decision on confidentiality in a mature minor rests on the judgement of the doctor, based on the age of the patient, his or her apparent maturity, whether in the view of the doctor the adolescent appears to be able to give a sound history, to understand the discussion and whether the patient appears willing and able to follow advice.

Most adolescents over the age of 16 conform to these criteria, as would many aged 15 years. Below the age of 15, the doctor must be on sure ground if he is not to inform parents as to some extent of his involvement with their child. At most ages it is wise to discuss with the adolescent, the advantages of sharing important health concerns with parents.

CHAPTER 30

GYNAECOLOGICAL CONDITIONS

VULVOVAGINITIS

Most infections are non-specific. Discharge is likely to occur for a short time following trauma. A normal increase in secretion occurs at puberty.

General measures such as regular daily bathing and toilet hygiene are important. The child should be taught to clean the perineum from front to back. Clean, well-fitted cotton underclothing, changed and boiled at least daily, are also important. Vaginal swabs and antibiotics are usually not indicated unless a specific infection such as gonorrhoea is suspected. Local acidification with dilute vinegar solution (10 mL in 500 mL warm water) will usually eradicate the problem. In children with persistent discharge, the following conditions should be considered :

- Foreign body which presents with an offensive blood-stained discharge. Examination under anaesthesia is usually sufficient for diagnosis and the foreign body can be removed at that time.
- Pinworm infestation.
- Trichomonas and moniliasis at adolescence.
- Gonorrhoea at any age.
- Sexual abuse.

FUSION OF THE LABIA AND IMPERFORATE HYMEN

A thin membrane between the labia is a frequent occurrence and is usually symptomless. Mothers should be shown how to apply dienoestrol cream 0.01% locally to the fused area for 10–14 days. This will usually result in separation. Failure to separate, thick membranes and imperforate hymen require consultation.

DYSMENORRHOEA

Acute dysmenorrhoea is managed with reassurance, analgesia and sedation. Antispasmodics are of no proven value. Ponstan is particularly useful. Persistent dysmenorrhoea requires gynaecological consultation.

MENORRHAGIA

Acute menorrhagia will require admission to hospital if there is heavy blood loss. Norethisterone (Primolut-n) 10 mg 2 hourly should then be given until bleeding stops or a maximum of six doses have been given. Then give 5 mg, t.d.s. for 1 week then 5 mg, b.d. for 2 weeks. Further bleeding will occur after this treatment is ceased. If the abnormal bleeding persists, gynaecological advice should be obtained and the possibility of a blood dyscrasia considered.

Recurrent menorrhagia requires gynaecological consultation. Menorrhagia within 2 years of the menarche is common and usually settles spontaneously. Give iron supplements to prevent anaemia but only use hormonal therapy if anaemia is occurring or blood loss is very heavy. If hormone therapy is required, use a 'high dose' pill not a 'low dose' pill.

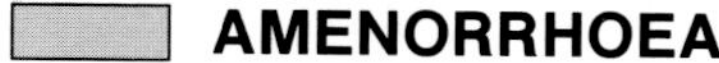

AMENORRHOEA

The age of menarche is variable. The range is from 11 to 16 years. For Australian-born girls the average age is 12.8 years and for foreign-born girls living in Australia the average age is 13.5 years. Assessment of amenorrhoea must primarily include a general physical examination to evaluate its various causes. It should be remembered that there is usually a delay of 2 years between the onset of pubertal breast development and the menarche.

Most girls presenting with delay in the onset of menstruation have no pathological cause. Girls who have delay in menarche beyond 16 years should be referred for investigation.

ORAL CONTRACEPTIVES

Except for adolescents who require high dose contraceptive pills, such as those with menorrhagia, those on antiepileptic medications, or those who have persistent breakthrough bleeding on lower dose preparations, the low dose preparation should be prescribed. Examples of appropriate pills are given below.

Low dose preparations	*High dose preparations*
Triquilar or Triphasil	Ovulen 1/50
Brevinor	Microgynon 50
Microgynon 30 or Nordette	Nordiol

CHAPTER 31

PAEDIATRIC PROCEDURES

All procedures performed on children have the potential to cause distress. Local anaesthetic agents applied subcutaneously (e.g. lignocaine 1%) or topically (e.g. EMLA cream) can lessen such distress.

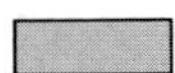

VENEPUNCTURE

The usual sites are:

- Antecubital fossa veins
- Hand or foot veins
- Scalp veins

External jugular puncture requires correct positioning and immobilization. At the end of the procedure the patient should be sat up and pressure applied to the puncture site. Femoral venepuncture carries a definite risk of serious complications in children, and should not be used. As infant's and children's veins are smaller, with less flow, aspiration may not be possible. Letting the blood flow out of a 21 gauge needle will often allow large volumes to be collected slowly. Intermittent relaxation and compression of the forearm or calf is often helpful.

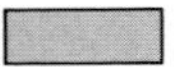

INSERTION OF INTRAVENOUS CANNULAS

In addition to the sites used in adults, useful sites in infants include the dorsum of the feet and scalp veins. Because of the smaller size, flashback into the chamber is often delayed, especially when inserting 24 gauge cannulas. This can be aided by removing the bung at the end of the cannula prior to insertion and cautious, slow advancement of the cannula. Priming the cannula with saline prior to insertion aids flashback.

Patience, comfortable position and good light are often the determinants of success. Grasping an infant's wrist between the index and middle fingers of the left hand and placing the thumb over the dorsal surface of the infant's fingers allows both compression and immobilization to be achieved with one hand. For scalp vein insertion a suitable area of hair is shaved to expose the veins. Immobilization of the cannula is best achieved with strapping secured to tincture of benzine applied to the scalp. Scalp veins should only be used when all other possible sites are exhausted. Note that shaved scalp hair usually regrows very slowly.

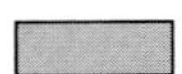

LUMBAR PUNCTURE

An experienced assistant is essential. The infant's spine must be flexed and movement must be minimal. The lateral position is routinely used. The spinous processes are usually readily palpable. The interspinous space at or below the level of the iliac crests is the preferred site. Failure is usually due to incorrect position of the patient or poor needle alignment. The most important factor is an experienced assistant with movement kept to a minimum.

Sedation is usually not necessary. However, local anaesthetic is helpful in all patients except neonates. The correct size to use is 2 cm for neonates, 3 cm for up to 6 or 9 months of age, 4 cm for up to 2–4 years, 5 cm between 4 and 10 years and a 6 cm for children older than 10 years. If in doubt use the longer needle. A 22 gauge needle is appropriate in most situations.

Pressure measurement is difficult in infants, and the CSF may seem to escape under high pressure in normal infants. The rate of flow is an unreliable guide to pressure. Ideally two tubes, each containing 1 mL of CSF should be collected for routine bacteriological and biochemical tests. A further 1 mL should be collected if viral studies are indicated.

ARTERIAL PUNCTURE

Arterial blood gas measurement is used when a true oxygen saturation is required. Often acid-base status can be adequately assessed by a capillary collection. Pre-heparinized 2 mL syringes will not auto-inject in most children. Gentle aspiration on withdrawing the needle is usually more successful than aspiration on insertion. In general only radial or brachial artery puncture should be attempted by resident staff. Femoral artery puncture is potentially dangerous and should never be attempted outside an intensive care situation.

SUPRAPUBIC ASPIRATION OF URINE

This is best performed when the child or infant has not voided for at least 1 h. The suprapubic skin area is prepared with 1 : 200 chlorhexidine in 70% alcohol. Insert a 23 gauge needle attached to a 2 mL syringe vertically through the abdominal wall at the mid-line 1–2 cm above the symphysis pubis. This usually corresponds to the skin crease above the pubis. The depth of insertion varies with the age of the child, in infants it is usually about 3–4 cm. Aspirate the urine while withdrawing the needle slowly. Local anaesthetic is not necessary.

URETHRAL CATHETERIZATION

Unlike suprapubic aspiration, catheterization almost always is successful in obtaining a urine sample. It is indicated where the child has recently voided or where one suprapubic aspiration has been attempted and has failed. In children over 12 months, catheterization is less distressing than suprapubic aspiration and should be attempted first. Catheterization requires at least one assistant to steady the child and hold the legs parted. The operator wearing gloves, cleans the area with a water-based preparation and drapes the area with sterile towels. For diagnostic catheterization a feeding tube, size 5 or 8, is used. Sterile lubricant aids insertion. A Foley catheter with inflatable balloon is used for indwelling catheters. Experience is needed to locate the urethral orifice in both male and female patients. In males the foreskin need not be fully retracted to successfully cannulate the orifice. The catheter is advanced with care until urine is obtained and then removed.

COLLECTION OF FUNGAL SPECIMENS

COLLECTION OF SKIN, NAILS AND HAIR

Scalp Lesions

Pluck broken hair stumps and scrape scales from near the advancing edge of the lesions with forceps or flat-edged tweezers. Infected hairs are more opaque and white than normal hairs. Do not scrape scalp lesions with a scalpel as hair and scales from above the invaded portion are likely to be collected and give a false negative result. Some infected hairs are so heavily invaded and digested by spores that they become twisted and fractured at the surface of the scalp. If this is the case, press the forceps firmly down and scrape into any scale present to collect broken fragments of infected hairs.

Acutely inflamed pustular lesions (kerion) should be swabbed for both mycological and bacterial culture. In addition, broken hair should be removed from the edge of the lesions. A round plastic hair brush (available from bacteriology) can be used to firmly stroke the surface of the lesions on the scalp. This can be transported to the laboratory in a Petri dish in a plastic bag and can then be inoculated directly onto agar.

Skin Lesions

Remove ointment or other local application with methylated spirits and allow to dry. Using a blunt scalpel, tweezers or a bone curette, firmly scrape the lesion, particularly at the advancing edge. If multiple lesions are present, choose the most recent, since old loose scale is less satisfactory. Small vellus hairs within the lesions should be epilated. Remove the tops of any fresh vesicles (in which the fungus is often plentiful) particularly in cases of vesicular tinea pedis.

In patients with suspected candidiasis the young 'satellite lesions' which have not exfoliated are more likely to yield positive results. Otherwise scrape the advancing scaly border of lesions. Use a moistened swab to collect material from inflamed lesions in flexures.

Nails

Pare and scrape the nails until crumbling, white degenerating portion is reached and collect any white debris beneath the nail. If chronic candidial paronychia is suspected, a swab moistened in sterile saline should be rolled firmly around the nail bed to force liquid from beneath the fold.

TRANSPORT

With the exception of swabs, specimens should be transported dry, wrapped in paper, in a Petri dish, or, if only a small quantity is available, between two glass slides which are taped together. Transport swabs in their plastic sleeve.

CHAPTER 32

ROYAL CHILDREN'S HOSPITAL ADMINISTRATIVE PROCEDURES

Hospital Medical Officers are reminded that details on hospital administrative procedures are in the Manual of Executive Instructions, Procedure Manual for Heads of Medical and Allied Health Departments, and Executive Memoranda. Several points of particular importance are outlined below.

VISITING TIMES AND REST TIME

Parents and guardians may visit inpatients on any day at any time. Visiting time for friends and other relatives is between 0800 and 1900 h. There is a daily rest period in the wards from 1200 to 1400 h.

ADMISSION TIME

Admission times for elective procedures are in accordance with the Admission and Discharge Policy and are generally in the afternoon except for day cases and where specific arrangements are made in response to patients' needs.

DISCHARGE TIME

This is in accordance with the Admission and Discharge Policy and patients should generally be discharged by 1130 h.

INTERPRETERS

Interpreters are on duty between the hours of 0830 and 1800 h on weekdays and 1300 and 2200 h on weekends and public holidays. The appropriate interpreter is obtained by contacting the Chief Interpreter — phone 5026 or 5998 or via the switchboard and requesting the specific language concerned. A Telephone Interpreter Service is also available through the switchboard outside the above hours.

NOTIFICATION OF CONSULTANTS

It is the responsibility of the resident to keep the registrar of the unit informed of all admissions and problems. It is the registrar's responsibility to decide when to contact the consultant of the unit. The following are guidelines:

- If the patient is severely ill
- If the patients is likely to die
- If it is considered that another consultant's opinion is necessary
- If the patient is admitted to the intensive care unit
- If surgery is contemplated

POSTMORTEM EXAMINATIONS

After a child's death, it is usual practice in this hospital for the parents to be interviewed by the consultant concerned or his registrar. At this interview, permission is usually requested for necropsy. If permission is granted, it is recorded in the patient's history and the Anatomical Pathology Department is advised. Also parents should be advised to contact a funeral director of their choice who will liaise with the mortuary attendant with respect to funeral arrangements.

The Pathology Department will perform necropsies on patients dying outside the hospital provided that the usual medical attendant provides a death certificate.

DEATH CERTIFICATES

These are kept in the Anatomical Pathology Department and should be filled out as soon as possible during office hours by the resident or registrar of the unit concerned. No death certificate is required for cases within the jurisdiction of the Coroner.

EMERGENCY PAGE SYSTEM

The person who recognizes a cardiac arrest, or any other medical or surgical emergency, is responsible for initiating the following procedure:
Call switchboard by dialling 777. State — 'Emergency in . . . '. Switchboard will place on visual page the following sequence of numbers, together with the audible emergency buzzer. All numbers, followed by:

1 A single number denoting the floor, i.e.
   0 = Casualty
   1 = first floor, etc
   10 = 10th floor.

2 Another single number denoting the wing, i.e.
   1 = North
   2 = South
   3 = East
   4 = West
   5 = South East Building
   6 = Entry Building.

There will be an audible page announcement stating '777 alert in . . . '.
For example: a cardiac arrest occurring in Ward 5 West will result in a visual page of the following sequence: *All numbers, then 5, then 4.*

The above procedure will take place regardless of time of day. All resident medical staff seeing an emergency visual page should proceed to that area immediately and, on arrival, the most senior doctor present will direct them. An ECG monitor and DC defibrillator are kept in the intensive care unit. This equipment will be transported to the emergency scene by intensive care staff.

CORONER'S CASES

A person dying will come under the jurisdiction of the Coroner if the death occurs in Victoria; or the body is in Victoria; or the cause of which occurred in Victoria; or if the dead person normally resided in Victoria at the time of death *and*

- Appears to have been unexpected, unnatural or violent or to have resulted, directly or indirectly, from accident or injury; or

- Occurs during an anaesthetic; or
- Occurs as a result of an anaesthetic and is not due to natural causes.
- Occurs in prescribed circumstances; or
- Of a person who immediately before death was a person held in care, or
- Of a person whose identity is unknown; or
- Occurs in Victoria where a notice under Section 19(1)(b) of the *Registration of Births, Deaths and Marriages Act* 1959 has not been signed; or
- Occurs at a place outside Victoria where the cause of death is not certified by a person who, under the law in that place, is a legally qualified medical practitioner.

All the above cases must be reported to the Coroner by notifying the Coroner's clerk at the time of death. Coroner's deposition forms are available in all wards. They are completed in duplicate — one copy accompanies the patient and the other copy is kept in the Department of Anatomical Pathology.

MEDICOLEGAL ISSUES

All questions regarding medicolegal matters should be referred to the Executive Officer or Fellow in Medical Administration. If they are unavailable the Director of Regional Paediatric Services or other senior executive staff should be contacted. Questions may arise concerning:

- Litigation
- Indemnity
- Child protection
- Family Court matters (custody and access)
- Freedom of information

CHAPTER 33

ROYAL CHILDREN'S HOSPITAL DEPARTMENTAL PROCEDURES

MICROBIOLOGY

LOCATION

- Bacteriology laboratories 7th floor South East — phone 5739
- Virology laboratory 8th floor South East — phone 5850

HOURS

- Bacteriology 0800–1800 h weekdays, 0900–1400 h Saturdays and public holidays.
- Virology 0800–1700 h weekdays, 0900–1200 h Saturdays. Closed public holidays.
- Additionally in Bacteriology only, one hospital scientist is on duty 1400–1800 h Saturdays, 0900–1400 h Sundays and on call at all times. A medical microbiologist is on call at any time.

SPECIMENS

Must be clearly labelled and presented with consideration for a high standard of hygiene. Specimens which are leaking or where the container is heavily contaminated will be discarded. Unlabelled or inaccurately labelled specimens will not be processed.

REPORTS

Are despatched between 1300 and 1400 h Monday–Saturday; 1700–1800 h Monday–Friday.

TELEPHONE INQUIRIES

Your co-operation is sought to limit telephone inquiries to a minimum and use only for an urgent report. The inquiry should be based on being able to provide the patient's full name, U.R. number, ward and the date the specimen was submitted. Consultation or discussion about interpretation, further investigation and treatment is welcomed.

TRANSPORT OF BLOOD SPECIMENS

Specimens of blood which are to be transported to the laboratory by a courier or ward assistant should be placed in a sealable specimen transport bag after checking to ensure that the cap is securely tightened. The bags must be transported upright to prevent spillage. The request form should be placed in the open sleeve of the bag. If request forms are soiled by blood they should be discarded and another written.

FAECES, SPUTUM, PUS AND URINE

After collection of these specimens into suitable containers, the lids should be securely tightened and any contamination cleaned from the outside of the containers. These specimens should be transported in plastic bags as above but must be kept upright. Couriers must not transport soiled specimens and should ensure that spillage does not occur during transport.

OTHER SPECIMENS

Other specimens including 'culture kits' for bacteriology, nasopharyngeal aspirates and fresh or fixed specimens for anatomical pathology, do not need to be transported in sealed bags. They should be placed in appropriate, clean or sterile containers with lids secured and transported with care.

LABORATORY CONSIDERATIONS

If the specimen is unlabelled, incompletely labelled, inadequate for the test requested or not accompanied by a request form it will be returned to the patient care area, if possible, or the doctor requesting the test will be notified and asked to come to the laboratory to correct the error, or if neither of these is possible the specimen will be discarded.

If the specimen tube is contaminated or leaking it may have to be discarded. The ward or department will be notified if this is necessary. If the request form is incomplete the ward or department will be notified and a report will not be issued until the appropriate information has been provided.

Contaminated request forms will be placed immediately in a plastic bag and photocopied if possible.

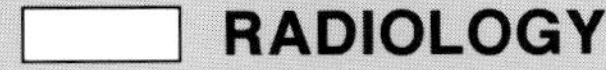

RADIOLOGY

SERVICE AVAILABILITY

All X-ray, ultrasound (US) and nuclear medicine (NM = radionuclide) services relevant to paediatric diagnostic imaging are available at all times. However, access to some of the more complex or higher radiation dose studies are limited to patient referrals from appropriate subspecialists and are outlined in booking procedures (see below). The radiologists welcome prior consultation regarding imaging protocols and discussion regarding the interpretation of subsequent findings.

Magnetic resonance imaging (MRI) is not available at the Royal Children's Hospital and access is strictly limited. All inquiries should be directed to the Director of Radiology.

Only urgent studies, required for immediate patient management decisions, are performed after hours (and arranged as outlined under bookings).

Every request for service must be accompanied by a fully completed request card or referral letter prior to commencing an examination. The referring doctor should be clearly identified (and beeper number included).

Axiom: The relevance and quality of an imaging investigation is directly related to the clinical information provided and the specificity of the questions being asked by the referring doctor.

STAFF AVAILABILITY

There is a staff radiologist and a medical imaging technologist (MIT = radiographer) available at all times. There is only one MIT in the hospital between 2030 and 0830 h each day. This can result in urgent after hours services requiring prioritizing.

In Hours

Monday–Friday 0830–1700 h contact radiologist or MIT via Radiology Receptionist (345 5255/5256). The beeper numbers for radiologists are listed in the Royal Children's Hospital internal telephone directory. A radiologist can generally be found in the Reporting Room of the department.

After Hours

Weekends and between 1700 and 0830 h other days contact is via the Royal Children's Hospital switchboard.

RADIOLOGISTS' REPORTS

If printed reports are not in a patient's records:

- Use a hospital computer terminal to access the Radiology database for all reports typed since 1986 (for procedure see below).
- If the computer file indicates the study has been done but the report is not yet available, you may obtain access to the radiologist's dictated report prior to typing (for procedure see below). Once typed and available on computer, reports are not retained in the dictation file.
- If reports are not obtainable by the above means consult a radiologist, or the Radiology Filing Room in hours.

Important: To obtain reports you must know patient(s) unit record number(s)

AVAILABILITY OF FILMS

Please keep all films with their master bag to minimize losses.

Inpatients

Master bags are kept in the Ward Room (S285) opposite the main waiting room. The films and film bags do not leave this room except under defined circumstances. Films and bags which are removed from this room are out of the control of Radiology and are effectively *lost*.

Exceptions: Intensive Care Unit and Orthopaedics retain their films in their wards; films may go to operating theatres, defined teaching seminars and some ward rounds.

Others (Including Outpatients)

Film bags are obtainable from the Filing Room (S271) only between the hours of 0800 and 1700 h Monday–Friday. You must be able to provide Radiology staff with the unit record numbers of patients whose films you wish to obtain.

BOOKINGS

Only in exceptional circumstances will a booking be made or a service provided without prior receipt of a completed request card or referral letter. One such exception is a mobile chest X-ray anywhere in the hospital to detect immediate life-threatening conditions (e.g. pneumothorax, haemothorax) during emergency patient resuscitation.

For purposes of booking, services fall into three groups according to their requirements and restrictions:

1 Plain X-rays.
   - **a** No booking required.
   - **b** Only urgent studies performed after hours (when availability of MIT staff is limited).
   - **c** In hours contact Radiology Reception (345 5355/5356).
   - **d** After hours contact on-duty MIT via Royal Children's Hospital switchboard.
   - **e** Mobile services (outside the department) are available only when transporting a patient to the department constitutes an unacceptable risk to that patient or because the patient must remain in isolation.

2 Services performed by or directly supervised by radiologists.
   - **a** Require either an appointment (non-urgent) or direct consultation with a staff radiologist (if required urgently). This includes all X-ray studies requiring administration of contrast of any sort, ultrasound and nuclear medicine.
   - **b** For appointments contact:

- US — 345 5319 (#5319)
- NM — 345 5259 (#5259):
- Others — 345 5255/5256 (#5255/5256)

3 Restricted availability — to appropriate subspecialists.
   - **a** Computerized tomography.
   - **b** Angiography.
   - **c** Myelography.
   - **d** MRI.
   - **e** Interventional.

Any doctor is welcome to discuss the indications for these investigations for her/his patients, but may be asked to seek subspecialist assistance to ensure the investigation is relevant and determine how it may best be performed. This is to ensure these higher radiation and/or invasive procedures (often requiring general anaesthesia) are used effectively.

Angiography, myelography and interventional bookings are all made directly with a staff radiologist. CT bookings should be made directly to 345 5268 (#5268). If no answer contact Radiology Reception 345 5255/5256). MRI bookings through the Director of Radiology.

SERVICE IN SURGICAL THEATRES

Prior bookings must be made for mobile X-rays and mobile fluoroscopy during surgery. In the absence of bookings anaesthetized patients may on occasions be kept waiting if MIT staff are not immediately available.

An emergency chest X-ray would be obtained as the highest priority on receipt of a telephone call only (to Radiology Reception in hours or via switchboard after hours) during emergency resuscitation.

GROUND FLOOR SERVICE

There is no imaging service provided in Emergency, General Clinic or Outpatients (exception: chest X-ray during resuscitation from an immediate life-threatening situation).

A mobile service following manipulation of fractures is available on the request of orthopaedic surgeons, their registrars and fellows.

COMPARISON X-RAY VIEWS

Although useful in particular circumstances the routine request for films of the opposite normal joint or bone will only be observed by radiographers after hours and only after a doctor has examined the films of the injured or abnormal parts.

CONFERENCES

There are eight or nine clinicoradiological conferences each week, mostly in the department, when units discuss current clinical problems with radiologists and sometimes pathologists. Lists of patients for conferences must be provided to the Filing Room at least 24 h before the conference.

TEACHING

If you are interested in the teaching programmes provided by the department please discuss them with a staff radiologist.

PROCEDURE FOR OBTAINING REPORTS FROM COMPUTER

1 After terminal is turned on wait for blinking cursor to appear.

2 Ensure there is an asterisk in the 'remote mode' box at the bottom of the screen (F4 function key). If this is not showing, press the F4 function key *once* to turn the asterisk on. If there are asterisks showing in the other boxes, press the corresponding function keys to turn them off.

3 Press *return* key until a colon (:) appears with the flashing cursor.

4 Type 'hello enquser.rchrad' and press *return*.

5 Type in the password and press *return.* The password can be obtained by contacting Radiology Department staff.

6 Despite the statement 'end of program' wait until the screen rolls over to a presentation titled 'Clinical Enquiry Patient Selection'
'Input'.
Enter the desired patient unit record number and press the *enter* key (*not the return key*).

7 Follow instructions using the eight grey function keys at the top of the keyboard (labelled F1 to F8), the functions of which are designated in the green boxes at the bottom of the screen.

8 When finished, press 'F8' twice to exit the program.

9 *Note:* Printouts of all reports are made only in Radiology, and distributed for inclusion in patient records.

PROCEDURE FOR OBTAINING REPORTS VIA TELEPHONE WHICH ARE NOT AVAILABLE FROM THE COMPUTER

Reports are removed from this system once typed into the computer.

1 Try the computer terminal first — voice reports are no longer available in this system once typed.

2 Use a phone with a 'tone' switch (currently Envoy — on the side) and dial 345 5273 (5273 from within the Royal Children's Hospital).

3 On receipt of the recorded message confirming you have successfully accessed the voice recording system, switch your phone into the tone mode and 'dial' the patient's unit record number.

4 This system is also available for patients without a Royal Children's Hospital unit record number if the Radiology number (R....) is known — in which case substitute 0 (zero) for R when dialling.

5 *Please remember to switch the phone back to 'dec' when finished.*

BIOCHEMISTRY

URGENT REQUESTS

When a test requires immediate or special attention, the registrar or resident responsible must contact the senior biochemist on duty and be prepared to justify the need for urgent work. The word *'urgent'* on a request form is not sufficient to justify diverting staff from existing work.

OUTPATIENTS

An outpatient blood collection centre is located on the 8th floor link and patients for biochemistry collections should be referred to this facility. The outpatient collection centre is open 0900–1700 h on weekdays.

INPATIENTS

Monday–Friday 0900–1700 h

Capillary blood collection rounds occur at 0900, 1100 and 1400 h. A request card may be sent to the outpatient blood collection centre or retained in the ward and a phone message given. Phone 5821 (answering service available before 0830 h).

Non-urgent requests accompanied by venous or arterial specimens should arrive before 1030 h. Unless notified by telephone by the resident concerned, the laboratory will assume that any request for specimen arriving after 1400 h will not require attention that day.

Monday–Friday 1700–0900 h

Minimum staff are on duty at all times for tests requiring immediate attention. All requests must be preceded by a telephone call to the laboratory.

Saturdays, Sundays and Public Holidays

- Mornings. Capillary blood collection rounds occur at 0900 and 1100 h. Because of reduced staffing, requests for capillary blood collections should, if at all possible, reach the laboratory by 0900 h. Requests accompanied by venous or arterial specimens should reach the laboratory by 1030 h.
- Other times. Minimum staff are on duty at all times for tests requiring immediate attention. All requests must be preceded by a telephone call to the laboratory.

TESTS ROUTINELY AVAILABLE AT TIMES OTHER THAN MONDAY–FRIDAY 0900–1700 h

- Acid–base/blood gases
- Ammonia
- Electrolytes
- Galactoscreen

- Aspartate aminotransferase (AST)
- Bilirubin
- Calcium
- Creatinine
- Digoxin (Saturday a.m. only)
- Glucose
- Magnesium
- Osmolality
- Theophylline
- Urea

All other tests require the approval of the Senior Biochemist on duty.

SPECIMEN REQUIREMENTS

Blood Tests

Arterial Po_2

Collect blood using syringe from special kit stored in ward refrigerator. Removal all bubbles, label and place in cold pack (at 4°C, not frozen). Transport to laboratory immediately. Arterial blood may also be used for acid base using the same kit, and other biochemical analyses.

Collection of capillary blood specimens by laboratory staff is restricted to patients less than 3 years of age, except by special arrangement. Capillary collections at specific times e.g. for drug levels cannot always be guaranteed. In such cases, it is the responsibility of the medical staff to make alternative arrangements.

Venous blood

For inpatients, it is the responsibility of medical staff to collect venous specimens. Outpatients may have venous specimens taken in the 8th floor outpatient collection centre.

In general

- For a single test a 1 mL specimen is required
- For two or three tests a 2 mL specimen is required
- For more than three tests 3–5 mL specimen is required.

Heparinized blood is preferred for most tests, and is always required for:

- Ammonia
- Enzymes related to metabolic disease
- Galactoscreen
- Galactose
- Galactose-1-phosphate
- Lead
- Parathormone
- Porphyrins
- Vitamin D

No anticoagulants other than heparin, in orange-capped tubes, should be used without prior consultation with the laboratory.

Blood tests requiring *consultation* before specimen collection:

- ACTH
- Cortisol
- Enzymes related to metabolic disease
- 17-Hydroxyprogesterone
- Isoenzymes
- Paracetamol
- Provocation tests, e.g. GTT, loading studies, etc.
- Pyruvate
- Vitamin D
- Ammonia
- Drug screen
- Insulin
- Lactate
- Parathormone
- Renin activity

Urine Tests

Random urine specimens

All random urine specimens should be delivered to the laboratory immediately after collection. For some, this is essential, namely:

- Cystine
- Homocystine
- Metabolic screen (amino acids, organic acids)
- pH
- Porpholbilinogen — must reach laboratory within 30 min, wrapped in foil
- Porphyrins (screen) — must be wrapped in foil

24 h urine collections

The appropriate bottle for collection will be provided on presentation of the request slip to the Biochemistry Department. During collection the specimen must be kept at 4°C in a refrigerator.

Clearance studies

Creatinine clearance — an accurately timed urine collection is required, plus a specimen of blood obtained during this period. Height and weight of the patient must be stated on the request card.

Metabolic screen (See also p. 142)

- Urine screen: 10 mL of fresh random specimen is required. Details of current medication and clinical notes must be provided. Investigations include chemical tests for pH, protein, reducing substances, glucose, blood and ketones plus amino acid profile and screen for methylmalonic acid. Organic acid or other profiles provided if clinical notes or other laboratory findings indicate the need for such studies.
- Blood screen (only required in special circumstances). For amino acids only — 1 mL blood.

Urgent metabolic screening requires consultation with the clinical staff of the Genetics Department and senior biochemist on duty.

Drug Screen

Requires serum or plasma (2 mL) and urine (20 mL). Clinical notes, with details regarding suspected toxic medications and drugs given therapeutically, must be provided. If an urgent drug screen is required, arrangements must be made with the screening laboratory (extension 5923 Monday–Friday 0900–1700 h) or after hours with the senior biochemist on duty.

DISTRIBUTION OF RESULTS

Ward Interim Reports

These summaries of all the most recent results from any given area are generated and delivered by couriers at 1400 h and 1800 h Monday–Friday and once daily at 1300 h on Saturdays, Sundays and public holidays.

Patient Cumulative Reports

These reports designed for insertion into the patient's medical records are generated mid-afternoon on all weekdays. They include all confirmed test results to that time and are distributed by 1730 h.

Patient Advance Reports

Fall into the following two groups:

1 *Automatic.* Printers linked to the Division of Pathology's computer are situated in the Intensive Care Unit, Neonatal Unit and in cardiac and diabetic wards. In these areas all results are printed out immediately they have been obtained.

2 *On request.* A printed advance report from any specimen or a cumulative report for any patient can be obtained on request at any time.

Telephone Reports

To ensure accurate reports, results are, in principle, not telephoned. Should difficulty be incurred in obtaining a result through the regular channels, the responsible medical officer should consult with the senior biochemist on duty by telephoning 5902 between 0900 and 1700 h on weekdays and 5906 after hours.

BIOCHEMISTRY REFERENCE RANGES

Reference ranges for a selected list of more commonly ordered biochemistry tests are included below. For ranges for other tests, consult printed reports or department's booklet *Reference Ranges in Clinical Biochemistry and Notes on Therapeutic Drug Monitoring.*

Reference ranges are derived from experience with patients of the Royal Children's Hospital supplemented by values from normal children and from the literature. Results within these ranges can be considered to be 'within normal limits'. Where possible, results are expressed in SI units.

ABBREVIATIONS

B	Blood (whole)	f	fasting
Erc	Erythrocytes	g	gram
F	Faeces	L	litre
Hb	Haemoglobin	Lkc	Leucocytes
P	Plasma	mol	mole
S	Serum	Pa	Pascal
U	Urine	m	metre
d	day	k	kilo 10^{-3}
h	hour	m	milli 10^{-3}
min	minute	μ	micro 10^{-6}
s	second	n	nano 10^{-9}
w	week	p	pico 10^{-12}
M	Month	f	femto 10^{-15}
IU	International Unit	y	year
a	arterial	c	capillary
v	venous		

Because of changes in laboratory methods, reference ranges are subject to revision. Therefore, if in doubt about the significance of a result, consult laboratory. Where possible, up-to-date reference ranges are quoted on reports.

BLOOD, SERUM AND PLASMA

Test	Arterial or venous specimens: vol. required (mL)	Age	Reference range(s)	Comments
Acid/base (P)	0.5 Not venous			Arterial or capillary samples only are suitable for pH, P_{CO_2}. Venous samples may be accepted for actual bicarbonate. Consult with lab.
pH		1 d 2 d–1 M > 1 M	7.30–7.46 7.32–7.46 7.34–7.43	
P_{CO_2}			32–45 mmHg	Higher values seen in newborn.
Base excess			– 4– + 3 mmol/L	Lower values seen in newborn.
Actual bicarbonate			18–25 mmol/L	
Albumin				See proteins.
Alkaline phosphatase – AP (SP)	0.5	0–2 y 2–10 y 10–16 y	100–350 U/L 100–300 U/L 100–350 U/L	Higher values may be seen during periods of rapid growth.
Amino acid screen				See Metabolic Screen (p. 191)
Amylase (SP)	0.5		8–85 U/L	
Aspartate amino-transferase – AST (SP)	0.5	< 1 y 1–3 y 3–16 y	20–80 U/L 15–60 U/L 10–45 U/L	Formerly SGOT. Upper limit of reference range, particularly in infancy, not well-defined.
Bilirubin – total (SP)	0.5	Full-term 0–24 h 24–48 h 3–5 d 1 M	 < 65 μmol/L < 115 μmol/L < 155 μmol/L < 10 μmol/L	Higher values in newborn due to increase in indirect (unconjugated) fraction. Even higher values in premature infants.
Calcium – ionized (P)	0.5	Adult	1.19–1.29 mmol/L	Whole blood specimen needed. Must be collected anaerobically, like blood gas. Consult laboratory for details.
Calcium – total (SP)	0.5	< 2 w 2 w–1 y > 1 y	1.90–2.70 mmol/L 2.10–2.70 mmol/L 2.10–2.60 mmol/L	Lower limit of normal range in neonates not well-defined.
Chloride	0.5		98–110 mmol/L	
Cholesterol – total (SP)	0.5	6 M 1 y 2–14 y	2.3–4.9 mmol/L 2.5–4.9 mmol/L 3.1–5.4 mmol/L	Reference ranges based on USA data. Australian National Heart Foundation recommends adult cholesterol < 5.5 mmol/L.
Creatine kinase – CK (SP)	0.5		40–240 units/L	Wrap in foil to keep dark. Higher values in newborn. Specimens on three separate occasions recommended when testing for carriers of Duchenne muscular dystrophy.

(Continued over)

BLOOD, SERUM AND PLASMA (Continued)

Test	*Arterial or venous specimens: vol. required (mL)*	*Age*	*Reference range(s)*	*Comments*
Creatinine (SP)	0.5	1 M–1 y 1–4 y 4–10 y 10–16 y	0.01–0.03 mmol/L 0.01–0.05 mmol/L 0.02–0.06 mmol/L 0.03–0.08 mmol/L	Reference range related to muscle mass.
Glucose f (SP)	0.5	2 d–1 M > 1 M	2.2–5.0 mmol/L 3.6–5.4 mmol/L	Lower values seen on day 1 and in premature infants. Therapy for hypoglycaemia should aim to keep the glucose concentration > 3mmol/L. The reference range for whole blood glucose is approximately 10% lower than that for plasma glucose.
Glutamyltransferase–GTT (SP)	0.5	0–1 M > 3 M	0–225 U/L < 40 U/L	Higher levels may be seen if on anticonvulsants, alcohol. Newborns have very high levels of GTT which rapidly decrease to adult levels by about 3 months.
Iron (SP)	2		9–27 μmol/L	
Iron binding capacity – total (SP)	2		45–72 μmol/L	
Liver function (SP)	1			See bilirubin, AST, GTT and proteins.
Magnesium (SP)	0.5		0.7–1.0 μmol/L	
Osmolality (SP)	1		265–295 mmol/L	
Phosphorus – inorganic (SP)	0.5	< 2 w 2 w–2 y 2–16 y	1.7–3.0 mmol/L 1.3–2.3 mmol/L 1.1–1.8 mmol/L	
Po_2 (P)	0.5 Arterial only	< 2 w > 2 w	55–100 mmHg 80–100 mmHg	
Potassium	0.5	2 d–2 w 2 w–3 M 3 M–1 y 1–16 y	3.7–6.0 mmol/L 3.7–5.7 mmol/L 3.5–5.1 mmol/L 3.5–5.0 mmol/L	Ranges quoted are based on arterial venous specimens. Capillary samples have higher potassium concentration (up to 0.6 mmol/L higher).
Proteins (S) Total protein	0.5	< 1 M 1 M–1 y 1–4 y 4–16 y	45–70 g/L 50–71 g/L 55–74 g/L 57–80 g/L	

(Continued over)

BLOOD, SERUM AND PLASMA (Continued)

Test	*Arterial or venous specimens: vol. required (mL)*	*Age*	*Reference range(s)*	*Comments*
Albumin		< 1 M	23–43 g/L	
		1 M–1 y	29–45 g/L	
		1–16 y	33–47 g/L	
Total globulins		< 1 M	10–31 g/L	Consult with immunology laboratory regarding specific globulin fractions.
		1 M–1 y	12–27 g/L	
		1–4 y	14–37 g/L	
		4–16 y	17–38 g/L	
Sodium	0.5		135–145 mmol/L	
Thyroid function (SP)	2			
Thyroxine total (TT4)		1–3 d	130–270 nmol/L	
		1–2 w	125–215 nmol/L	
		2–4 w	105–215 nmol/L	
		1–4 M	90–190 nmol/L	
		4 M–1 y	70–175 nmol/L	
			70–155 nmol/L	
free (FT4)		Adult	9–26 pmol/L	Higher values in infants.
T3 Resin uptake (T3 RU)		< 1 M	70–115%	
		1–4 M	70–110%	
		4 M–1 y	70–110%	
		> 1 y	75–115%	
Free thyroxine index (FTI)		< 1 M	80–210%	
		1–4 M	70–180%	
		4 M–1 y	60–160%	
		> 1 y	60–155%	
Triiodothyronine (T3)		Adult	1.0–2.7 nmol/L	Higher values in infants and children.
Thyroxine binding globulin (TBG)		Adult	12–28 mg/L	
Thyroid stimulating hormone (TSH)		1–3 d	< 40 mU/L	
		3–7 d	< 25 mU/L	
		7–14 d	< 10 mU/L	
		> 14 d	< 5 mU/L	
Triglycerides f (P)	0.5	Adult	0.9–2.0 mmol/L	*Note:* fasting essential
Urea (SP)	0.5	< 1 M	1.3–5.7 mmol/L	Related to protein intake. Lower values in breast fed infants and newborns.
		1 M–4 y	1.3–6.6 mmol/L	
		> 4 y	2.1–6.5 mmol/L	
Uric acid (SP)	0.5	Prepubertal	0.13–0.39 mmol/L	Higher values may be seen in first 2 years and following onset of puberty.
Zinc (SP)	2	11–22 μmol/L		

URINE

Test	*Specimens: vol. required (mL)*	*Age*	*Reference range(s)*	*Comments*
Calcium	24 h		< 0.12 mmol/kg per day	Include weight of patient on request card. Specimen must be collected into special bottle containing acid.
Calcium/creatinine ratio	Random	> 2 y	< 0.7 mmol/day	
Creatinine clearance	24 h		1.4–2.4 mL/s per 1.73 m^2	Plasma sample for creatinine required during urine collection period. Height and weight must be recorded on request card. See special note in general instructions.
Drug screen	Random (20 mL)			
Potassium	Random		Variable (mmol/L)	Many factors determine excretion rates, e.g. intake, renal function, hormonal influences and drug therapy.
Sodium	Random		Variable (mmol/L)	Many factors influence urinary sodium concentration. This test is of value in differentiating causes of hyponatraemia.

SWEAT

Test	*Specimens: vol. required (mL)*	*Age*	*Reference range(s)*	*Comments*
Sodium chloride	–	Prepubertal	< 50 mmol/L < 50 mmol/L	At least 100 mg of sweat must be collected. If sodium is > 50 mmol/L and chloride is > 70 mmol/L, result is definitely abnormal. All other results outside reference ranges are doubtful. Higher values may be seen in normal adolescents and adults.

SERUM DRUG LEVELS

Test	*Arterial or venous specimens: vol. required (mL)*	*Reference range(s)*	*Comments*
Carbamazepine (SP)	1	20–50 μmol/L (therapeutic)	
Chloramphenicol (SP)	0.5	Peak 20–30 mg/L (therapeutic)	
Clonazepam (SP)	1	60–150 nmol/L (therapeutic)	Therapeutic range not well-defined.
Cyclosporin (B)	1.0	ng/mL	Collect sample in EDTA. Consult laboratory re. therapeutic range.
Digoxin (SP)	1	Low < 0.6 nmol/L Borderline low 0.6–1.0 nmol/L Therapeutic range 1.0–2.5 nmol/L Borderline high 2.5–3.0 nmol/L High > 3.0 nmol/L	
Ethosuximide (SP)	1	0.30–0.70 mmol/L (therapeutic)	Therapeutic range not well-defined.
Gentamicin (SP)	0.5	Peak 5–10 mg/L Trough < 2 mg/L (therapeutic)	
Nitrazepam (SP)	1		Consult with laboratory regarding therapeutic range.
Paracetamol (SP)	0.5		Only measured in suspected overdose – consult laboratory.
Phenobarbitone (SP)	1	80–120 μmol/L (therapeutic)	
Phenytoin (SP)	1	40–80 μmol/L (therapeutic)	
Primidone (SP)	1		Only the phenobarbitone metabolite measured, as this usually gives sufficient information for therapeutic monitoring.
Salicylate (SP)	0.5	0.7–2.00 nmol/L (therapeutic)	
Theophylline (SP)	0.5	Neonatal apnoea 40–80 μmol/L (therapeutic) Asthma 55–110 μmol/L (therapeutic-peak)	
Thiopentone (SP)	0.5	150–200 μmol/L (for anaesthesia)	
Tobramycin (SP)	0.5	Peak 5–10 mg/L Trough < 2 mg/L (therapeutic)	
Valproate (SP)	0.5	0.30–0.70 mmol/L (therapeutic)	
Vancomycin (SP)	0.5	Peak 25–40 mg/L Trough < 10 mg/L (therapeutic)	

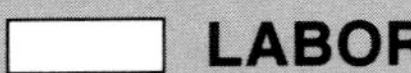

LABORATORY HAEMATOLOGY

Telephone inquiries 5823, Secretary 5822, Lab. Manager 5825, Director 5827. The department is situated on the 8th floor of the main block. It provides a wide range of haematology, coagulation and blood bank services.

HOURS

A 24 h service is provided for 5 nights a week. On Friday night and Saturday nights, after midnight, the department is on call from home for *urgent* specimens *only*.

Weekdays	*Service available*
0800–1700 h	Full range of tests
1700–0800 h	Urgent tests only
Weekends	
0001–0900 h	*On call from home*
0900–1800 h	Limited service
1800–2400 h	Urgent tests only

BLOOD COLLECTION

A combined pathology service is available for collection of capillary blood specimens from both inpatients and outpatients. The collection area is situated in the 8th floor link. Requests for ward collections should reach there before the rounds at 0900, 1100 and 1400 h. A request card may be sent to the collection rooms or retained in the ward and a phone message given. Phone 5821 (answering service available before 0830 h).

Venous blood collection by ward staff is required for some specimens and is preferred from children over 3 years of age. Venous blood collection from outpatients is performed in the pathology outpatient rooms.

SPECIMEN REQUIREMENTS

Capillary Blood

Capillary blood collections can be made for the tests listed below. For children 3 years of age and over venous specimens are preferable.

- FBE (coulter parameters)
- Differential count and film report
- Reticulocyte count
- IM screen
- G6PD screen
- Thrombotest

Results

Reports are issued routinely at 1200 and 1800 h. If a test is required to be performed urgently the laboratory must be phoned to indicate this need. Results for urgent FBE are usually available within 2 h of receipt of the specimen.

Phone calls regarding results frequently interrupt us when carrying out the tests and should be avoided if possible.

Tests Available During Non-Routine Hours

The following tests can be provided by the after hours service. Any other test will only be done during these times by special arrangement.

- Blood grouping and cross-matching
- Coombs' test
- FBE and differential
- G6PD screen
- PT, APTT, XDP, fibrinogen.

HAEMATOLOGY REFERENCE RANGES

	Haemoglobin (g/L)	*Haematocrit (L/L)*	*Reticulocytes × 10^9/L (%)*
Birth	110–170	0/30–0/40	
28 week gestation	120–180	0.35–0.50	
34 week gestation	140–200	0.40–0.55	
38 week gestation	135–195	0.42–0.60	200–300 (2.6)
40 week gestation			
1 week	135–205	0.42–0.62	< 5 (0)
2 weeks	125–205	0.40–0.62	< 5 (0)
1 month	100–180	0.31–0.55	
2 months	90–135	0.27–0.40	
3 months	95–140	0.29–0.41	5–250
6–24 months	105–140	0.33–0.42	10–100 (0.5–1.5)
2–5 years	115–140	0.35–0.42	10–100 (0.5–1.5)
6–11 years	115–155	0.35–0.48	10–100 (0.5–1.5)
12–18 years (male)	130–160	0.37–0.48	10–100 (0.5–1.5)
12–18 years (female)	120–160	0.36–0.48	10–100 (0.5–1.5)

RED CELL INDICES

	MCV (fL)	*MCH (pg)*	*MCHC (g/L)*
Birth			
28–37 week gestation	120		320–360
38–40 week gestation	110		320–360
1 week	110		320–360
1 month	90	24–34	320–360
2 months	80	24–24	320–360
3–12 months	70	24–31	320–360
Older	84–94	24–31	320–360

NORMAL WHITE CELL LEVELS

Age	*Total* ($\times 10^9$/L)	*Neutrophils* ($\times 10^9$/L) (%)	*Lymphocytes* ($\times 10^9$/L) (%)	*Monocytes* ($\times 10^9$/L) (%)	*Platelets* ($\times 10^9$/L)
Birth	9.0–30	6.0–26 (60)	2.0–11.0 (30)	1.1 (7)	150–400
1 wk	5–21	1.5–10 (45)	2.0–17.0 (40)	1.1 (9)	150–400
6 months	6–17.5	1.0–8.5 (30)	4.0–13.5 (60)	0.6 (5)	150–400
2 years	6–17.5	1.5–8.5 (33)	3.0–9.5 (60)	0.5 (5)	150–400
6 years	6–14.5	1.5–8.0 (50)	1.5–7.0 (42)	0.4 (5)	150–400
10 years	4.5–13.5	1.8–8.0 (54)	1.5–6.5 (38)	0.4 (4)	150–400
16 years	4.5–13.5	1.8–8.0 (60)	1.0–4.8 (33)	0.3 (4)	150–400

ESR 0–6 mm in 1 h (micro Westergren)

HAEMOGLOBIN ELECTROPHORESIS

Hb F Birth (40 week gestation)	60–90%
2 months	30–55%
3 months	15–30%
4 months	5–15%
6 months	2–5.0%
1 year	0.2–2.0%
Hb $A_2 > 1$ year	1.5–3.5%

ERYTHROPOIETIC FACTORS

Serum iron	9–27 μmol/L
Total iron binding capacity	45–72 μmol/L
Percentage saturation	16–33%
Serum ferritin	
$<$ 1 year	10–300 μg/L
$>$ 1 year	16–300 μg/L
Folate	
Serum	$>$ 4 μmol/L
Red cell	$>$ 270 μmol/L
Whole blood	$>$ 110 μmol/L
Vitamin B_{12}	150–590 pmol/L

COAGULATION

Bleeding time (Ivy)	2.0–7.0 min
Prothrombin time (PT)	10–14 s
Activated partial thromboplastin time (APTT)	27–40 s
D – Dimers	$<$ 10 μg/mL
Fibrinogen $<$ 6 months	1.5–4.0 g/L
$>$ 6 months	2.0–4.0 g/L

APPENDIX 1

DRUGS USED IN PAEDIATRICS LISTED BY GENERIC NAME

The following list contains the drugs most commonly used in paediatric practice. This list is by no means complete. It specifically does not include any antineoplastic agents nor any radioisotopes. While every effort has been made to check the drug doses in this list, it is still possible that errors may have been missed. Furthermore, dosage schedules are continually being revised and side effects recognized. For these reasons the reader is strongly advised to consult the drug companies' printed information before administering any of the drugs listed below. The Royal Children's Hospital Pharmacopoeia provides further information about drug usage in paediatrics.

Acetazolamide 2–7.5 mg/kg per dose (max. 350 mg) 8 hourly oral.

Acetylcysteine *Paracetamol poisoning* (up to 24 h after ingestion): 150 mg/kg oral or i.v. over 15 min stat, then 15 mg/kg per h for 72 h.

Activated charcoal See charcoal.

Acyclovir 5 mg/kg per dose 8 hourly i.v. over 1 h. *Encephalitis:* 10 mg/kg per dose 8 hourly i.v. over 1 h.

Adrenaline *Croup:* 1% (L isomer) or 2.25% (racaemic) 0.05 mL/kg per dose by inhalation; or 1 in 1000 (0.1%) 0.5 mL/kg per dose (max. 5 mL) by inhalation. *Cardiac arrest:* 0.1 mL/kg of 1 in 10 000 i.v. or intracardiac or via ETT (up to 1 mL/kg per dose if no response). *Anaphylaxis:* 0.05–0.1 mL/kg per dose of 1 in 10 000 i.v. *Infusion:* see p. 212.

Agarol See paraffin and phenolphthalein.

Albendazole 400 mg/dose 12 hourly for 3 days. *Enterobiasis:* 400 mg once, repeated after 2–4 weeks.

Albumin 25% *Undiluted:* 2–4 mL/kg. *Five per cent in 5%D or saline:* 10–20 mL/kg.

Aldactone See spironolactone.

Alginic acid See Gaviscon.

Allopurinol 2.5 mg/kg per dose 6 hourly oral.

Aluminium hydroxide 5–50 mg/kg per dose t.i.d. with meals. Gel (64 mg/mL) 0.1 mL/kg per dose 6 hourly oral.

Amiloride 0.2 mg/kg per dose (max. 5 mg/dose) 12 hourly oral.

Aminocaproic acid 100 mg/kg stat, then 30 mg/kg per h until bleeding stops (max. 18 g/m^2 per day) oral or i.v. *Prophylaxis:* 70 mg/kg per dose 6 hourly.

Aminophylline (100 mg aminophylline = 80 mg theophylline) *Load:* 10 mg/kg i.v. over 1 h. *Maintenance 1st week of life:* 2.5 mg/kg per dose 12 hourly. *Second week of life:* 4 mg/kg per dose 12 hourly. *Three weeks to 12 months:* (0.12 × age in weeks) + 3 mg/kg per dose 8 hourly. *One to 9 years:* 1.1 mg/kg per h. *Ten + years:* 0.7 mg/kg per h. *Note:* with 50 mg/kg in 50 mL, 1 mL/h = 1 mg/kg per h. Theophylline level 60–80 μmol/L (neonate), 60–110 (asthma), done on request at Royal Children's Hospital (× 0.18 = μg/mL).

Amitriptyline *Enuresis:* 1.0–1.5 mg/kg nocte.

Amoxycillin 10–20 mg/kg per dose 8 hourly i.v., i.m. or oral. *Severe infection:* 50 mg/kg per dose i.v. 12 hourly (1st week of life), 6 hourly (2–4 weeks), 4 hourly (4 + weeks).

Amoxycillin and clavulanic acid Dose as for amoxycillin.

Amphotericin B 0.25 mg/kg i.v. over 3–6 h daily, increasing by 0.25 mg/kg per day to max. 0.5–1 mg/kg per day (protect from light). *Oral:* 100 mg 6 hourly treatment, 50 mg 6 hourly prophylaxis.

Ampicillin 15–25 mg/kg per dose 6 hourly i.v., i.m. or oral. *Severe infection:* 50 mg/kg per dose i.v. 12 hourly (1st week of life), 6 hourly (2–4 weeks), 4 hourly (4 + weeks).

Antacid See Mylanta.

Anthaquinone See Sennoside.

Antidiuretic hormone See vasopressin.

Antivenom (box jellyfish, funnel-web spider, sea snake, tiger snake, death adder, taipan, brown snake, black snake, tick) Dose depends on amount of venom injected, not size of patient. Higher doses needed for multiple bites, severe symptoms or delayed administration. Give adrenaline 0.01 mg/kg (max. 0.25 mg) s.c. and promethazine 0.1 mg/kg i.v. Initial dose antivenom usually 1–2 amp diluted 1/10 in Hartmann's solution i.v. over 30 min. Monitor PT, PTT, fibrinogen, platelets. Give antivenom repeatedly if symptoms or coagulopathy persist.

Antivenom, redback spider 1 amp i.m., repeat in 2 h if required. *Severe envenomation:* 2 amps diluted 1/10 in Hartmann's solution i.v. over 30 min.

Antivenom, stonefish 1000 units (2 mL) per puncture i.m. *Severe envenomation:* 1000 units/puncture diluted 1/10 in Hartmann's solution i.v. over 30 min.

Aramine See metaraminol.

Arginine HCl mg = BE × wt(kg) × 70 (give half this) i.v. over 2 h.

Artane See benzhexol.

Ascorbic acid *Scurvy:* 100 mg/dose 8 hourly oral for 10 days. *Urine acidification:* 10–30 mg/kg per dose 6 hourly oral.

Aspirin 15 mg/kg per dose 6 hourly oral. *Antiplatelet:* 5 mg/kg daily. *Arthritis:* 60 mg/kg per dose 12 hourly for 3 days, then 30 mg/kg per dose 12 hourly; > 25 kg 600–900 mg/dose 6 hourly. *Kawasaki:* 50 mg/kg per dose 12 hourly 14 days (monitor levels), then 4 mg/kg daily. Salicylate level (arthritis) 0.7–2.0 mmol/L (× 13.81 = mg/100 mL), done on request.

Atenolol 1–2 mg/kg per dose 12–24 hourly oral; 0.05 mg/kg per dose every 5 min till response (max. four doses) i.v., then 0.2–1 mg/kg per dose 12–24 hourly.

Atracurium 0.5 mg/kg stat, then 5–10 μg/kg per min i.v.

Atropine *Premed or reversal:* 0.02 mg/kg (max. 0.6 mg) i.v. or i.m. *Organophosphate poisoning:* 0.05 mg/kg i.v., then 0.02–0.05 mg/kg per dose every 15–60 min until atropinized (continue 12–24 h). *Colic:* Royal Children's Hospital mixture (12 μg/mL) 2.5–5 mL oral before feeds (max. 15 mL/day). See also colic mixture.

Atrovent See ipratropium.

Augmentin See amoxycillin and clavulanic acid.

Azathioprine 25–75 mg/m^2 (approx. 1–3 mg/kg) daily.

Aztreonam 30 mg/kg per dose 8 hourly. *Severe infection:* 50 mg/kg per dose 12 hourly (1st week of life), 8 hourly (2–4 weeks), 6 hourly (4 + weeks) i.v.

Baclofen 0.1 mg/kg per dose 8 hourly oral, increasing by 0.1 mg/kg per dose every 3 days. Effective dose about 0.5 mg/kg per dose 8 hourly (max. 1 mg/kg per dose 8 hourly). *Intrathecal infusion:* 2–3 μg/kg per day.

Beclomethasone 200–200 μg/day

Benzhexol Slow increase to 0.1–0.2 mg/kg daily oral.

Benztropine 0.02 mg/kg stat i.m. or i.v., repeated after 15 min if required; 0.02–0.1 mg/kg per dose 12–24 hourly oral.

Benzylpenicillin See penicillin G.

Bethanecol *Oral:* 0.2 mg/kg per dose 6–8 hourly. s.c.: 0.05 mg/kg per dose 6–8 hourly.

Bicarbonate *Under 5 kg:* mmol deficit = BE × wt/2 (give half this) slow i.v. *Over 5 kg:* mmol deficit = BE × wt/3 (give half this) slow i.v.

Bisacodyl Under 12 months 2.5 mg p.r., 1–5 years 5 mg p.r. or 5–10 mg oral, over 5 years 10 mg p.r. or 10–20 mg oral.

Bismuth subcitrate, colloidal (De-Nol) *H. pylori:* > 5 years old, One tablet (107.7 mg) 6 hourly for 4 weeks (with amoxycillin and metronidazole). Avoid milk.

Blood products See albumin, cryoprecipitate, Factor VIII, fresh frozen plasma, packed cells, platelets and prothombinex.

Bretylium 5 mg/kg i.v. over 1 h, then 5–15 μg/kg per min.

Bupivacaine *Max. dose:* 2 mg/kg.

Bupivacaine with adrenaline *Max. dose:* 3 mg/kg.

Calcium carbonate 168 mg/mL (Titralac) 5 mL 8–12 hourly oral.

Calcium chloride 10% (0.7 mmol/mL Ca) 0.2 mL/kg (max. 10 mL) slow i.v. stat. Requirement 2 mL/kg per day. *Inotrope:* 0.5–2 mmol/kg per day (0.03–0.12 mL/kg per h).

Calcium edetate (EDTA) 25 mg/kg per dose 12 hourly i.m. or i.v. over 1 h for 5 days.

Calcium gluconate 10% (0.22 mmol/mL Ca) 0.5 mL/kg (max. 20 mL) slow i.v. stat. Requirement 5 mL/kg per day. *Inotrope:* 0.5–2 mmol/kg per day (0.1–0.4 mL/kg per h).

Canrenoate See potassium canrenoate.

Captopril 0.1–1.0 mg/kg per dose 8 hourly oral.

Carbamazepine 2 mg/kg per dose 8 hourly oral, increasing over 2 weeks to about 5 mg/kg per dose (max. 10 mg/kg per dose) 8 hourly. Level 20–50 μmol/L (× 0.24 = μg/mL), done Mondays, Wednesdays and Fridays at Royal Children's Hospital.
Carbimazole 0.25 mg/kg per dose (max. 15 mg/dose) 8 hourly oral for 2 weeks, then 0.1 mg/kg per dose 8–12 hourly.
Carnitine 35 mg/kg per dose 8 hourly oral or i.v.
Cefaclor (Ceclor) 10–15 mg/kg per dose (max. 500 mg) 8 hourly oral.
Cefazolin See cephazolin.
Cefotaxime 30 mg/kg per dose 6 hourly. *Severe infection:* 50 mg/kg per dose i.v. 12 hourly (preterm), 8 hourly (1st week of life), 6 hourly (2–4 weeks), 4–6 hourly (4 + weeks).
Cefoxitin (Mefoxin) 20–40 mg/kg per dose (max. 3 g/dose) 6 hourly i.v.
Ceftazidime 30 mg/kg per dose 8 hourly. *Severe infection:* 50 mg/kg per dose 12 hourly (1st week of life), 8 hourly (4 + weeks) i.v. or i.m.
Ceftriaxone 30 mg/kg per dose 12–24 hourly. Severe infection: 50 mg/kg per dose daily (1st week of life), 12 hourly (2 + weeks) i.v., or i.m. (in 1% lignocaine).
Cephalothin 10–20 mg/kg per dose 6 hourly i.v. or i.m. *Irrigation fluid:* 2 g/L (2 mg/mL).
Cephazolin (Kefzol) 30 mg/kg 8 hourly i.v.
Charcoal (activated) *Check bowel sounds present:* 0.25 g/kg per dose hourly n.g. (*Laxative:* colonic lavage solution or magnesium sulfate n.g., or Coloxyl suppository).
Chloral hydrate *Hypnotic:* 50 mg/kg (max. 1 g) stat. *Sedative:* 6 mg/kg per dose 6 hourly oral.
Chlorazepate *Over 9 years:* 7.5 mg/dose 8–12 hourly oral, gradually increasing to max. 60 mg/day.
Chloramphenicol 40 mg/kg stat, then 25 mg/kg per dose (max. 1 g/dose) i.v., i.m. or oral. *First week of life:* daily. Two to 4 weeks: 12 hourly. 5 + weeks: 8 hourly for 5 days, then 6 hourly. Level 20–30 mg/L peak, < 15 mg/L trough, on request at Royal Children's Hospital.
Chlormethiazole *i.v. (0.8%):* 1–2 mL/kg (8–16 mg/kg) i.v. over 15 min, then 0.05–0.15 mL/kg per h (3.3–10 mg/kg per h).
Chloroquine 10 mg/kg oral stat, or 5 mg/kg after 6 h then 5 mg/kg for 2 days. *Prophylaxis:* 5 mg/kg oral once a week.
Chlorothiazide 10 mg/kg per dose 12–24 hourly oral.
Chlorpheniramine and phenylephine Chlorpheniramine 0.05 mg/kg per dose and phenylephine 0.1 mg/kg per dose 6–8 hourly oral.
Chlorpromazine *Sedation, head injury:* 0.5 mg/kg per dose slow i.v., i.m. or oral (usual max. 2 mg/kg per day). *After cardiac surgery:* 0.05 mg/kg i.v. (may be repeated).
Cholestyramine *Resin:* 0.05–0.1 g/kg per dose 8 hourly oral.
Cimetidine 5–10 mg/kg per dose (usual max. 200 mg/dose) 6 hourly i.v. or oral.
Ciprofloxacin 5–10 mg/kg per dose 12 hourly i.v. or oral. Reduce dose of theophylline.
Cisapride 0.2 mg/kg per dose (max. 5–10 mg) 6 hourly oral before meals and at bedtime.
Citravescent See sodium citrotartrate.
Clavulanic acid with amoxycillin or ticarcillin Dose as for amoxycillin or ticarcillin.
Clindamycin 5–10 mg/kg per dose 6 hourly i.v. over 30 min, i.m. or oral.
Clobazam *Over 3 years:* 5–20 mg/dose 8–12 hourly oral.
Clonazepam *Status (may be repeated):* neonates 0.25 mg, children 0.5 mg, adults 1 mg i.v. *Maintenance:* 0.01 mg/kg per dose (up to 0.03 mg/kg per dose) 8 hourly oral.
Clonidine 5 μg/kg i.v., 1–4 μg/kg per dose 8 hourly oral. *Migraine:* start with 0.5 μg/kg per dose 12 hourly oral.
Codeine *Analgesic:* 0.5 mg/kg per dose 4 hourly oral. *Antitussive:* 0.25 mg/kg per dose 6 hourly.
Cogentin See benztropine.
Colonic lavage solution *Poisoning:* if bowel sounds present, 30 mL/kg per h, n.g. for 4–8 h (until rectal effluent clear).
Coloxyl (dioctyl sodium sulfosuccinate, poloxalkol) *Drops:* one drop/month of age 8 hourly (< 3 years). *Tablets:* 0.5–1.0 mg/kg per dose 8–24 hourly oral. *Tablets with danthon:* over 12 years one to two tablets daily. Suppository: under 1 year half suppository, over 1 year one suppository. *Enema* (5 mL 18% poloxalkol diluted to 120 mL): neonate 30 mL, 1–12 months 60 mL, > 12 months 60–120 mL.
Corticotrophin See ACTH.
Cortisone acetate *Physiological:* 0.2 mg/kg per dose 8 hourly oral.

Cosyntropin See tetracosactrin zinc injection.
Cotrimoxazole (trimethoprim 1 mg + sulfamethoxazole 5 mg) Trimethoprim 2.5 mg/kg per dose 12 hourly oral.
Cromolyn sodium See sodium cromoglycate.
Cryoprecipitate (Factor VIII about 5 units/mL and 100 units/bag, fibrinogen about 10 mg/mL and 200 mg/bag) *Low Factor VIII:* 1 unit/kg increases activity 2% (half-life 12 h); usual dose 5 mL/kg or 1 bag/4 kg 12 hourly i.v. for one to two infusions (muscle, joint), three to six infusions (hip, forearm, retroperitoneal, oropharynx), seven to 14 infusions (intracranial). *Low fibrinogen:* usual dose 5 mL/kg or 1 bag/4 kg i.v.
Curare See tubocurarine.
Cyclosporin 1–3 μg/kg per min i.v. for 24–48 h, then 5–8 mg/kg per dose 12 hourly reducing by 1 mg/kg per dose each month to 3–4 mg/kg per dose oral. Trough level by fluorescent polarization on whole blood (done Tuesdays and Fridays at the Royal Children's Hospital): 200–450 ng/mL (marrow), 350–875 ng/mL (kidney), 800–1200 ng/mL (heart, liver).
Cyclosporine See cyclosporin.
Cyproheptadine 0.1 mg/kg per dose 8–12 hourly oral.
Cyproterone acetate 25–50 mg/m^2 per dose 8–12 hourly oral.
Danthon 1–6 years 25 mg, 7–12 years 50 mg, adult 100 mg stat.
Dantrolene 1 mg/kg per min until improves (max. 10 mg/kg), then 1–2 mg/kg per dose 6 hourly for 1–3 days i.v. or oral.
DDAVP See desmopressin.
Deferoxamine See desferrioxamine.
Desferrioxamine *Antidote:* 10–15 mg/kg per h i.v. for 12 h. *Thalassaemia:* 500 mg/unit blood and 1–3 g in 5 mL s.c. over 10 h 5–6 nights per week.
Desmopressin (DDAVP) 5–10 μg (0.05–0.1 mL)/dose 12–24 hourly nasal. *Low Factor VIII:* 0.3 μg/kg in 1 mL/kg saline i.v. over 1 h 12–24 hourly.
Dexamethasone 0.1–0.25 mg/kg per dose 6 hourly oral or i.v. *BPD:* 0.1 mg/kg per dose 6 hourly for 3 days, then 8 hourly 3 days, 12 hourly 3 days, 24 hourly 3 days, 48 hourly 7 days. *Severe croup:* 0.6 mg/kg (max. 12 mg) i.m. stat, then 0.15 mg/kg per dose 6 hourly oral. Dexamethasone has no mineralocorticoid action, but 1 mg = 32 mg hydrocortisone in glucocorticoid action.
Dexamphetamine 0.2 mg/kg daily (need permit).
Dexchlorpheniramine 0.05 mg/kg per dose 8 hourly oral.
Dextran 70 *6% solution:* 10 mL/kg per dose (up to 20 mL/kg on the first day, then not more than 10 mL/kg per day).
Dextrose (glucose) *Hypoglycaemia:* 1 mL/kg 50% D i.v. *Hyperkalaemia:* 0.1 units/kg insulin + 2 mL/kg 50% D i.v. *Neonates:* 4 mg/kg per min day 1, increase to 8 mg/kg per min (up to 12 mg/kg per min with hypoglycaemia). Infusion rate (mL/h) = (6 × wt × mg/kg per min)/%dextrose. Dose (mg/kg per min) = (mL/h × %dextrose)/(6 × wt).
Diazepam 0.2 mg/kg per dose i.v. 0.2–0.5 mg/kg per dose 8–12 hourly oral or p.r. Do not give by i.v. infusion (binds to PVC).
Diazoxide 2–5 mg/kg stat by rapid i.v. injection (repeat once p.r.n.), then 2–5 mg/kg per dose i.v. 6 hourly. Severe hypotension may occur.
Diclofenac 1 mg/kg per dose 8–12 hourly.
Dicyclomine 0.5 mg/kg per dose (max. 15 mg/dose) 6 hourly oral.
Digoxin 15 μg/kg stat and 5 μg/kg after 6 hourly, then 5 μg/kg per dose 12 hourly slow i.v. or oral. Level 0.5–2.5 nmol/L (× 0.78 = ng/mL), done Monday–Saturday at Royal Children's Hospital hourly.
Digoxin FAB antibodies Dose (to nearest 40 mg) = serum digoxin (nmol/L) × wt (kg) × 0.26, or mg ingested × 0.8.
Dimercaprol (BAL) 4 mg/kg per dose i.m. 4 hourly for 2 days, then 3 mg/kg per dose 6 hourly 2 days, then 3 mg/kg per dose 12 hourly 7 days.
Dinoprostone See prostaglandin E_2.
Dioctyl sodium sulfosuccinate See Coloxyl.
Diphenhydramine 1.25 mg/kg per dose 6 hourly oral.
Diphenylmethane See bisacodyl.
Dipyriadamole 1–2 mg/kg per dose 8 hourly oral.
Disopyramide 5 mg/kg stat, then 2–5 mg/kg per dose 6 hourly oral. Level 9–15 μmol/L (× 0.3395 = μg/mL), on request.
Dobutamine Infusion: see p. 212.
Docusate See Coloxyl.
Domperidone 0.2–0.4 mg/kg per dose 4–8 hourly oral; 4 mg/kg per day rectal.
Dopamine *Infusion:* see p. 212.
Doxapram 5 mg/kg i.v. over 1 h, then 0.5–1.0 mg/kg per h.

Doxepin 0.2–2 mg/kg per dose 8 hourly oral.
Doxycycline *Over 7 years:* 2.5 mg/kg per dose 12 hourly for two doses, then daily.
Droperidol 0.1 mg/kg per dose slow i.v., 0.15 mg/kg per dose i.m.
Edrophonium Test dose 20 μg/kg, then 100 μg/kg i.v.
EDTA See calcium edetate.
Enalapril 0.2–1.0 mg/kg daily oral.
Epinephrine See adrenaline.
Epoprostenol (prostacyclin, PGI_2) 0.01 μg/kg per min i.v. Pulmonary vasodilation: 0.01 μg/kg per min epoprost = 5 μg/kg per min nitroglycerine = 2 μg/kg per min nitroprusside = 0.1 μg/kg per min PGE_1 approx.
Epsilon aminocaproic acid See aminocaproic acid.
Ergotamine *Over 10 years:* 2 mg sublingual stat, then 1 mg/h (max. 6 mg/episode, 10 mg/week). *Suppository* (1–2 mg): 1 stat, repeat once after 1 h if required.
Erythromycin 10–20 mg/kg per dose 6–8 hourly slow i.v. or oral.
Ethamsylate 10 mg/kg 6 hourly oral, i.m. or i.v.
Ethinyloestradiol *Adult:* 20 μg daily for 21 days each month.
Ethosuximide 2.5 mg/kg per dose 6 hourly oral, increasing by 50% each week to max. 10 mg/kg per dose 6 hourly.
Etidronate See sodium etidronate.
Factor VIII concentrate (vial 200–250 u) Joint 20 u/kg, psoas 30 u/kg, cerebral 50 u/kg.
Fat emulsion 20% 1 g/kg per day = 0.21 mL/kg per h i.v.
Fentanyl 1–2 μg/kg per dose i.m. or i.v., infuse 2–4 μg/kg per h. *Ventilated:* 5–10 μg/kg stat or 50 μg/kg over 1 h, infuse 5–10 μg/kg per h (amp 100 μg/2 mL at 0.1–0.2 mL/kg per h).
Ferrous gluconate (Fergon 300 mg/5 mL) Prophylaxis 0.3 mL/kg daily, treatment 1 mL/kg daily oral.
Ferrous sulfate (Ferrogradumet 350 mg = 105 mg iron) Prophylaxis 2 mg/kg per day, treatment 6 mg/kg per day iron.
Flagyl See metronidazole.
Flecainide 2 mg/kg per dose 12 hourly oral or i.v. over 10 min. Increase slowly (2 weeks) to 5 mg/kg per dose 12 hourly if required.
Flucloxacillin 25–50 mg/kg per dose 12 hourly (1st week of life), 8 hourly (2–4 weeks), 4–6 hourly (over 4 weeks) i.v. or oral.
Fludrocortisone 0.05–0.2 mg daily oral.
Flumazenil 5 μg/kg stat i.v. repeated every 60 s to max. total 40 μg/kg, then 2–10 μg/kg per h i.v.
9α-fluorohydrocortisone See fludrocortisone.
Folic acid *Treatment:* 0.25 mg/kg daily i.v., i.m., oral.
Folinic acid 5–15 mg i.v., i.m. or oral 6 hourly for 36–48 h.
Fresh frozen plasma Contains all clotting factors; 10–20 mL/kg i.v.
Frusemide Usually 0.5–1.0 mg/kg per dose 6–12 hourly (daily if preterm) i.m., i.v. or oral. Up to 5 mg/kg per dose in resistant cases. *i.v. infusion:* 0.1–1.0 mg/kg per h.
Furosemide See frusemide.
Fusidic acid 20 mg/kg stat, then 10–15 mg/kg 8 hourly i.v. over 30 min or oral. Level 40–400 μmol/L (× 0.52 = μg/mL), done on request.
Gammaglobulin See immunoglobulin.
Gammahydroxybutyrate 40–100 mg/kg i.v. stat (40 mg/kg for short anaesthetic).
Gaviscon *Infants:* 1–2 g powder with feed 4 hourly. *Under 12 years:* liquid 5–10 mL, or granules half sachet after meals. *Over 12 years:* liquid 10–20 mL, or granules one sachet after meals.
Gentamicin 2.5 mg/kg per dose (max. 100 mg/dose) i.v. daily (< 30 week gestation), 18 hourly (30–35 week gestation), 12 hourly (1st week of life), 8 hourly (2 + weeks).
Glucagon 1 unit = 1 mg. 0.2 units/kg i.v. stat, then 0.005–0.01 unit/kg per h.
Glucose See dextrose.
Glucose electrolyte solution See oral glucose solution.
Glyceryl trinitrate *Sublingual:* 0.01–0.015 mg/kg per dose. *i.v.:* see nitroglycerine.
Gonadorelin 100 μg/dose i.v.
Griseofulvin 10–15 mg/kg daily oral.
Griseofulvin (ultramicrosize) 5 mg/kg daily oral.
Haemaccel 10–20 mL/kg stat (may be repeated). Half-life 2 h.
Haloperidol Start 0.5 mg daily, increase up to 0.025 mg/kg per dose 12 hourly i.v. or oral.
Heparin 1 mg = 100 units. *Low dose:* 75 units/kg i.v. stat, then 10–15 units/kg per h i.v. (500 units/kg in 50 mL at 1 mL/h = 10 units/kg per h). *Full dose:* 200 units/kg stat, then 15–30 units/kg per h. *Extracorporeal circuits:* 10–20 units/kg per h prefilter, 2–5 units/kg per h postfilter.

Heparin calcium *Low dose:* 75 units/kg per dose s.c. 12 hourly.
Hydralazine *i.v. or i.m.:* 0.25–0.5 mg/kg stat, then 0.1–0.2 mg/kg per dose 4–6 hourly. *Oral:* 0.2 mg/kg per dose, gradually increasing to max. 2.0 mg/kg per dose 12 hourly.
Hydrochloric acid Use solution of 150 mmol/L, give i.v. by central line only. Dose (mL) = BE × wt × 2.2 (give half this). Max. rate = 1.33 mL/kg per h.
Hydrochlorothiazide 1 mg/kg per dose 12–24 hourly oral.
Hydrocortisone sodium succinate 2–4 mg/kg per dose 3–6 hourly i.m. or i.v., tapering over several days. *Physiological:* 0.2 mg/kg per dose 8 hourly i.m. or i.v.
Hydroxycobalamin (Vitamin B_{12}) 20 μg/kg per dose, daily for 7 days then weekly (treatment), monthly (prophylaxis), i.m. (not i.v.).
Hyoscine 0.01 mg/kg per dose 6 hourly, i.m. or i.v.
Hyoscine *N*-butyl bromide 0.5 mg/kg per dose 6–8 hourly i.v., i.m. or oral.
Ibuprofen 2.5–10 mg/kg per dose 6 hourly.
Imipramine 0.5 mg/kg per dose 8 hourly oral. *Enuresis:* 5–6 years 25 mg nocte, 7–10 years 50 mg, over 10 years 50–75 mg.
Immunoglobulin, hepatitis B 400 units i.m. within 5 days of needle stick, repeated in 30 days; 100 units i.m. within 24 h birth to baby of hepatitis B carrier.
Immunoglobulin, zoster Prevention of chicken pox in immunocompromised, 0.4–1.2 mL/kg i.m.
Indomethacin *PDA:* 0.1 mg/kg daily for 6 days oral or i.v. over 1 h (? higher dose if > 14 days old). *Arthritis:* 12.5 mg 12 hourly, increasing to 25 mg 8 hourly oral.
Insulin 0.05–0.2 units/kg p.r.n., or 0.1 units/kg per h in 20% *Haemaccel*; later 1 units/10 g dextrose i.v. *Hyperkalaemia:* 0.1 units/kg insulin and 2 mL/kg 50% D i.v. *TPN:* 5–25 units/250 g dextrose.
Intal See sodium cromoglycate.
Intralipid 20% 1 g/kg per day = 0.21 mL/kg per h i.v.
Ipecacuanha syrup 1–2 mL/kg (max. 30 mL) stat oral, NG.
Ipratropium *Respiratory solution:* 0.25–1.0 mL diluted to 2 mL 4–6 hourly. Aerosol: 2–4 puffs 6–8 hourly.
Iron See ferrous gluconate, ferrous sulfate.
Iron dextran (Fe 50 mg/mL) No. mL = 0.05 × wt in kg × (15 — Hb in g%) i.m. i.v. infusion dangerous.
Isoniazid 10–15 mg/kg daily.
Isoprenaline See p. 212. Ampoules (1 : 5000, 0.2 mg/mL) give max. concentration of 10 mg/50 mL.
Isoproterenol See isoprenaline.
Kefzol See cephazolin.
Ketamine 1–2 mg/kg i.v., 5–10 mg/kg i.m. *Infusion:* anaesthesia 10–20 μg/kg per min, analgesia 4 μg/kg per min.
Konakion See phytomenadione.
Labetalol 2 mg/kg per dose 12 hourly oral. Increase weekly to max. 20 mg/kg per dose 12 hourly if required.
Lactulose 50% (Duphalac) *Laxative:* 0.5 mL/kg per dose 12–24 hourly oral. *Hepatic coma:* 1 mL/kg per dose 6 hourly oral.
Latamoxef (Moxalactam) 25–50 mg/kg per dose 6 hourly i.v., i.m.
Leucovorin See folinic acid.
Levothyroxine sodium See thyroxine.
Lidocaine See lignocaine.
Lignocaine *i.v.:* 1 mg/kg stat (0.1 mL/kg of 1%), then 15–50 μg/kg per min (see p. 212). *Nerve block:* without adrenaline 4 mg/kg, with adrenaline 7 mg/kg. *Topical spray:* 3–4 mg/kg (Xylocaine 10% spray pack gives approx. 10 mg per puff).
Liothyronine (triiodothyronine) 0.2–0.4 μg/kg per dose i.v. 4–12 hourly.
Lithium carbonate 5–10 mg/kg per dose 12 hourly to maintain trough serum level 0.8–1.6 mmol/L (> 2 mmol/L toxic).
Loperamide 5–8 years 1 mg/dose, > 8 years 2 mg/dose 8 hourly.
Magnesium chloride 0.48 g/5 mL (1 mmol/mL Mg); 0.4 mmol (0.4 mL)/kg per dose 12 hourly slow i.v.
Magnesium hydroxide mixture (Royal Children's Hospital) 0–6 months 2.5–5 mL, 6 months–5 years 5–10 mL. See also Mylanta.
Magnesium sulfate *Deficiency:* 50% magnesium sulfate (2 mmol/mL) 0.2 mL/kg per dose 12 hourly i.m. or slow i.v. *Tachyarrhythmias from digoxin:* 50% magnesium sulfate 0.1 mL/kg i.v. over 10 min, then infuse 0.4 mL/kg over 6 h, then 0.8 mL/kg over 18 h (keep serum mg 1.5–2.0 mmol/L). *As laxative:* 0.5 g/kg per dose (max. 15 g) as 10% solution 8 hourly for 2 days oral.
Mannitol 0.25–0.5 g/kg per dose i.v. (1–2 mL/kg of 25%) 2 hourly p.r.n., provided serum osmolality < 330 mmol/L.
Marcain See bupivacaine.
Mebendazole 100 mg/dose 12 hourly for

3 days. *Enterobiasis:* 100 mg once, repeated after 2–4 weeks.

Medroxyprogesterone 5 mg daily for 5–10 days/month oral.

Mefenamic acid *Adults:* 500 mg/dose 8 hourly oral for 5 days.

Menadione See menaphthone sodium bisulfate.

Menaphthone sodium bisulfate *Children:* 5–10 mg daily oral.

Meperidine See pethidine.

Metaproterenol See orciprenaline.

Metaraminol 0.01 mg/kg stat (repeat p.r.n.), then 0.1–1.0 μg/kg per min and titrate dose against BP.

Methenamine mandelate 15 mg/kg per dose 6 hourly oral.

Methohexital sodium See methohexitone.

Methohexitone 1.5–2.0 mg/kg per dose i.v.

Methyldopa Start with 2.5 mg/kg per dose 8 hourly oral.

Methylene blue 1–2 mg/kg per dose i.v.

Methylphenidate 0.2 mg/kg daily, increasing to 0.5 mg/kg per dose 12 hourly if needed. Usual maintenance dose 0.7 mg/kg daily.

Methylprednisolone *Asthma:* 0.5–1.0 mg/kg per dose 6 hourly for 24 h, 12 hourly for the next 24 h, then 1.0 mg/kg daily. *Spinal cord injury:* 30 mg/kg stat, then 5 mg/kg per h for 2 days. 1 mg = hydrocortisone 0.5 mg in mineralocorticoid action, 5 mg in glucocorticoid.

4-Methylpyrazole 10 mg/kg stat i.v. over 1 h, then 5 mg/kg per dose 12 hourly i.v. over 30 min for four doses.

Metolazone 0.1 mg/kg daily oral. Up to 0.5 mg/kg daily short term for severe oedema or ascites.

Metoprolol 0.1 mg/kg i.v. over 5 min, repeated every 5 min to max. of 0.3 mg/kg, then 1–5 μg/kg per min; 1 mg/kg per dose 6–12 hourly oral.

Metronidazole 15 mg/kg stat, then 7.5 mg/kg per dose 12 hourly in neonate (1st maintenance dose 48 h after load in pre-term, 24 h in term baby), 8 hourly (4 + weeks) i.v., i.m. or oral. Level 60–300 μmol/mL (× 0.17 = μg/mL), done on request.

Mexiletine *i.v. infusion:* 5 mg/kg over 15 min, then 5–20 μg/kg per min. *Oral:* 10 mg/kg stat, then 5 mg/kg per dose 8 hourly commencing 2 h after loading dose.

Miconazole 7.5–15 mg/kg per dose 8 hourly i.v. over 1 h.

Microlax enema < 12 months 1.25 mL, 1–2 years 2.5 mL, > 2 years 5 mL.

Midazolam *Sedation:* usually 0.1–0.2 mg/kg i.v. or i.m., but up to 0.5 mg/kg used safely in children. *Anaesthesia:* 0.5 mg/kg, then 2 μg/kg per min (3 mg/kg in 50 mL at 2 mL/h) i.v.

Mineral oil See paraffin liquid.

Misoprostol (synthetic PGE$_1$) 4 μg/kg per dose 6 hourly oral.

Morphine 0.1–0.2 mg/kg per dose i.v., 0.2 mg/kg per dose i.m. (half-life 2–4 h). *Infusion:* 0.5 mg/kg in 50 mL 5%D at 1–5 mL/h (10–50 μg/kg per h).

Moxalactam See latamoxef.

Mylanta (aluminium hydroxide and magnesium hydroxide 40 mg/mL) 0.5 mL/kg per dose 3 hourly oral if gastric pH < 5.

Nalidixic acid 12.5 mg/kg per dose 6 hourly oral.

Naloxone *Opiate intoxication (including newborn):* 0.1 mg/kg (max. 2 mg) stat i.v. or intratracheal, then 0.01 mg/kg per h i.v. *Postoperative depression:* 0.002 mg/kg per dose repeated every 2 min, then 0.01 mg/kg per h, i.v.

Naproxen 5–7.5 mg/kg per dose 12 hourly oral.

Neostigmine 0.07 mg/kg per dose i.v. *Suggested dilution in babies:* neostigmine (0.5 mg/mL) 1 mL + atropine (0.6 mg/mL) 0.25 mL diluted to 7 mL, give 1 mL/kg i.v.

Niclosamide 40 mg/kg daily oral.

Nicotinic acid *Hypercholesterolaemia and hypertriglyceridaemia:* 5 mg/kg per dose 8 hourly, gradually increase to 20–30 mg/kg per dose 8 hourly oral.

Nifedipine 0.25–1.0 mg/kg 6–12 hourly oral or sublingual.

Nimodipine 15 μg/kg per h for 2 h, then 15–45 μg/kg per h, i.v.

Nitrazepam 1.25–5 mg/dose 12 hourly. *Hypnotic:* 2.5–5 mg.

Nitrofurantoin 1.5 mg/kg per dose (max. 100 mg) 6 hourly oral. *Prophylaxis:* 2.5 mg/kg at night.

Nitroglycerine *Infusion:* see p. 212. Use polyethylene-lined syringe and tubing (not PVC). *Pulmonary vasodilation:* 5 μg/kg per min nitroglycerine = 2 μg/kg per min nitroprusside = 0.1 μg/kg per min PGE$_1$.

Nitroprusside *Infusion:* see p. 212. Protect from light. Used for > 24 h, max. rate 4 μg/kg per min. Max total dose 70 mg/kg with normal renal function (or sodium thiocyanate

< 1725 μmol/L, × 0.058 = mg/L). *Pulmonary vasodilation:* 5 μg/kg per min nitroglycerine = 2 μg/kg per min nitroprusside = 0.1 μg/kg per min PGE_1 approx.

Noradrenaline *Infusion:* see p. 212.

Norepinephrine See noradrenaline.

Norethindrone See norethisterone.

Norethisterone *Menorrhagia:* 10 mg 3 hourly until bleeding stops, then 5 mg 6 hourly for 1 week, then 5 mg 8 hourly for 2 weeks.

Norfloxacin 10 mg/kg per dose 12 hourly oral.

Normacol granules 6 months–5 years half teaspoon 12 hourly, 6–10 years one teaspoon 12 hourly, over 10 years 1 teaspoon 8 hourly.

Nortriptyline 0.5 mg/kg per dose 8 hourly oral.

Nystatin 500 000 units (one tablet) 6–8 hourly n.g. or oral. *Neonates:* 100 000 units (1 mL) 8 hourly.

Oestrogen See ethinyloestradiol.

Omnopon See papaveretum.

Oral glucose solution *Not dehydrated:* one heaped teaspoon sucrose in a large cup of water (4% sucrose = 2% glucose); do not add salt. *Dehydrated:* one sachet of Gastrolyte in 200 mL water; give frequent small sips, or infuse though a nasogastric tube.

Oral rehydration solution (ORS) See oral glucose solution.

Orciprenaline *Oral:* 0.25–0.5 mg/kg per dose 6 hourly. Respiratory solution (2%): 0.5 mL/dose diluted to 2 mL 3–6 hourly (mild), 1.0 mL/dose diluted to 2 mL (moderate), undiluted continuously (severe, in ICU). *Aerosol:* two puffs 4–6 hourly.

Ornipressin (POR 8) 5 units in 30 mL saline, max. total dose 0.5 units/kg s.c.

Oxandrolone 0.1 mg/kg daily oral.

Packed cells 4 mL/kg raises Hb 1 g%.

Pancreatic enzymes *With meals:* 1–3 Cotazyme-S Forte cap, 1–5 Pancrease cap oral.

Pancuronium *ICU:* 0.1 mg/kg i.v. p.r.n. *Theatre:* 0.1 mg/kg i.v. stat, then 0.02 mg/kg p.r.n.

Papaveretum (Omnopon) 0.2 mg/kg per dose i.v., 0.4 mg/kg per dose i.m. (half-life 2–4 h).

Papaveretum (20 mg/mL) and hyoscine (0.4 mg/mL) 0.4 mg/kg (P) + 0.008 mg/kg (hourly) = 0.02 mL/kg per dose i.m.

Paracetamol 15 mg/kg per dose 4 hourly oral or p.r.

Paraffin liquid 1 mL/kg daily oral.

Paraffin (65%) and agar 6 months–2 years 5 mL, 3–5 years 5–10 mL, over 5 years 10 mL 8–24 hourly oral.

Paraffin and phenolphthalein (Agarol) 6 months–2 years 2.5 mL, 3–5 years 2.5–5 mL, over 5 years 5 mL 8–24 hourly oral.

Paraldehyde *i.m.:* 0.2 mL/kg stat, then 0.1 mL/kg per dose 4–6 hourly. *i.v.:* 0.2 mL/kg over 15 min, then 0.02 mL/kg per h. *Rectal or n.g.:* 0.3 mL/kg per dose diluted 1 : 10.

Penicillamine 62.5 mg/day, gradually increasing to max. 7.5 mg/kg per dose 8 hourly oral.

Penicillin, benzathine co (Bicillin 1 200 000 units) 0–2 years half vial, 3–6 years three-quarters of a vial, > 6 years one vial i.m. once.

Penicillin G (benzyl) *Serious infection:* 100 000 units (60 mg)/kg per dose i.v. 12 hourly (1st week of life), 6 hourly (2–4 weeks), 4 hourly (> 4 weeks). Usually 50 000 units (30 mg)/kg per dose 4–6 hourly.

Penicillin, procaine 25 000–50 000 units (25–50 mg)/kg 12–24 hourly i.m.

Penicillin V (phenoxymethylpenicillin) 7.5–15 mg/kg per dose 6 hourly oral. *Prophylaxis:* 12.5 mg/kg per dose 12 hourly oral.

Pentavite (Vitamins A,B,C,D) *Neonates:* 12 drops daily, oral. *0–6 years:* 2.5–5 mL daily. *Over 6 years:* 5 mL daily.

Pethidine 0.5–1.0 mg/kg per dose i.v., 1–1.5 mg/kg per dose i.m. (half-life 2–4 h). *Infusion:* 5 mg/kg in 50 mL heparin–5%D at 1–3 mL/h (100–300 μg/kg per h).

Pheniramine 0.5 mg/kg per dose 6 hourly oral.

Phenobarbital See phenobarbitone.

Phenobarbitone See also colic mixture. *Loading dose in emergency:* 20–30 mg/kg i.v. or i.m. stat. *Maintenance dose:* 5 mg/kg daily i.v., i.m. or oral. Level 80–120 μmol/L (× 0.23 = μg/mL) done Monday, Wednesday and Friday morning at the Royal Children's Hospital.

Phenoperidine 0.01–0.02 mg/kg per dose i.v.

Phenoxybenzamine 0.2 mg/kg daily oral. *Cardiac surgery:* 1 mg/kg i.v. over 1 h stat, then 0.5 mg/kg per dose 8–12 hourly i.v. over 30 min or oral.

Phenoxymethylpenicillin See penicillin V.

Phentolamine 0.1 mg/kg stat, then 5–50 μg/kg per min i.v.

Phenylephrine 5 μg/kg stat, then 1–5 μg/kg per min i.v.
Phenytoin *Loading dose in emergency:* 15–20 mg/kg i.v. over 1 h. *Maintenance:* 2 mg/kg per dose 12 hourly (preterm), 4 mg/kg per dose 12 hourly (1st week of life), 6 hourly (2–12 months), 8 hourly (1–4 years), 12 hourly (12 years). Level 40–80 μmol/L (× 0.25 = μg/L), done Monday, Wednesday and Friday morning at the Royal Children's Hospital.
Phosphate, potassium (1 mmol/mL) 1 mmol/kg per day i.v. infusion.
Phosphate, sodium (500 mg tablet) 0.5–1 g 8 hourly oral.
Physostigmine 0.02 mg/kg i.v. every 5 min till response (max. 0.1 mg/kg), then 0.5–2.0 μg/kg per min.
Phytomenadione 0.3 mg/kg (max. 10 mg), i.m. or slow i.v. *Prophylaxis in neonates:* 1 mg i.m.
Phytonadione See phytomenadione.
Piperacillin 50 mg/kg per dose i.v. 6–8 hourly (1st week of life), 4–6 hourly (2 + weeks).
Piperazine 75 mg/kg (max. 4 g) oral daily for 2 days (ascaris), 7 days (pinworm).
Pizotifen 1–3 mg/day oral. Usually 0.5 mg morning, 1 mg night.
Platelets 10 mL/kg i.v. stat, then daily if necessary.
Poloxalkol See Coloxyl.
POR 8 See ornipressin.
Potassium Max. i.v. 0.5 mmol/kg per h (0.25 mmol/kg per h in neonates). Requirement 2–4 mmol/kg per day; 1 g KCl = 13.3 mmol potassium.
Potassium canrenoate 3 mg/kg daily i.v.
Pralidoxime 25–50 mg/kg over 30 min, then up to 10 mg/kg per h.
Prazosin 0.005 mg/kg test dose, then 0.025–0.1 mg/kg per dose 6 hourly oral.
Prednisolone Initially 1 mg/kg per dose 8 hourly oral. See also methylprednisolone.
Primidone 5–10 mg/kg per dose 12 hourly oral.
Probenicid 25 mg/kg stat, then 10 mg/kg per dose 6 hourly oral.
Procainamide 3–6 mg/kg (max. 100 mg) i.v. over 15 min, then 20–80 μg/kg per min (max. 80 mg/h); 2.5–7.5 mg/kg 4 hourly oral.
Prochlorperazine 0.25 mg/kg (max. 12.5 mg) stat, then 0.1 mg/kg per dose 8 hourly i.m., i.v. or oral. Not to be used if < 10 kg.
Promethazine 0.5 mg/kg per dose 6–8 hourly i.v., i.m. or oral.
Propantheline bromide 0.3 mg/kg per dose 6 hourly oral.
Propofol 1–3 mg/kg stat, then 4–6 mg/kg per h i.v.
Propranolol 0.02–0.1 mg/kg per dose i.v. over 10 min stat (repeat p.r.n.), then 6 hourly. Oral 0.2–0.5 mg/kg per dose 6 hourly, increase to max. 1.5 mg/kg per dose 6 hourly.
Prostacyclin See epoprostenol.
Prostaglandin E_1 0.01 μg/kg per min (*Arch. Dis. Child* 1984; **59:** 1020); *< 16 kg:* put 30 μg/kg in 50 mL saline, run at 1 mL/h; *> 16 kg:* put 500 μg in 830/wt mL saline, run at 1 mL/h (e.g. 20 kg child, 500 μg in 41.5 mL saline at 1 mL/h). *Pulmonary vasodilation:* 5 μg/kg per min nitroglycerine = 2 μg/kg per min nitroprusside = 0.1 μg/kg per min PGE_1 approx.
Prostaglandin E_2 25 μg/kg per h (less after 1 week) oral.
Protamine i.v. 1 mg/100 units heparin stat (or 1 mg/25 mL pump blood), repeat dose protamine 1 mg/kg bodyweight. Heparin 1 mg = 100 u (half-life 1–2 h).
Prothrombinex (Factors II, IX and X 250 units/10 mL) 1 mL/kg slow i.v. daily. Risk of thrombosis in acute liver failure.
Protirelin 200 μg i.v. stat.
Pseudoephedrine 1 mg/kg per dose 6 hourly oral.
Pyridostigmine 1 mg/kg daily, increase to 1–4 mg/kg per dose 6–12 hourly oral. *Timespan:* 1–3 180 mg tablets 12–24 hourly in adult.
Pyridoxine *With isoniazid:* 5–10 mg daily i.v. or oral. *Neonatal fitting:* 50–100 mg daily i.v. or oral. *Sideroblastic anaemia:* 2–8 mg/kg daily i.v. or oral.
Quinalbarbitone Sedative 5 mg/kg. Premed 10 mg/kg.
Quinidine 12 mg/kg stat, then 6 mg/kg/dose 4–6 hourly oral.
Quinine 20 mg/kg i.v. over 4 h or i.m., then 7.5 mg/kg per dose 8 hourly i.v. over 1 h or i.m. for 2–3 days, then 10 mg/kg per dose 8 hourly oral for 5 days.
Ranitidine 1 mg/kg per dose slow i.v. 6–8 hourly; 3 mg/kg per dose 8–12 hourly oral.
Resonium See sodium polystyrene sulfonate.
Riboflavine 5–10 mg daily oral.
Rifampicin 10–15 mg/kg (max. 600 mg) daily oral on an empty stomach (monitor AST). *Prophylaxis:* 5 mg/kg per dose 12 hourly for

4 doses (< 4 weeks), 10 mg/kg per dose (max. 600 mg/dose) 12 hourly × 4 (> 4 weeks).
Rolitetracycline (Reverin) See tetracycline.
Salbutamol 0.1–0.15 mg/kg per dose 6 hourly oral. *Respiratory solution (0.5%):* 0.5 mL/dose diluted to 4 mL 3–6 hourly (mild), 1.0 mL/dose diluted to 4 mL 1–2 hourly (moderate), undiluted continuously (severe, in ICU). *Aerosol:* one to two puffs 4–6 hourly if over 8 years. *i.v.:* 5 μg/kg stat. *Infusion:* see p. 212.
Scopolamine See hyoscine.
Secobarbital sodium See quinalbarbitone.
Sennoside *Tablets 7.5 mg, once daily:* 6 months–2 years half to one tablet, 3–10 years one to two tablets, over 10 years two to four tablets. *Granules 22.5 mg/teaspoon, 12–24 hourly:* under 6 months quarter–half teaspoon, 6 months–2 years half to one teaspoon, 3–10 years one to two teaspoons.
Sodium *Deficit:* mL of 20% NaCl = w × 0.2 × (140 − serum Na); do not increase serum Na faster than 2 mmol/L per h. Requirement 2–6 mmol/kg per day; 1 g NaCl = 17.1 mmol Na.
Sodium bicarbonate See bicarbonate.
Sodium citrotartrate 2–4 g/dose in 50 mL water 8–12 hourly.
Sodium cromoglycate (Intal) One cap 6–8 hourly by inhalation, 2 mL solution 6–8 hourly by inhalation, aerosol one to two puffs 6–8 hourly.
Sodium etidronate 5–20 mg/kg daily (no food for 2 h before and after dose).
Sodium nitrite 3% solution: 0.2 mL/kg i.v. over 5 min.
Sodium nitroprusside See nitroprusside.
Sodium polystyrene sulfonate (Resonium) 1 g/kg per dose 4 hourly n.g. (give lactulose) or p.r.
Sodium thiosulfate 1 mL/kg 25% solution i.v. over 10 min.
Somatotropin 0.1–0.2 U/kg s.c. daily on 4–7 days per week.
Sotalol *i.v.:* 0.5–1.5 mg/kg per dose over 10 min 6 hourly. *Oral:* 1–2 mg/kg per dose 8 hourly (increase up to 4 mg/kg per dose 8 hourly).
Spironolactone 0–10 kg 6.25 mg/dose 12 hourly, 11–20 kg 12.5 mg/dose, 21–40 kg 25 mg/dose 12 hourly, over 40 kg 25 mg/dose 8 hourly, oral. *i.v.:* see potassium canrenoate.
Stemetil See prochlorperazine.
Streptokinase (SK) 4000 U/kg over 30 min, then 1500 U/kg per h (up to 2000 U/kg per h if required); check fibrinogen > 200 mg/dL 4 hourly. Stop heparin and aspirin during SK, give heparin after SK. *Local infusion:* 50 U/kg per h (continue low-dose heparin).
Streptomycin 20–30 mg/kg i.m. daily.
Succinyl choline See suxamethonium.
Sucralfate 1 g tablet 0–2 years quarter tablet 6 hourly, 3–12 years half tablet 6 hourly, over 12 years 1 tablet 6 hourly oral.
Sulfasalazine *Active disease:* 10–15 mg/kg per dose 6 hourly oral. *Remission:* 5–7.5 mg/kg per dose 6 hourly oral.
Suxamethonium 1 mg/kg per dose i.v., 3 mg/kg per dose i.m. (higher doses in neonates).
Tacrine (THA) 0.5–2 mg/kg per dose 3 hourly i.v.
Terbutaline *Oral:* 75 μg/kg per dose 6 hourly. *s.c.:* 5 μg/kg per dose. *i.v.:* 2 μg/kg stat over 5 min, then 5 μg/kg per h. *Respiratory solution* (10 mg/mL): 0.5 mL/dose diluted to 2 mL 3–6 hourly (mild), 1.0 mL/dose diluted to 2 mL 1–2 hourly (moderate), undiluted continuously (severe, in ICU). *Aerosol:* one to two puffs 4–6 hourly if over 8 years.
Testosterone esters 100–250 mg i.m. every 2–4 weeks.
Testosterone implant 8 mg/kg (rounded to nearest 100 mg). *Testosterone level:* < 16 years 5–10 nmol/L, > 16 years 10–30 nmol/L.
Testosterone undecanoate 40–120 mg daily oral.
Tetracosactrin zinc injection (Synacthen Depot) 0.5–1.0 mg i.m. alternate days or twice weekly (monitor response).
Tetracycline *Over 7 years:* 250–500 mg/dose 6 hourly oral. *Rolitetracycline (Reverin)* 10 mg/kg per dose (max. 275 mg) daily slow i.v.
Theophylline (80 mg theophylline = 100 mg aminophylline) Loading dose 8 mg/kg oral. *Maintenance 1st week of life:* 2 mg/kg per dose 12 hourly. *Second week of life:* 3 mg/kg per dose 12 hourly. *Three weeks to 12 months:* (0.1 × age in weeks) + 3 mg/kg per dose 8 hourly. *One to 9 years:* 6 mg/kg per dose 6 hourly, or 10 mg/kg per dose slow release 12 hourly. *Ten + years:* 4 mg/kg per dose 6 hourly, or 7 mg/kg per dose 12 hourly slow release. Level 60–80 μmol/L (neonate), 60–110 (asthma), done immediately at Royal Children's Hospital (× 0.18 = μg/mL).
Thiabendazole 25 mg/kg per dose 12 hourly oral for 3 days.
Thiamine See Vitamin B_1.
Thiopentone 3–5 mg/kg slowly stat (beware hypotension), then 1–5 mg/kg per h,

i.v. Level 150–200 μmol/L (× 0.24 = μg/mL), done on request.
Thioridazine 0.5 mg/kg per dose 6–8 hourly oral or i.m.
Thiosulfate See sodium thiosulfate.
Thiothixene *Over 12 years:* initially 1 mg/dose 8 hourly oral, gradually increase. *Adults:* 10–60 mg/day.
Thyroxine *Infants:* 25 μg daily, gradually increasing to 3–5 μg/kg per day oral. *Adults:* 100–200 μg daily.
Ticarcillin 50 mg/kg per dose i.v. 6–8 hourly (1st week of life), 4–6 hourly (2 + weeks).
Ticarcillin and clavulanic acid Dose as for ticarcillin.
Tinidazole *Giardia:* 50 mg/kg (max. 2 g) stat, repeated after 48 h. *Amoebic dysentery:* 50 mg/kg (max. 2 g) daily for 3 days.
Tissue plasminogen activator 0.2 mg/kg over 2 min, then 1 mg/kg for 1 h, then 0.5 mg/kg for 2 h i.v. (keep fibrinogen > 100 mg/dL). *Local IA infusion:* 0.05 mg/kg per h for 4–8 h.
Tobramycin 2.5 mg/kg per dose (max. 100 mg/dose) i.v. daily (< 30 weeks gestation), 18 hourly (30–35 weeks gestation), 12 hourly (1st week of life), 8 hourly (2 + weeks). Level 5–10 mg/L peak, < 2 trough, done Monday–Friday Royal Children's Hospital.
Tocainide 10 mg/kg per dose 8–12 hourly i.v. over 30 min or oral.
Tocopherol See Vitamin E.
Tolazoline 1–2 mg/kg slowly stat (beware hypotension), then 2–6 μg/kg per min (0.12–0.36 mg/kg per h) i.v. *Note:* 1–2 mg/kg per h too much (*Pediatrics* 1986; **77:** 307).
Tranexamic acid 15–20 mg/kg per dose (max. 1 g) 8 hourly oral.
Trifluoperazine 1 mg/dose 12–24 hourly oral.
Trihexyphenidyl See benzhexol.
Triiodothyronine See liothyronine.
Trimeprazine (Vallergan) *Antihistamine:* 0.1–0.25 mg/kg per dose 6 hourly i.m. *Sedation:* 0.5–1.0 mg/kg per dose i.m., 3–4 mg/kg per dose oral.
Trimethoprim 3–4 mg/kg per dose (usual max. 150 mg) 12 hourly, or 6–8 mg/kg (usual max. 300 mg) daily oral or i.v.
Trimethoprim-sulfamethoxazole See cotrimoxazole.
Triprolidine/pseudoephedrine *Mixture* (1.25 mg/30 mg in 5 mL): 0.25 mL/kg per dose 8 hourly oral. *Tablets* (2.5 mg/60 mg): 6–12 years half tablet, > 12 years one tablet 8 hourly oral.
Tubocurarine *ICU:* 0.6 mg/kg i.v. p.r.n. *Theatre:* 0.6 mg/kg i.v. stat, then 0.15 mg/kg per dose.
Valium See diazepam.
Vallergan See trimeprazine.
Valproate 5–25 mg/kg per dose (max. 500 mg/dose) 8–12 hourly i.v., oral. Level 0.3–0.7 mmol/L (× 144 = μg/mL), done Fridays.
Vancomycin *20 mg/kg per dose (max. 500 mg) i.v. over 2 h:* daily (preterm), 12 hourly (1st week of life), 8 hourly (2 + weeks). *Oral:* 5 mg/kg per dose 6 hourly. Peak level 25–40 mg/L, trough < 10 mg/L, done Mondays–Fridays Royal Children's Hospital.
Vasopressin *Aqueous:* put 1–2 units in 1 L fluid, and replace urine output + 10% i.v.; or 2–10 units i.m. or s.c. 8 hourly. *Brain death:* 0.00033 units/kg per min (1 units/kg in 50 mL at 1 mL/h) + adrenaline 0.1–0.2 μg/kg per min. *Oily:* 2.5–5 units i.m. every 2–4 days. *GI hge (aqueous solution):* 0.4 units/min i.v. in adult; 0.1 units/min selective IA in adult. See also desmopressin.
Vecuronium 0.1 mg/kg stat, then 1–10 μg/kg per min i.v..
Verapamil 0.1–0.2 mg/kg i.v. over 10 min, then 5 μg/kg per min. *Oral:* 0–2 years 5–20 mg/dose 8–12 hourly, over 2 years 10–40 mg/dose 8 hourly.
Vitamin A, B, C, D compound See Pentavite.
Vitamin A + D (Royal Children's Hospital 12 000 units A, 2000 units D/mL) 1 mL/day.
Vitamin B group *Amp:* i.v. over 30 min. *Tablets:* 1–2/day.
Vitamin B_{12} See hydroxycobalamin.
Vitamin C See ascorbic acid.
Vitamin D *Nutritional rickets:* ergocalciferol (D_2) 10 000 units daily for 30 days, oral. *Renal rickets or hypoparathyroidism:* calcitriol (1,25-OH D_3) start 0.01 μg/kg per day; dihydrotachysterol (1-OH D_2) 20 μg/kg per day; ergocalciferol (D_2): 50 000–300 000 units/day.
Vitamin E (Copherol E) *Preterm babies:* 40 units (two drops) daily oral. 1 unit = 1 mg.
Vitamin K_1 *Oral:* 5–10 mg daily. *Parenteral:* see phytomenadione.
Vitaprem (Royal Children's Hospital) (Pentavite, folate, B_{12}, C) 1 mL daily oral.
Warfarin 0.1–0.2 mg/kg daily oral. INR usually 2–2.5 mg/kg for prophylaxis, 2–3 mg/kg for treatment.
Xylocaine See lignocaine.
Zinc sulfate Adult dose is 220 mg capsules 8 hourly oral.

DRUG INFUSION TABLE

	0.15 mg/kg in 50 mL	*0.3 mg/kg in 50 mL*	*0.6 mg/kg in 50 mL*	*1.5 mg/kg in 50 mL*	*3 mg/kg in 50 mL*	*6 mg/kg in 50 mL*	*15 mg/kg in 50 mL*	*30 mg/kg in 50 mL*	*60 mg/kg in 50 mL*
μg/kg per min	mL/h								
0.05	1	mL/h							
0.1	2	1	mL/h						
0.2	4	2	1						
0.3	6	3	1.5						
0.4	8	4	2	mL/h					
0.5	10	5		1					
0.6	12	6	3						
0.7	14	7							
0.8	16	8	4						
0.9	18	9			mL/h				
1.0	20	10	5	2	1				
1.5		15		3	1.5	mL/h			
2.0		30	10	4	2	1			
3.0				6	3	1.5			
4.0			20	8	4	2	mL/h		
5.0				10	5		1		
6.0				12	6	3			
7.0				14	7				
8.0				16	8	4			
9.0				18	9			mL/h	
10.0				20	10	5	2	1	
12.0					12	6			
14.0					14	7			
15.0					15		3	1.5	mL/h
20.0					20	10	4	2	1
25.0							5		
30.0						15	6	3	1.5
40.0						20	8	4	2
50.0							10	5	
100.0							20	10	5
150.0								15	
200.0								20	10

Noradrenaline

Morphine

Salbutamol Dobutamine Dopamine

Tolazoline

Lignocaine

Nitroglycerine-tridelset

Thiopentone

Adrenaline Isoprenaline

Ketamine

Nitroprusside
Max. hours of infusion
10
8
7
7
6

Calculation of the composition of drug infusion (50 mL syringe pump).

1 Select desired drug dosage to be delivered in μg/kg per min.

2 Select infusion rate of syringe pump in mL/h (from centre of table).

3 Calculate number of milligrams of drug to be mixed in 50 mL syringe.

For example: 10 kg child, 0.1–2 μg/kg per min, infusion 1–20 mL/h; put 0.3 mg/kg (= 3 mg) in 50 mL.

1 mg/kg per h = 16.7 μg/kg per min = 50 mg/kg in 50 mL at 1 mL/h; 1 mg/kg in 50 mL at 1 mL/h = 0.02 mg/kg per h = 0.33 μg/kg per min.

APPENDIX 2

APPROXIMATE PULSE RATE, RESPIRATORY RATE AND BLOOD PRESSURE OF NORMAL CHILDREN

Age	*Pulse rate/min*	*Respirations/min*	*BP*	*Systole 98%*	*Diastole 98%*
At birth–6 months	120–140	45	90/60	104	78
6 months–3 years	110	30	90/60	104	78
4 –7 years	95	25	95/70	116	80
8–10 years	85	20	100/70	125	84
11–12 years	80	20	105/75	132	86

APPENDIX 3

GROWTH CHARTS AND PUBERTAL STAGING

GIRLS IN UTERO 24 – 42 WKS
POST NATAL 0 – 3 YEARS

Reproduced with permission of the Kabi Pharmacia Growth Service

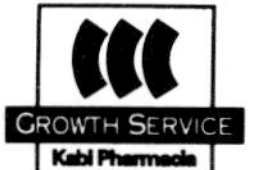

INTRAUTERINE GROWTH CURVES (COMPOSITE MALE/FEMALE)

Measuring techniques: (as for ages 0–36 months – see over page)

Additional Notes: Gestational ages are recorded in completed weeks from the first day of the mother's last menstrual period. Foetal growth is influenced by many factors including age, body weight, height, parity, ethnic origin of the mother and sex of the foetus. Corrections for some of these factors are found in the quoted reference.

Data Source: W.H. Kitchen et al *Revised intrauterine growth curves for an Australian hospital population.* Aust. Paediatr. J. *(1983) 19:157–161.*

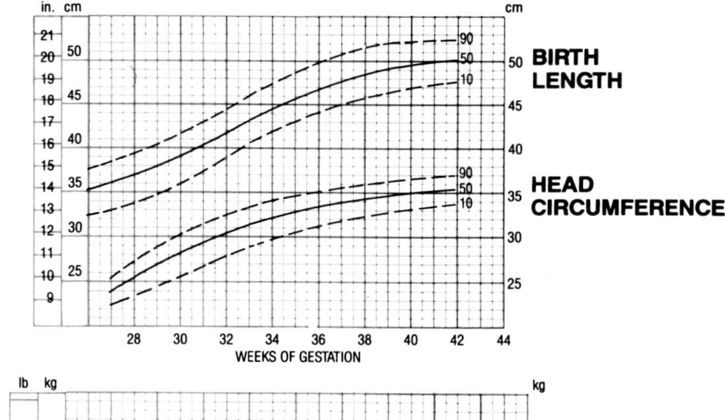

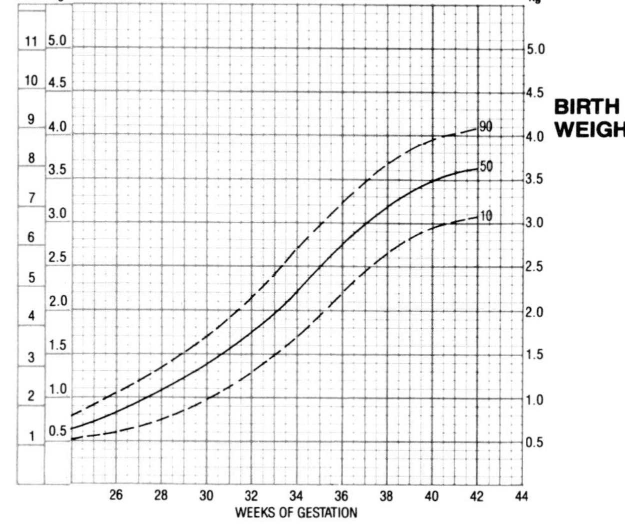

Designed by the Department of Endocrinology, The Adelaide Children's Hospital, 1989.

GIRLS 0–3 YEARS
LENGTH PERCENTILE CHART

Reproduced with permission of the Kabi Pharmacia Growth Service

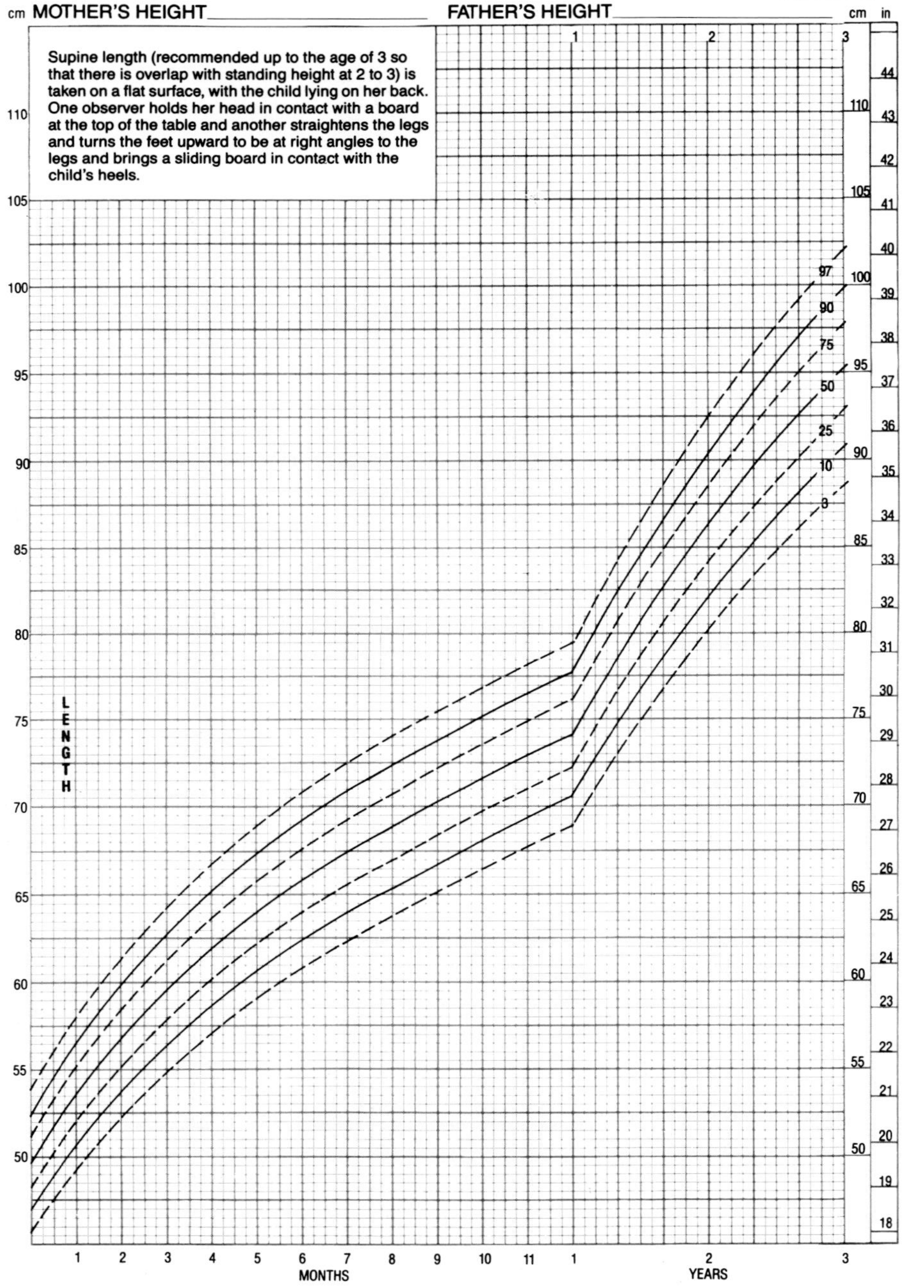

MOTHER'S HEIGHT__________ FATHER'S HEIGHT__________

Supine length (recommended up to the age of 3 so that there is overlap with standing height at 2 to 3) is taken on a flat surface, with the child lying on her back. One observer holds her head in contact with a board at the top of the table and another straightens the legs and turns the feet upward to be at right angles to the legs and brings a sliding board in contact with the child's heels.

cm: 110, 105, 100, 95, 90, 85, 80, 75, 70, 65, 60, 55, 50

in: 44, 43, 42, 41, 40, 39, 38, 37, 36, 35, 34, 33, 32, 31, 30, 29, 28, 27, 26, 25, 24, 23, 22, 21, 20, 19, 18

LENGTH

Percentiles: 97, 90, 75, 50, 25, 10, 3

1 2 3 4 5 6 7 8 9 10 11 MONTHS

1 2 3 YEARS

Data Source: Hamill P.V.V. NCHS growth curves for children. DHEW publication (PHS) 78–1650.

GIRLS 0–3 YEARS
WEIGHT PERCENTILE CHART

Reproduced with permission of the Kabi Pharmacia Growth Service

Weight should be taken in the nude, or as near thereto as possible. If a surgical gown or minimum underclothing (vest and pants) is worn, then its estimated weight (about 0.1 kg) must be subtracted before weight is recorded. Weights are conveniently recorded to the last completed 0.1 kg above the age of six months. The bladder should be empty.

DATE	AGE	LENGTH	WEIGHT	HEAD CIRCUM.

SIMPLIFIED CALCULATION OF BODY SURFACE AREA (BSA)

$$\text{BSA (m}^2) = \sqrt{\frac{\text{Ht (cm)} \times \text{Wt (kg)}}{3600}}$$

Ref: Mosteller R.D.
Simplified calculation of body surface area
N.Engl. J.Med. 1987; 317:1098.

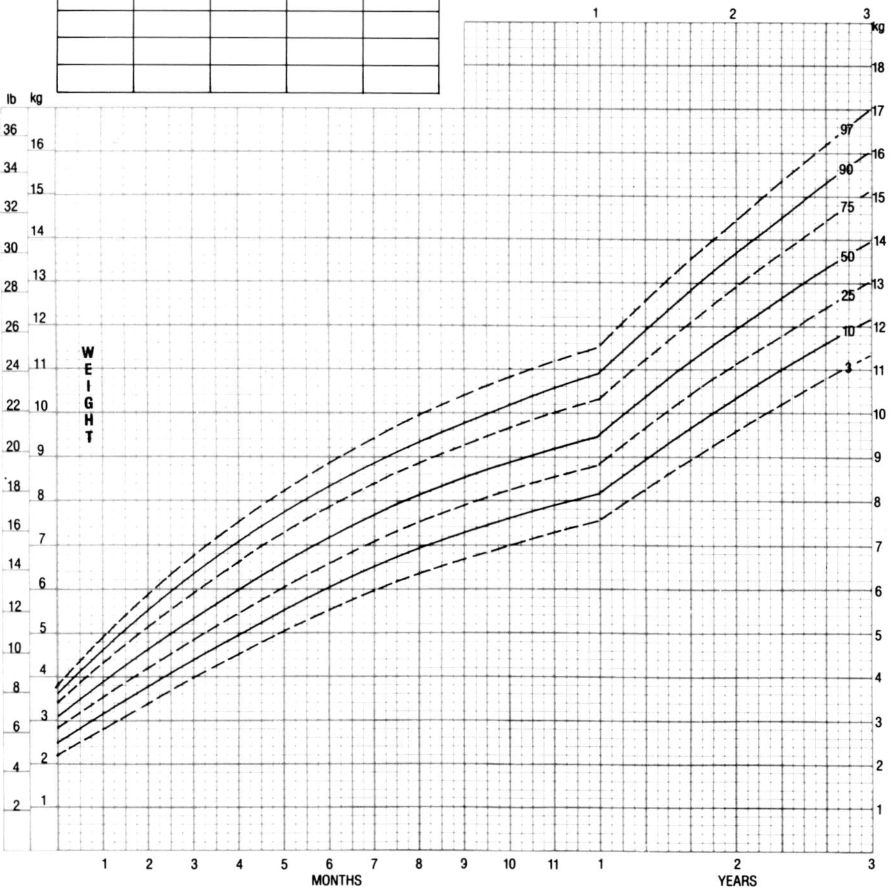

lb kg

WEIGHT

97 90 75 50 25 10 3

1 2 3 4 5 6 7 8 9 10 11 1 2 3

MONTHS YEARS

Data Source: Hamill P.V.V. NCHS growth curves for children. DHEW publication (PHS) 78–1650.

HEAD CIRCUMFERENCE
GIRLS
In utero 28–40 weeks, 0–12 months

Reproduced with permission of the Kabi Pharmacia Growth Service

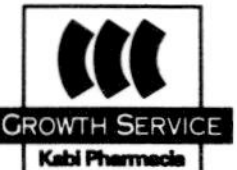

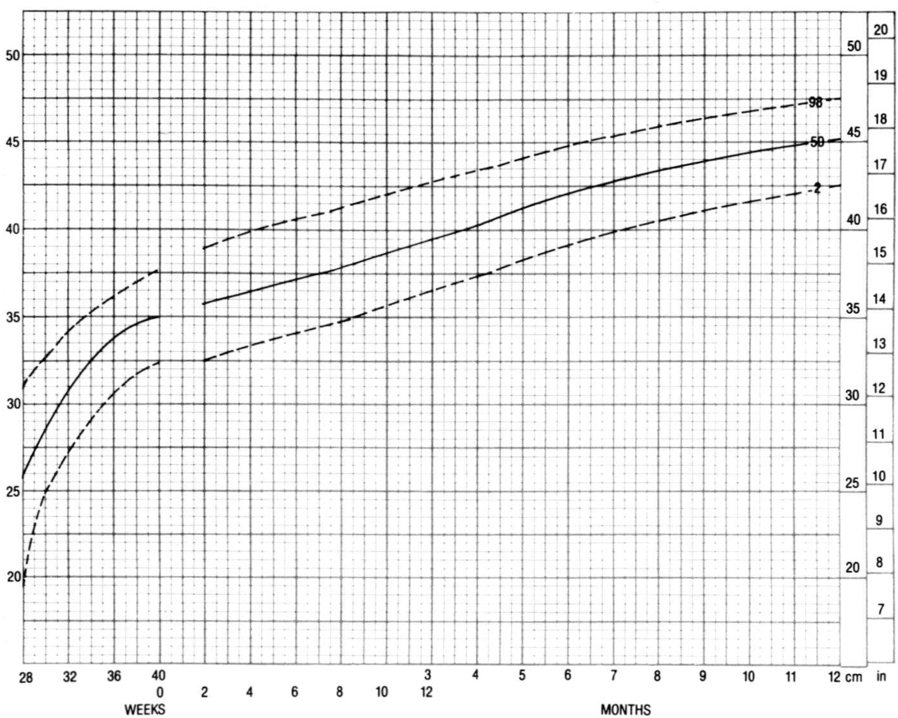

1–3 years

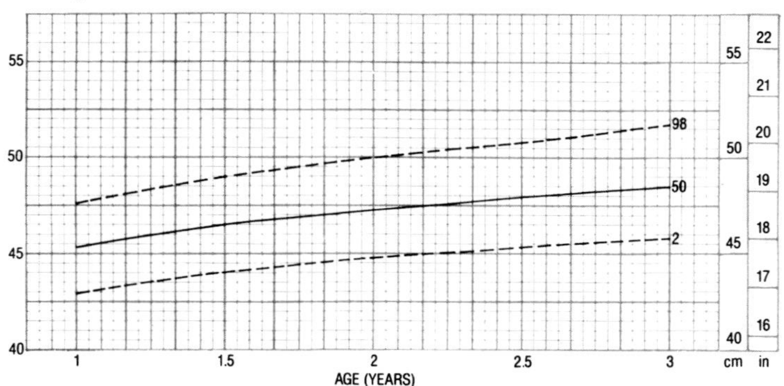

MEASURING TECHNIQUE HEAD CIRCUMFERENCE

The tape should be placed over the eyebrows, above the ears and over the most prominent part of the occiput taking a direct route. A paper tape is preferable to plastic which stretches unacceptably. Record to nearest 0.1 cm.

SOURCES

Head circumference 0–3 years from NSW Health Commission Publication (Jones DL and Hemphill W, 1974).

Head circumference 28–40 weeks gestation from Kitchen WH Aust. Paediatr. J. *(1983) 19:157–161).*

BOYS IN UTERO 24 – 42 WKS POST NATAL 0 – 3 YEARS

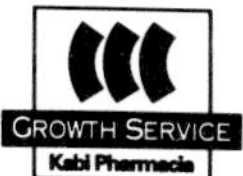

INTRAUTERINE GROWTH CURVES (COMPOSITE MALE/FEMALE)

Measuring techniques: (as for ages 0–36 months – see over page)

Additional Notes: Gestational ages are recorded in completed weeks from the first day of the mother's last menstrual period. Foetal growth is influenced by many factors including age, body weight, height, parity, ethnic origin of the mother and sex of the foetus. Corrections for some of these factors are found in the quoted reference.

Data Source: *W.H. Kitchen et al Revised intrauterine growth curves for an Australian hospital population.* Aust. Paediatr. J. *(1983) 19:157–161.*

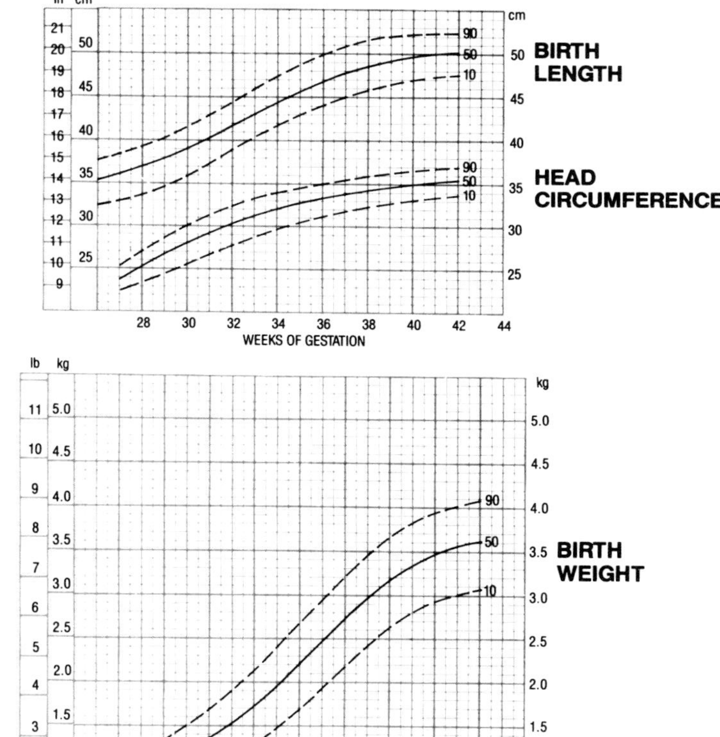

Designed by the Department of Endocrinology, The Adelaide Children's Hospital, 1989.

BOYS 0–3 YEARS
LENGTH PERCENTILE CHART

Reproduced with permission of the Kabi Pharmacia Growth Service

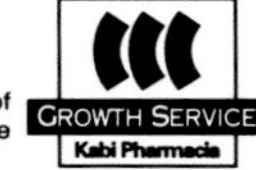

cm MOTHER'S HEIGHT__________ FATHER'S HEIGHT__________ cm in

Supine length (recommended up to the age of 3 so that there is overlap with standing height at 2 to 3) is taken on a flat surface, with the child lying on his back. One observer holds his head in contact with a board at the top of the table and another straightens the legs and turns the feet upward to be at right angles to the legs and brings a sliding board in contact with the child's heels.

LENGTH

97
90
75
50
25
10
3

cm: 50 55 60 65 70 75 80 85 90 95 100 105 110

in: 18 19 20 21 22 23 24 25 26 27 28 29 30 31 32 33 34 35 36 37 38 39 40 41 42 43 44

1 2 3 4 5 6 7 8 9 10 11 1 2 3

MONTHS YEARS

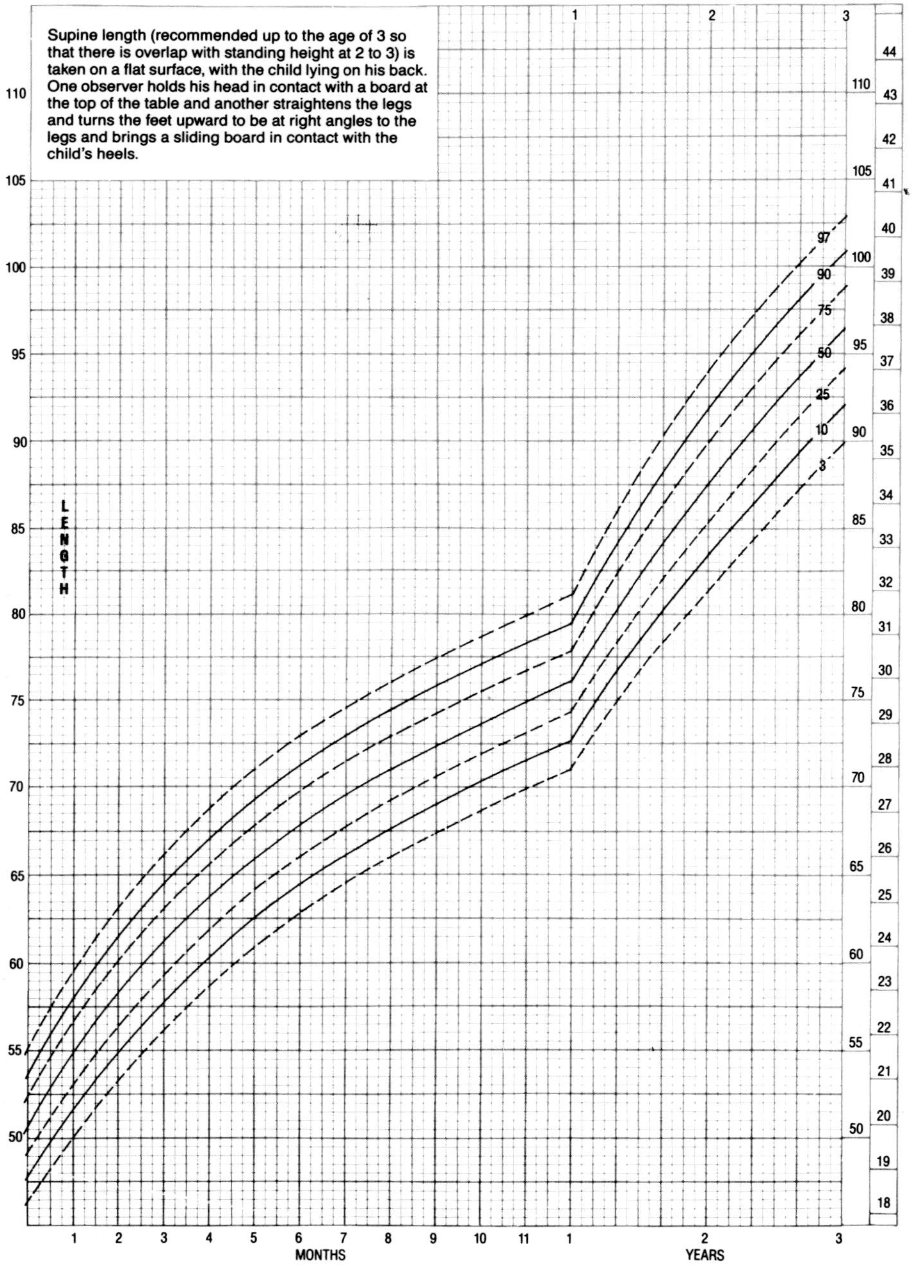

Data Source: Hamill P.V.V. NCHS growth curves for children. DHEW publication (PHS) 78–1650.

BOYS 0–3 YEARS
WEIGHT PERCENTILE CHART

Reproduced with permission of the Kabi Pharmacia Growth Service

GROWTH SERVICE
Kabi Pharmacia

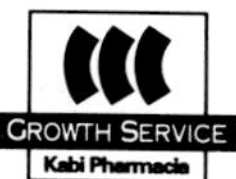

Weight should be taken in the nude, or as near thereto as possible. If a surgical gown or minimum underclothing (vest and pants) is worn, then its estimated weight (about 0.1 kg) must be subtracted before weight is recorded. Weights are conveniently recorded to the last completed 0.1 kg above the age of six months. The bladder should be empty.

DATE	AGE	LENGTH	WEIGHT	HEAD CIRCUM.

SIMPLIFIED CALCULATION OF BODY SURFACE AREA (BSA)

$$\text{BSA (m}^2\text{)} = \sqrt{\frac{\text{Ht (cm)} \times \text{Wt (kg)}}{3600}}$$

Ref: Mosteller R.D.
Simplified calculation of body surface area
N.Engl. J.Med. 1987; 317:1098.

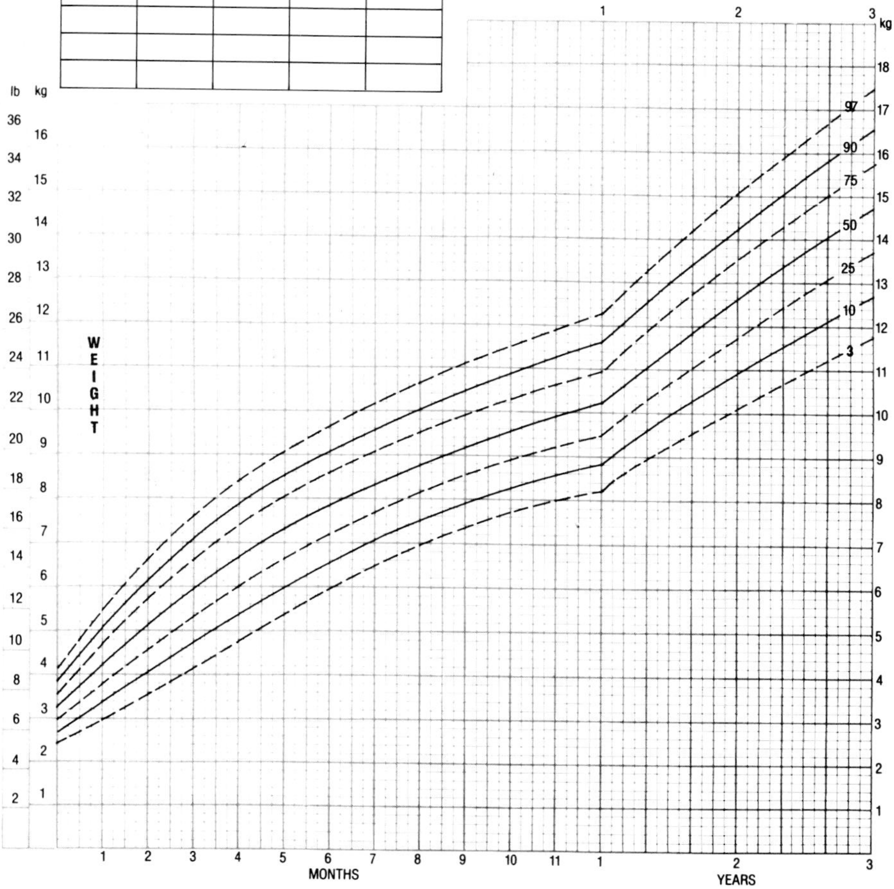
lb
kg
WEIGHT
97
90
75
50
25
10
3
1 2 3 4 5 6 7 8 9 10 11 1
MONTHS
2 3
YEARS

Data Source: Hamill P.V.V. NCHS growth curves for children. DHEW publication (PHS) 78–1650.

Reproduced with permission of the Kabi Pharmacia Growth Service

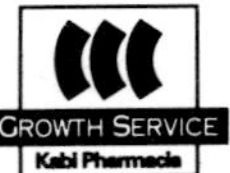

HEAD CIRCUMFERENCE BOYS

In utero 28–40 weeks, 0–12 months

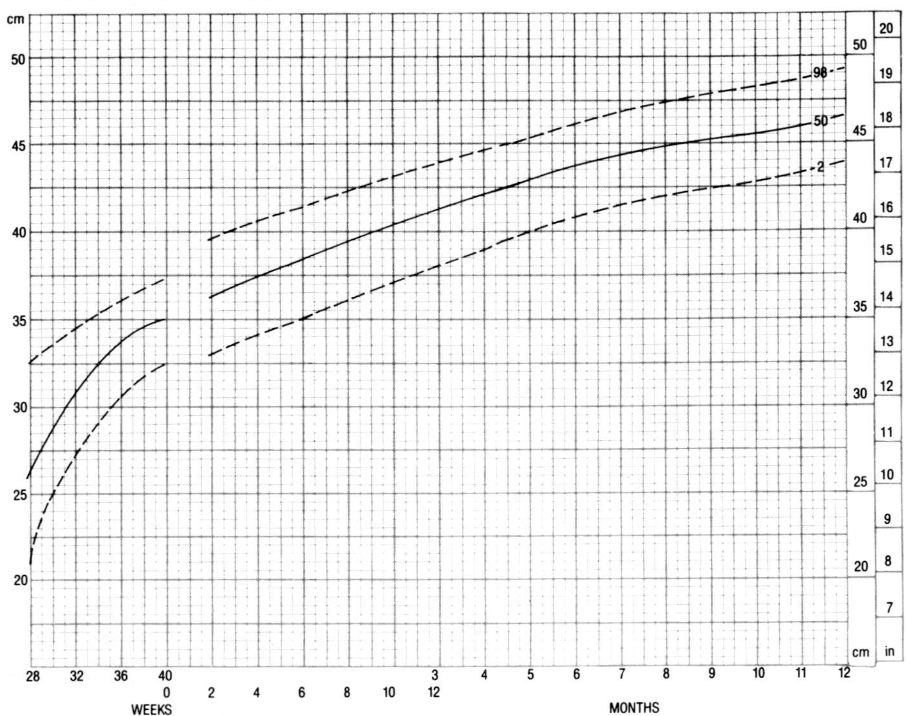

1–3 years

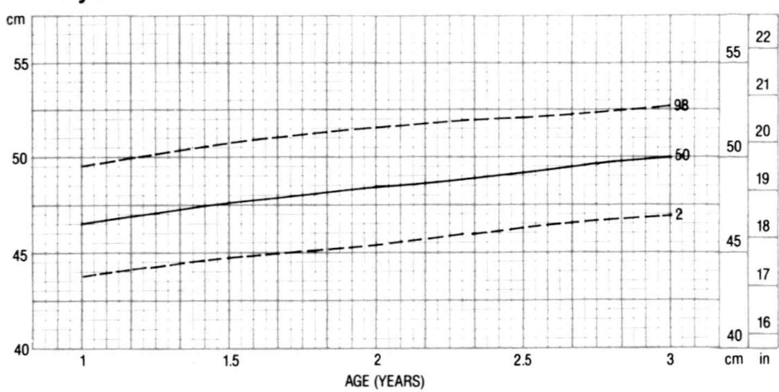

MEASURING TECHNIQUE HEAD CIRCUMFERENCE

The tape should be placed over the eyebrows, above the ears and over the most prominent part of the occiput taking a direct route. A paper tape is preferable to plastic which stretches unacceptably. Record to nearest 0.1 cm.

SOURCES

Head circumference 0–3 years from NSW Health Commission Publication (Jones DL and Hemphill W, 1974).

Head circumference 28–40 weeks gestation from Kitchen WH Aust. Paediatr. J. *(1983) 19:157–161).*

GIRLS: 2 TO 18 YEARS
HEIGHT PERCENTILE

Reproduced with permission of the Kabi Pharmacia Growth Service

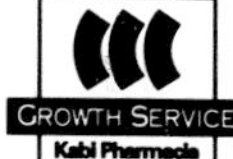

MOTHER'S HEIGHT________________ FATHER'S HEIGHT________________

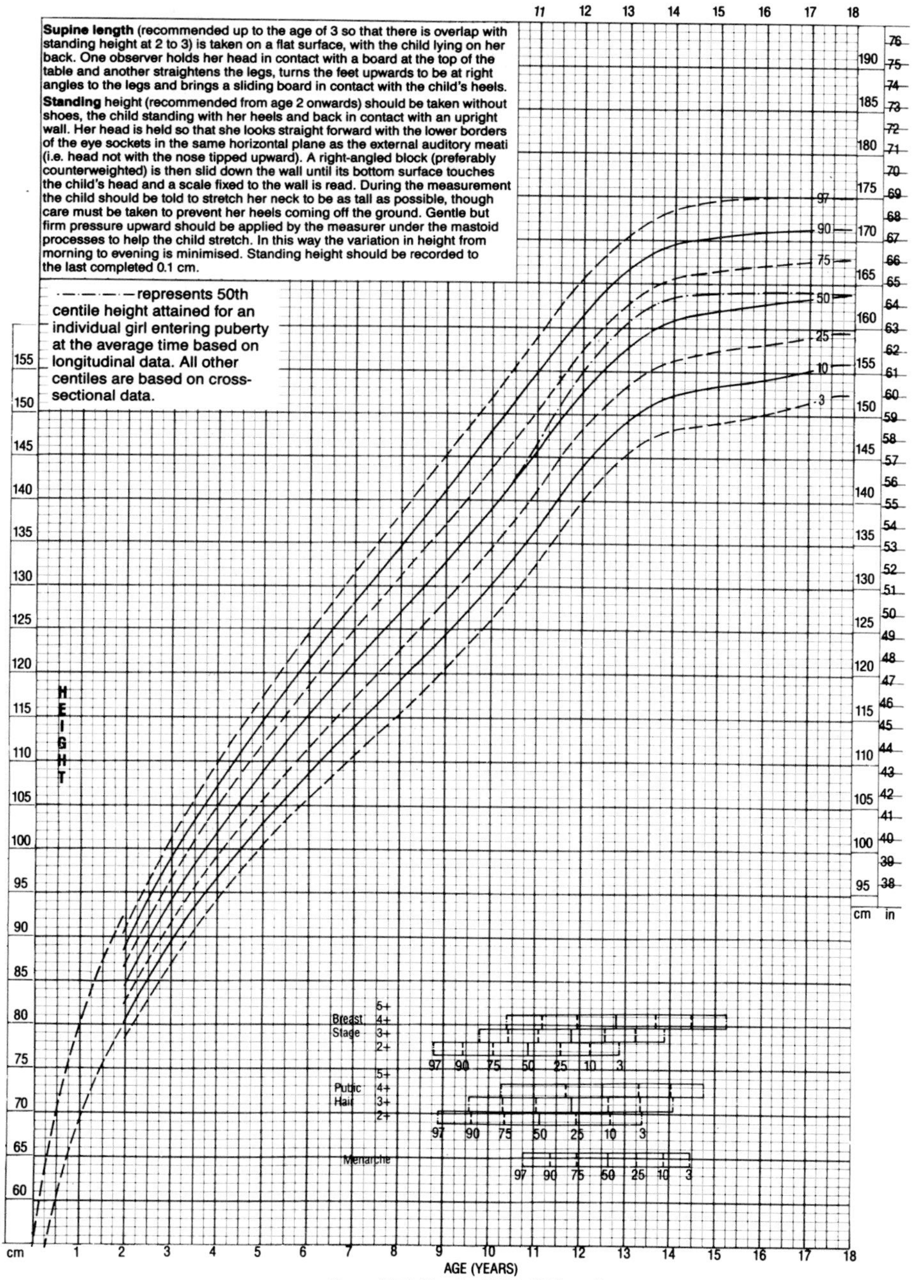

Supine length (recommended up to the age of 3 so that there is overlap with standing height at 2 to 3) is taken on a flat surface, with the child lying on her back. One observer holds her head in contact with a board at the top of the table and another straightens the legs, turns the feet upwards to be at right angles to the legs and brings a sliding board in contact with the child's heels.

Standing height (recommended from age 2 onwards) should be taken without shoes, the child standing with her heels and back in contact with an upright wall. Her head is held so that she looks straight forward with the lower borders of the eye sockets in the same horizontal plane as the external auditory meati (i.e. head not with the nose tipped upward). A right-angled block (preferably counterweighted) is then slid down the wall until its bottom surface touches the child's head and a scale fixed to the wall is read. During the measurement the child should be told to stretch her neck to be as tall as possible, though care must be taken to prevent her heels coming off the ground. Gentle but firm pressure upward should be applied by the measurer under the mastoid processes to help the child stretch. In this way the variation in height from morning to evening is minimised. Standing height should be recorded to the last completed 0.1 cm.

-·-·-·-·- represents 50th centile height attained for an individual girl entering puberty at the average time based on longitudinal data. All other centiles are based on cross-sectional data.

HEIGHT

cm: 60, 65, 70, 75, 80, 85, 90, 95, 100, 105, 110, 115, 120, 125, 130, 135, 140, 145, 150, 155, 160, 165, 170, 175, 180, 185, 190

in: 38, 39, 40, 41, 42, 43, 44, 45, 46, 47, 48, 49, 50, 51, 52, 53, 54, 55, 56, 57, 58, 59, 60, 61, 62, 63, 64, 65, 66, 67, 68, 69, 70, 71, 72, 73, 74, 75, 76

Centiles: 97, 90, 75, 50, 25, 10, 3

Breast Stage: 2+, 3+, 4+, 5+ — 97 90 75 50 25 10 3

Pubic Hair: 2+, 3+, 4+, 5+ — 97 90 75 50 25 10 3

Menarche — 97 90 75 50 25 10 3

1 2 3 4 5 6 7 8 9 10 11 12 13 14 15 16 17 18

AGE (YEARS)

Source: Adapted from Hamill P.V.V.: NCHS growth curves for children. DHEW publication (PHS) 78–1650

GIRLS: 2 TO 18 YEARS WEIGHT PERCENTILE

Reproduced with permission of the Kabi Pharmacia Growth Service

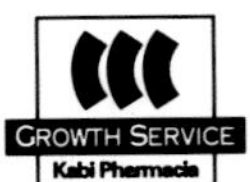

Weight should be taken in the nude, or as near thereto as possible. If a surgical gown or minimum underclothing (vest and pants) is worn, then its estimated weight (about 0.1 kg) must be subtracted before weight is recorded. Weights are conventionally recorded to the last completed 0.1 kg above the age of six months. The bladder should be empty.

					PUBERTAL STAGES		
DATE	AGE	HEIGHT	WEIGHT	HEAD CIRCUM.	BREAST	PUBIC HAIR	MEN-ARCHE

SIMPLIFIED CALCULATION OF BODY SURFACE AREA (BSA)

$$BSA\ (m^2) = \sqrt{\frac{Ht\ (cm) \times Wt\ (kg)}{3600}}$$

Ref: Mosteller R.D.
Simplified calculation of body surface area
N.Engl. J.Med. 1987; 317:1098.

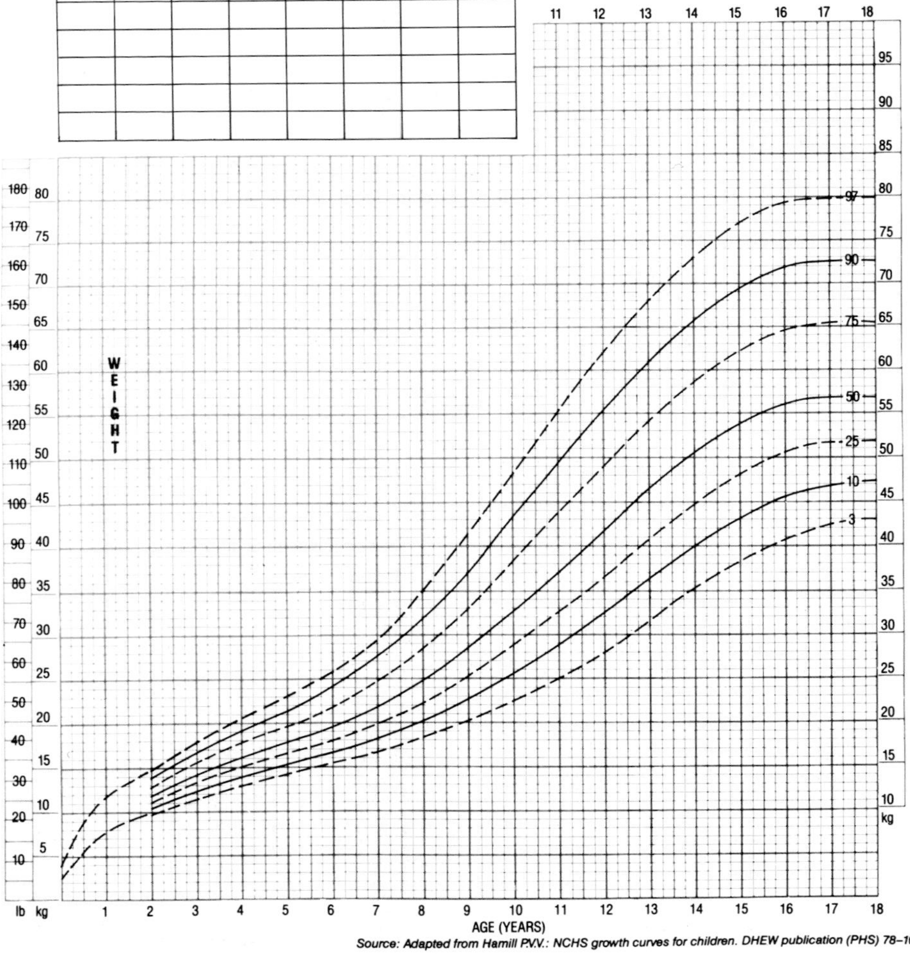

WEIGHT

AGE (YEARS)

Source: Adapted from Hamill P.V.V.: NCHS growth curves for children. DHEW publication (PHS) 78–1650

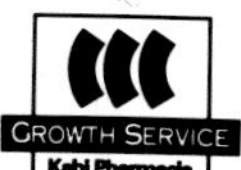

Reproduced with permission of the Kabi Pharmacia Growth Service

HEAD CIRCUMFERENCE, GIRLS

Head Circumference: The tape should be placed over the eyebrows, above the ears and over the most prominent part of the occiput taking a direct route. A paper tape is preferable to plastic, which stretches unacceptably under tension. The maximum measurement should be recorded to the nearest 0.1 cm.

Data Source: *2–5 yr. Jones DL (1973) NSW Health Comm. Publ. 5–18 yr Nellhaus G. Pediatrics (1968) 41:106–114*

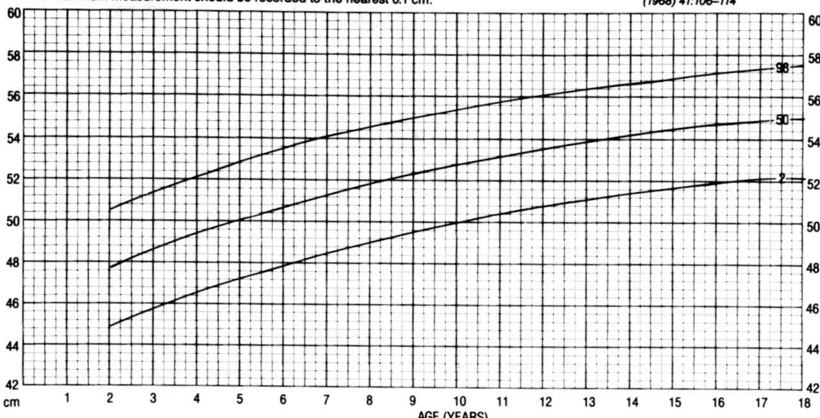

HEIGHT VELOCITY, GIRLS

The standards are appropriate for velocity calculated over a whole year period, not less, since a smaller period requires wider limits (the 3rd and 97th centiles for whole year being roughly appropriate for the 10th and 90th centiles over six months). The yearly velocity should be plotted at the mid-point of a year. The centiles given in black are appropriate to children of average maturational tempo, who have their peak velocity at the average age for this event. The red line is the 50th centile line for the child who is two years early in maturity and age at peak height velocity, and the blue line refers to a child who is 50th centile in velocity but two years late. The arrows mark the 3rd and 97th centiles at peak velocity for early and late maturers.

Centiles for girls maturing at average time — 97, 50, 3

97 and 3 centiles at peak height velocity for ∧ ∨

Early (+2SD) maturers

Late (−2SD) maturers

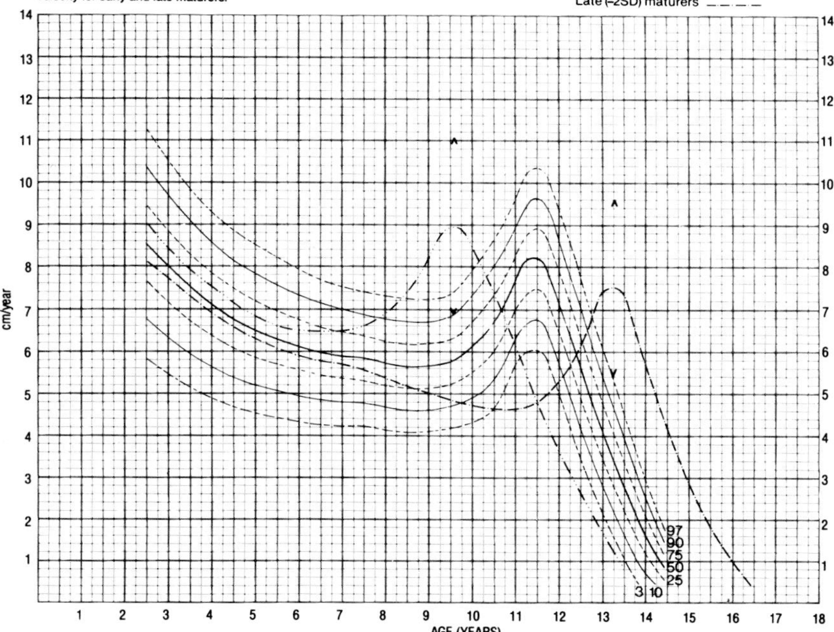

Data Source: Tanner J, Davis PSW, *Journal of Pediatrics* 1985:107

BOYS: 2 TO 18 YEARS HEIGHT PERCENTILE

Reproduced with permission of the Kabi Pharmacia Growth Service

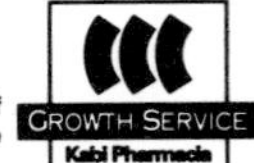

MOTHER'S HEIGHT__________ FATHER'S HEIGHT__________

Supine length (recommended up to the age of 3 so that there is overlap with standing height at 2 to 3) is taken on a flat surface, with the child lying on his back. One observer holds his head in contact with a board at the top of the table and another straightens the legs, turns the feet upwards to be at right angles to the legs and brings a sliding board in contact with the child's heels.

Standing height (recommended from age 2 onwards) should be taken without shoes, the child standing with his heels and back in contact with an upright wall. His head is held so that he looks straight forward with the lower borders of the eye sockets in the same horizontal plane as the external auditory meati (i.e. head not with the nose tipped upward). A right-angled block (preferably counterweighted) is then slid down the wall until its bottom surface touches the child's head and a scale fixed to the wall is read. During the measurement the child should be told to stretch his neck to be as tall as possible, though care must be taken to prevent his heels coming off the ground. Gentle but firm pressure upward should be applied by the measurer under the mastoid processes to help the child stretch. In this way the variation in height from morning to evening is minimised. Standing height should be recorded to the last completed 0.1 cm.

·—·—·— represents 50th centile height attained for an individual boy entering puberty at the average time based on longitudinal data. All other centiles are based on cross-sectional data.

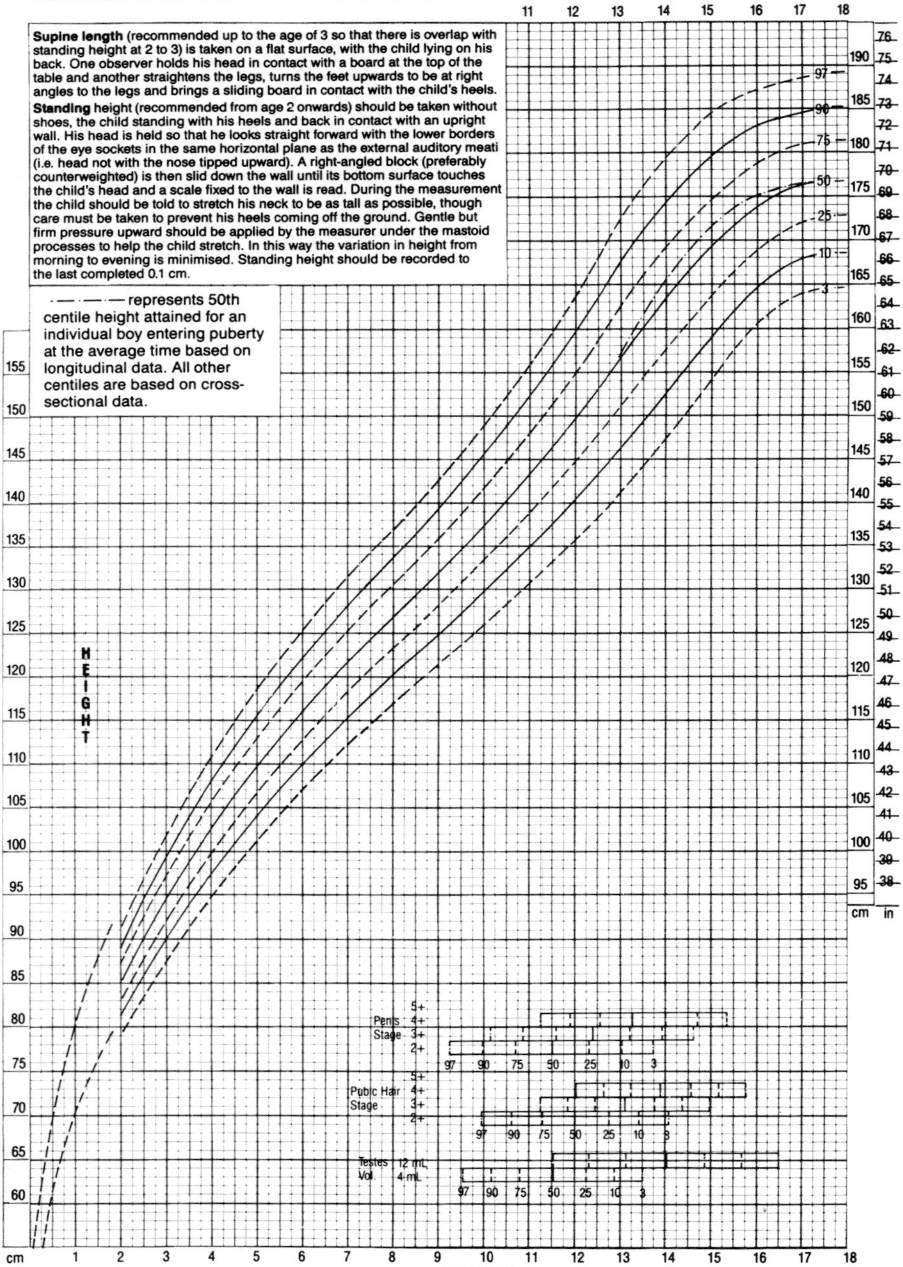

HEIGHT

cm: 60 65 70 75 80 85 90 95 100 105 110 115 120 125 130 135 140 145 150 155 160 165 170 175 180 185 190

in: 38 39 40 41 42 43 44 45 46 47 48 49 50 51 52 53 54 55 56 57 58 59 60 61 62 63 64 65 66 67 68 69 70 71 72 73 74 75 76

Centiles: 97 90 75 50 25 10 3

Penis Stage: 2+ 3+ 4+ 5+ (97 90 75 50 25 10 3)

Pubic Hair Stage: 2+ 3+ 4+ 5+ (97 90 75 50 25 10 3)

Testes Vol. 4 mL 12 mL (97 90 75 50 25 10 3)

AGE (YEARS): 1 2 3 4 5 6 7 8 9 10 11 12 13 14 15 16 17 18

Source: Adapted from Hamill P.V.V.: NCHS growth curves for children. DHEW publication (PHS) 78–1650

BOYS: 2 TO 18 YEARS WEIGHT PERCENTILE

Reproduced with permission of the Kabi Pharmacia Growth Service

Weight should be taken in the nude, or as near thereto as possible. If a surgical gown or minimum underclothing (vest and pants) is worn, then its estimated weight (about 0.1 kg) must be subtracted before weight is recorded. Weights are conventionally recorded to the last completed 0.1 kg above the age of six months. The bladder should be empty.

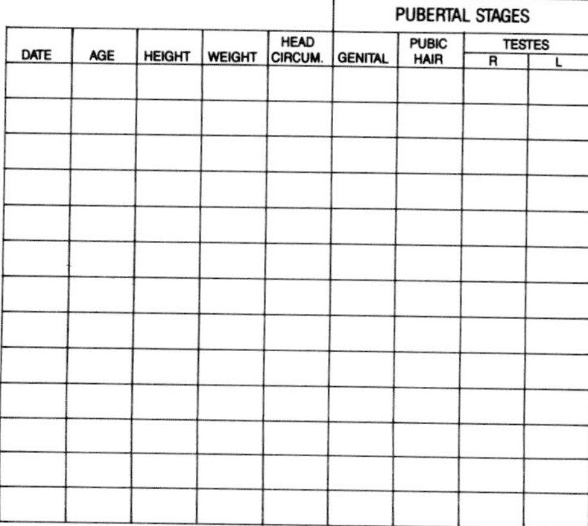

DATE	AGE	HEIGHT	WEIGHT	HEAD CIRCUM.	PUBERTAL STAGES: GENITAL	PUBIC HAIR	TESTES R	TESTES L

SIMPLIFIED CALCULATION OF BODY SURFACE AREA (BSA)

$$\text{BSA (m}^2) = \sqrt{\frac{\text{Ht (cm)} \times \text{Wt (kg)}}{3600}}$$

Ref: Mosteller R.D.
Simplified calculation of body surface area
N.Engl. J.Med. 1987; 317:1098.

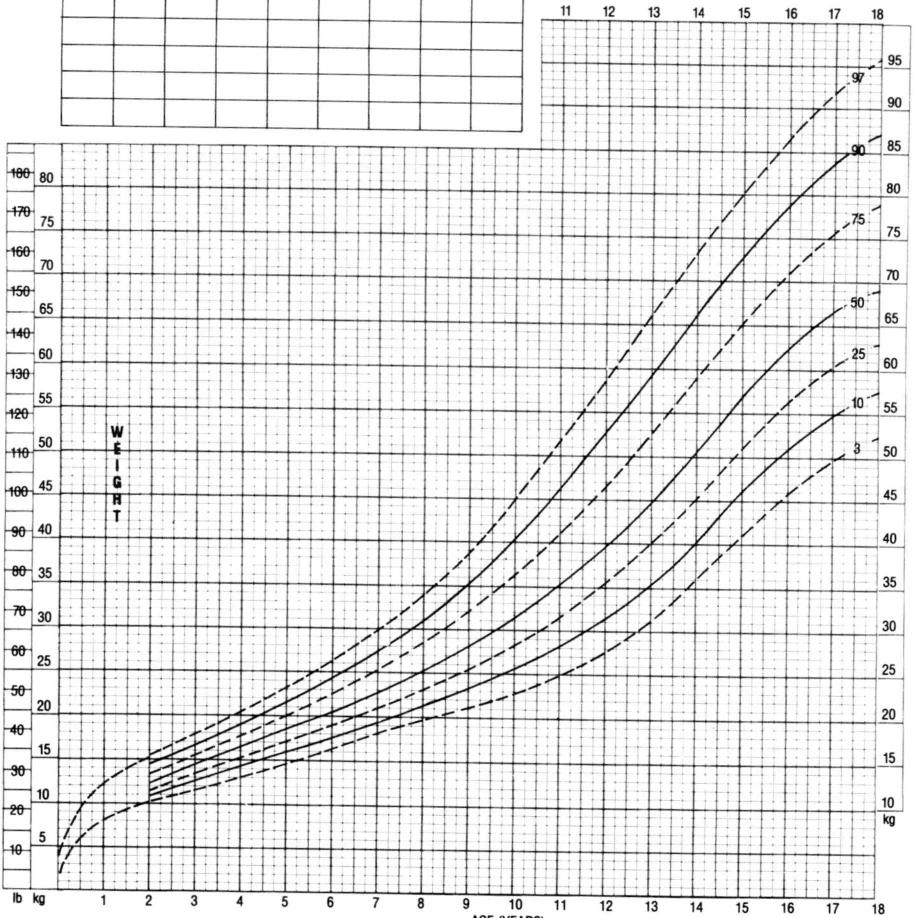

WEIGHT

lb kg

AGE (YEARS)

Source: Adapted from Hamill P.V.V.: NCHS growth curves for children. DHEW publication (PHS) 78–1650

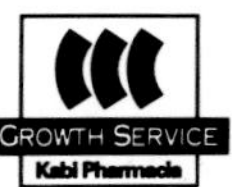

Reproduced with permission of the Kabi Pharmacia Growth Service

HEAD CIRCUMFERENCE, BOYS

Head Circumference: The tape should be placed over the eyebrows, above the ears and over the most prominent part of the occiput taking a direct route. A paper tape is preferable to plastic, which stretches unacceptably under tension. The maximum measurement should be recorded to the nearest 0.1 cm.

Data Source: 2–5 yr. Jones DL (1973) NSW Health Comm. Publ. 5–18 yr Nellhaus G. Pediatrics (1968) 41:106–114

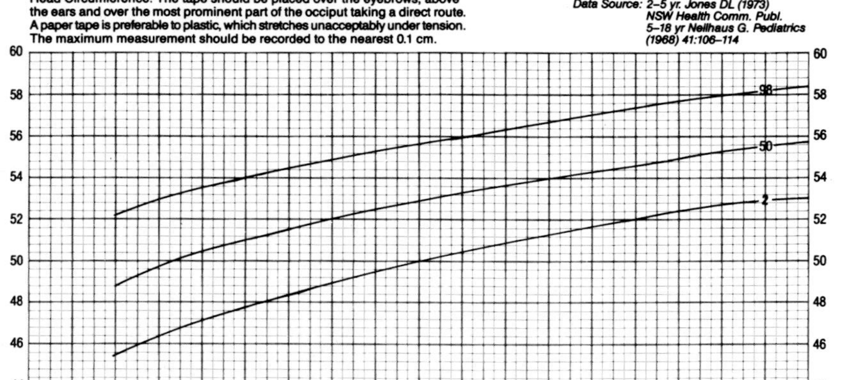

HEIGHT VELOCITY, BOYS

The standards are appropriate for velocity calculated over a whole year period, not less, since a small period requires wider limits (the 3rd and 97th centiles for whole year being roughly appropriate for the 10th and 90th centiles over six months). The yearly velocity should be plotted at the mid-point of a year. The centiles given in black are appropriate to children of average maturational tempo, who have their peak velocity at the average age for this event. The red line is the 50th centile line for the child who is two years early in maturity and age at peak height velocity, and the green line refers to a child who is 50th centile in velocity but two years late. The arrows mark the 3rd and 97th centiles at peak velocity for early and late maturers.

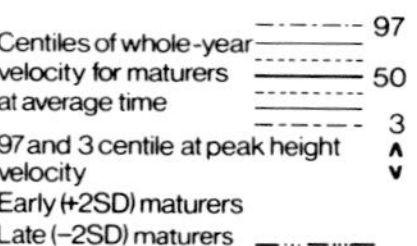

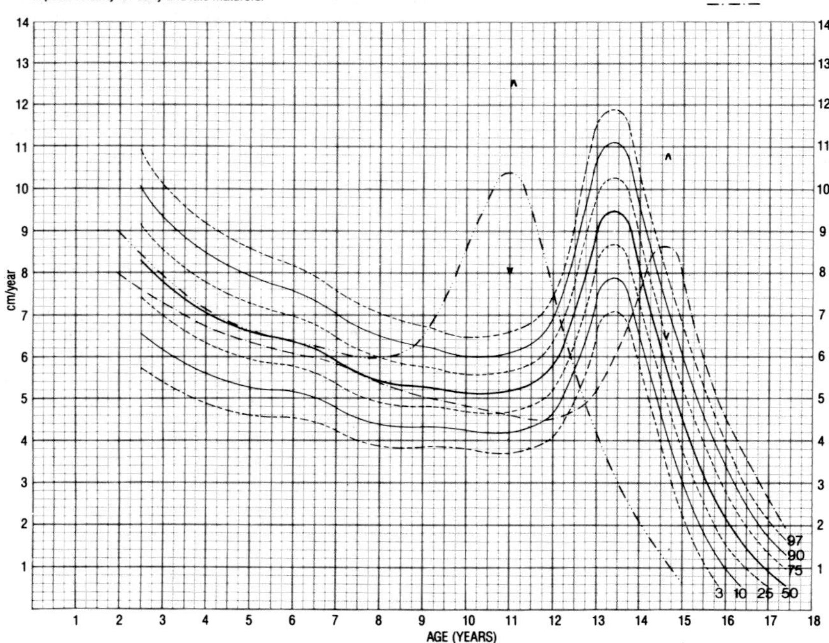

Data Source: Tanner J, Davis PSW, *Journal of Pediatrics* 1985:107

GIRLS 2–18

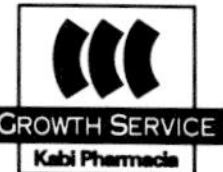

Breast Development

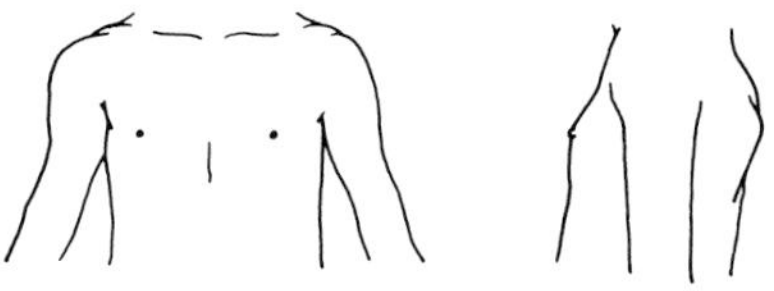

Stage 1 – prepubertal

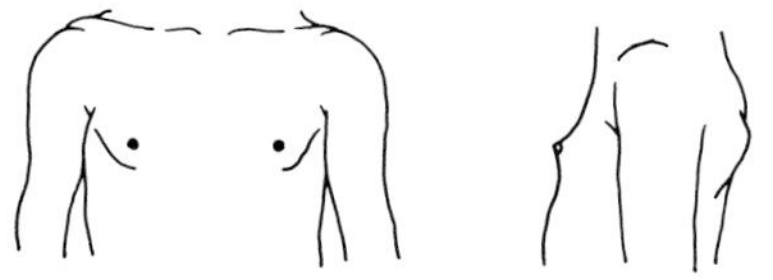

Stage 2 – elevation of breasts and papilla

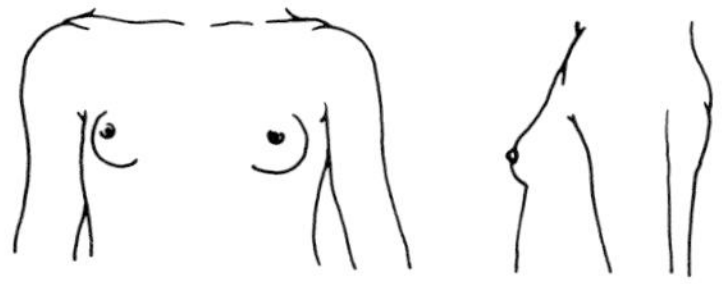

Stage 3 – further elevation and areola but no separation of contours

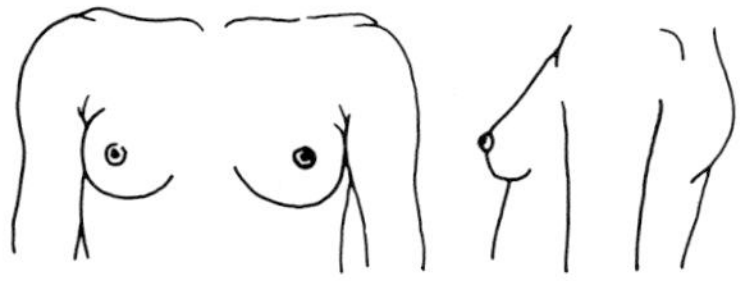

Stage 4 – areola and papilla form a secondary mound above level of the breast

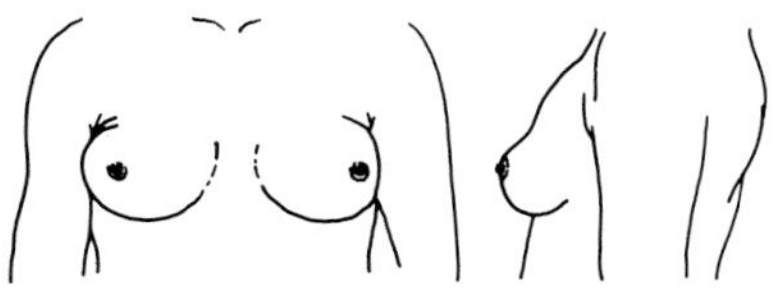

Stage 5 – areola recesses to the general contour of the breast

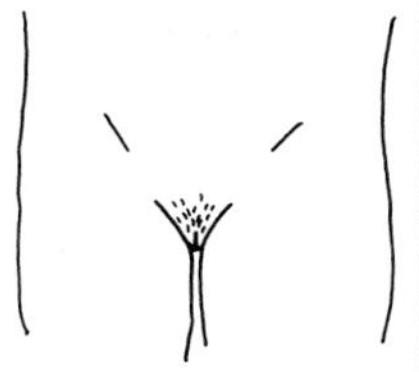

Pubic Hair Stage 2

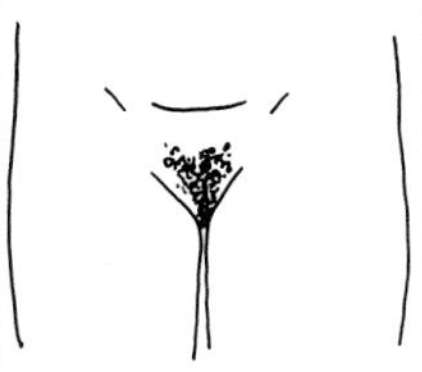

Pubic Hair Stage 3

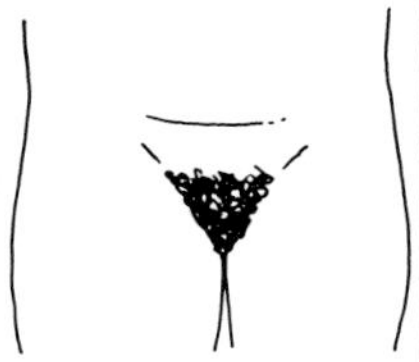

Pubic Hair Stage 4

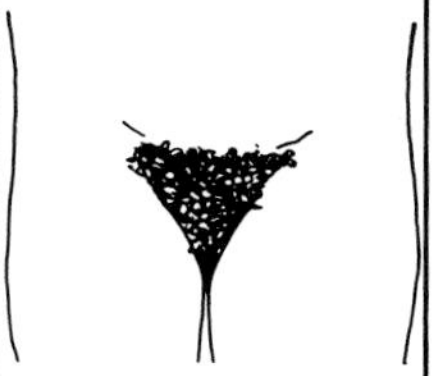

Pubic Hair Stage 5

STAGES OF PUBERTY

Ages of attainment of successive stages of pubertal sexual development are given in the height centile chart overpage. The stage Pubic Hair 2+ represents the state of a child who shows the pubic hair appearance stage 2 but not stage 3 (see below). The centiles for age at which this state is normally seen are given, the 97th centile being considered as the early limit, the 3rd centile as the late limit. The child's puberty stages may be plotted at successive ages (Tanner, *Growth at Adolescence*, 2nd Ed., 1962).

Pubic hair:

Stage 1. Pre-adolescent. The vellus over the pubes is not further developed than that over the abdominal wall, i.e. no pubic hair.

Stage 2. Sparse growth of long, slightly pigmented downy hair, straight or slightly curled, chiefly along labia.

Stage 3. Considerably darker, coarser and more curled. The hair spreads sparsely over the junction of the pubes.

Stage 4. Hair now adult in type, but area covered is still considerably smaller than in the adult. No spread to the medial surface of thighs.

Stage 5. Adult in quantity and type with distribution of the horizontal (or classically 'feminine') pattern. Spread to medial surface of thighs but not up linea alba or elsewhere above the base of the inverse triangle (spread up linea alba occurs late and is rated stage 6).

Designed by the Department of Endocrinology, The Adelaide Children's Hospital, 1989.

BOYS 2–18

Reproduced with permission of the Kabi Pharmacia Growth Service

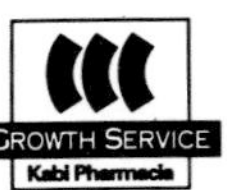

Genital and Pubic Hair Stages

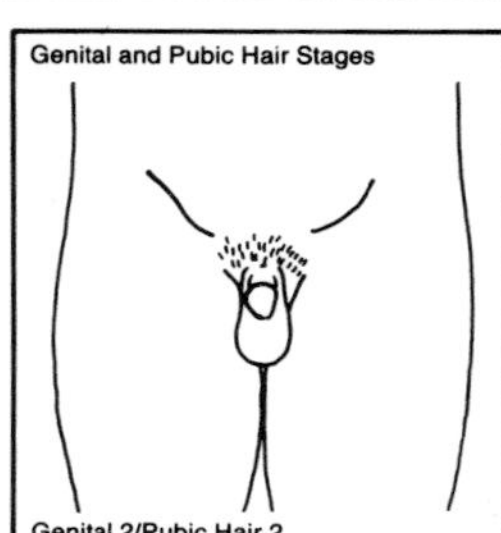

Genital 2/Pubic Hair 2

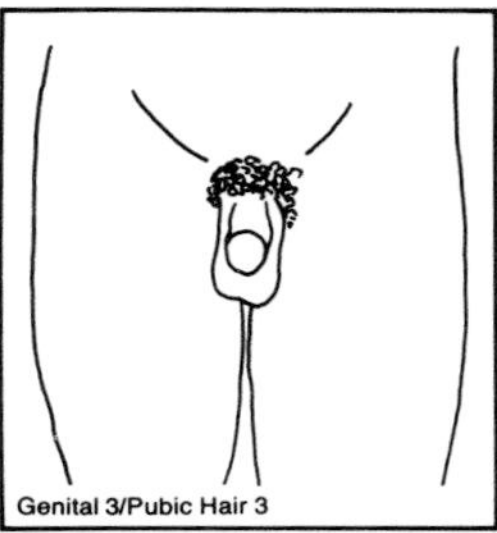

Genital 3/Pubic Hair 3

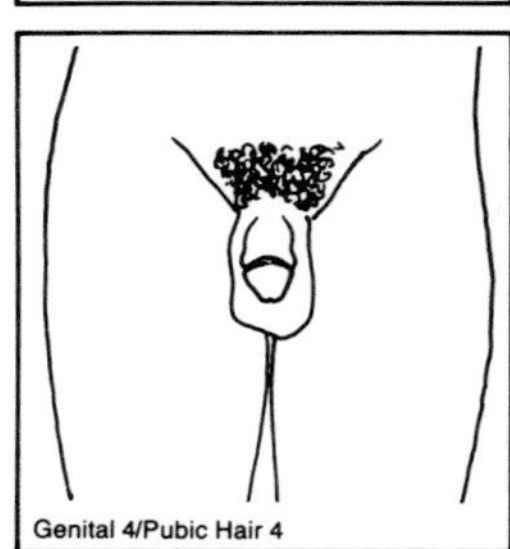

Genital 4/Pubic Hair 4

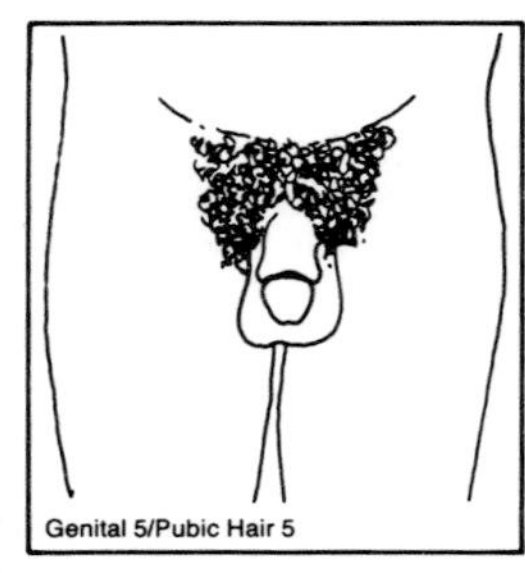

Genital 5/Pubic Hair 5

STAGES OF PUBERTY

Ages of attainment of successive stages of pubertal sexual development are given in the height centile chart overpage. The stage Pubic Hair 2+ represents the state of a child who shows the pubic hair appearance stage 2 but not stage 3 (see below). The centiles for age at which this state is normally seen are given, the 97th centile being considered as the early limit, the 3rd centile as the late limit. The child's puberty stages may be plotted at successive ages (Tanner, *Growth at Adolescence*, 2nd Ed., 1962). Testis sizes are judged by comparison with the Prader orchidometer (Zachmann, Prader, Kind, Haflinger and Budliger, *Helv. Paed. Acta.* 29, 61–72, 1974).

Genital (penis) development:

Stage 1. Pre-adolescent, testes, scrotum and penis are of about the same size and proportion as in early childhood.

Stage 2. Enlargement of scrotum and testes. Skin of scrotum reddens and changes in texture. Little or no enlargement of penis at this stage.

Stage 3. Enlargement of the penis which occurs at first mainly in length. Further growth of the testes and scrotum.

Stage 4. Increased size of penis with growth in breadth and development of glans. Testes and scrotum larger; scrotal skin darkened.

Stage 5. Genitalia adult in size and shape.

Pubic hair:

Stage 1. Pre-adolescent. The vellus over the pubes is not further developed than that over the abdominal wall, i.e. no pubic hair.

Stage 2. Sparse growth of long, slightly pigmented downy hair, straight or slightly curled at the base of the penis.

Stage 3. Considerably darker, coarser and more curled. The hair spreads sparsely over the junction of the pubes.

Stage 4. Hair now adult in type, but area covered is still considerably smaller than in the adult. No spread to the medial surface of thighs.

Stage 5. Adult in quantity and type with distribution of the horizontal (or classically 'feminine') pattern. Spread to medial surface of thighs but not up linea alba or elsewhere above the base of the inverse triangle (spread up linea alba occurs late and is rated stage 6).

Stretched Penile Length

Measured from the pubo-penile skin junction to the tip of the glans (Schonfeld and Beebe, *J. of Urology* 48, 759–777, 1942).

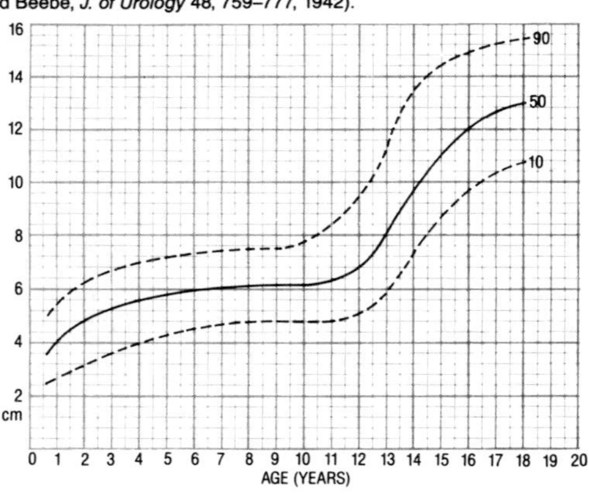

Designed by the Department of Endocrinology, The Adelaide Children's Hospital, 1989.

INDEX

D

E

F

G

H